# Severe Acute Malnutrition

# Severe Acute Malnutrition

**Praveen Kumar** MD
Professor
Department of Pediatrics
Lady Hardinge Medical College and
Kalawati Saran Children's Hospital
New Delhi

**Piyush Gupta** MD, FIAP, FNNF, FAMS
Professor
Department of Pediatrics
University College of Medical Sciences
New Delhi

CBS

## CBS Publishers & Distributors Pvt Ltd

New Delhi • Bengaluru • Chennai • Kochi • Kolkata • Mumbai
Hyderabad • Nagpur • Patna • Pune • Vijayawada

## Severe Acute Malnutrition

ISBN: 978-93-86478-08-5

Copyright © Authors

**First Edition: 2017**

Published by Satish Kumar Jain and Produced by Varun Jain for
**CBS Publishers & Distributors** Pvt Ltd
4819/XI Prahlad Street, 24 Ansari Road, Daryaganj, New Delhi 110 002, India.
Ph: 23289259, 23266861, 23266867    Fax: 011-23243014    Website: www.cbspd.com
e-mail: delhi@cbspd.com; cbspubs@airtelmail.in.
*Corporate Office:* 204 FIE, Industrial Area, Patparganj, Delhi 110 092, India
Ph: 4934 4934    Fax: 4934 4935    e-mail: publishing@cbspd.com; publicity@cbspd.com

*Branches*

- **Bengaluru:** Seema House 2975, 17th Cross, K.R. Road,
  Banasankari 2nd Stage, Bengaluru 560 070, Karnataka, India
  Ph: +91-80-26771678/79    Fax: +91-80-26771680    e-mail: bangalore@cbspd.com
- **Chennai:** 7, Subbaraya Street, Shenoy Nagar, Chennai 600 030, Tamil Nadu, India
  Ph: +91-44-26260666, 26208620    Fax: +91-44-42032115    e-mail: chennai@cbspd.com
- **Kochi:** Ashana House, No. 39/1904, AM Thomas Road, Valanjambalam, Ernakulam 682 018, Kochi, Kerala, India
  Ph: +91-484-4059061-65    Fax: +91-484-4059065    e-mail: kochi@cbspd.com
- **Kolkata:** No. 6/B, Ground Floor, Rameswar Shaw Road, Kolkata-700014 (West Bengal), India
  Ph: +91-33-2289-1126, 2289-1127, 2289-1128    e-mail: kolkata@cbspd.com
- **Mumbai:** 83-C, Dr E Moses Road, Worli, Mumbai-400018, Maharashtra, India
  Ph: +91-22-24902340/41    Fax: +91-22-24902342    e-mail: mumbai@cbspd.com

*Representatives*

- **Hyderabad** 0-9885175004
- **Nagpur** 0-9021734563
- **Patna** 0-9334159340
- **Pune** 0-9623451994
- **Vijayawada** 0-9000660880

*Printed at* Goyal Offset Printers, GT Karnal Road, Industrial Area, Delhi, India

*to*
*all those*
*working tirelessly*
*to prevent and manage*
*severe acute malnutrition*

# Preface

Malnutrition is a major contributor to under-five mortality in developing countries including India. During last 10 years, National Health Mission has taken several steps for preventing deaths due to severe acute malnutrition (SAM). There are more than one thousand dedicated treatment centers for treatment of severe acute malnutrition. Heath workers who are working for child survival need sound knowledge about physiological changes and treatment modalities for children with severe acute malnutrition. To achieve this, UNICEF has been supporting workshops for various cadres of health functionaries in states with high prevalence of undernutrition in India. Interestingly, the idea of this book dawned upon us in a running train while travelling together to conduct one of these workshops at Gwalior.

At present no book is available which provides comprehensive information about management of children with SAM. This book seeks to fill this gap. We have put together current evidence on management of malnutrition in 16 chapters, ranging from the epidemiology to prevention of malnutrition. This book also has chapters on moderate acute malnutrition and stunting which are not easily available elsewhere. Throughout the book we have used malnutrition to imply undernutrition; though as per traditional teaching it includes both undernutrition and overnutrition. The language is simple and we hope, easy to follow. All the chapters are backed by sound evidence and references are cited for all data, figures, and facts in the text. A numbered list is provided at the end of each chapter. So it will be easy to trace the source of information for the reader.

The book is primarily meant for the postgraduate students of pediatrics, nutrition, and community medicine; though we are sure that medical students, nurses, paramedical workers, program officers, and policy makers will be equally benefitted. We hope the readers will find solutions to many of their problems related to SAM; and also serve to generate more queries, paving way for future research. We hope it serves as a useful reference to the people working for the benefit of severely malnourished children.

We are indebted to all the contributors for completing this difficult task in a short time. They are the stalwarts in this field and remain the backbone of this venture.

We extend our gratitude to Mr Satish Jain, Managing Director, CBS for his belief in this project and Mr YN Arjuna, Senior Vice president–Publishing for invaluable suggestions in the format and layout. We thank Ms Ritu Chawla for her dedication and commitment during preparation of the typescript, Ms Jyoti Kaur for DTP work, Mr Neeraj Prasad for preparing graphics and cover design, and Ms Anju Kumari for secretarial assistance.

Praveen Kumar
Piyush Gupta

# Contributors

**AK Patwari** MD, DCH, MNAMS, FIAP, FAMS
Professor and Head
Department of Pediatrics
Hamdard Institute of Medical Sciences and
Research
New Delhi
Email: *akpatwari@gmail.com*

**AK Rawat** MD
Professor and Head
Department of Pediatrics
Bundelkhand Medical College
Sagar
Madhya Pradesh
Email: *drakrawat01@rediffmail.com*

**Abhishek Vijay Raut** MD DNB
Associate Professor
Dr. Sushila Nayar, School of Public Health
Department of Community Medicine
Mahatma Gandhi Institute of Medical
Sciences
Sewagram Wardha
Maharashtra
Email: *abhishekvraut@gmail.com*

**Ajay Gaur** MD, PhD, FIAP
Professor and Head
Department of Pediatrics
GR Medical College
Gwalior
Madhya Pradesh
Email: *drajaygaur@gmail.com*

**Amir Maroof Khan** MD
Associate Professor
Department of Community Medicine
University College of Medical Sciences
New Delhi
Email: *khanamirmaroof@gmail.com*

**Bhavna Dhingra** MD DNB
Assistant Professor
Department of Pediatrics
All India Institute of Medical Sciences
Bhopal, Madhya Pradesh
Email: *drbdhingra@gmail.com*

**JP Dadhich** MD
National Coordinator
Breastfeeding Promotion Network of India
(BPNI)
Pitampura, Delhi
Email: *jpdadhich@gmail.com*

**Karanveer Singh** MD
Nutrition Specialist
Child Development and Nutrition
UNICEF, Delhi
Email: *drkaranveers@gmail.com*

**Kirtisudha Mishra** MD DNB
Associate Professor
Department of Pediatrics
Chacha Nehru Bal Chikitsalaya, Delhi
Email: *kirtisen@gmail.com*

**Neha Sareen** MSc, PhD
Research Scientist
Department of Human Nutrition
All India Institute of Medical Sciences
New Delhi
Email: *nehasareen088@gmail.com*

**Nidhi Bedi** MD
Assistant Professor
Department of Pediatrics
Vardhman Mahavir Medical College and
Safdarjung Hospital
New Delhi
Email: *drnidhibedi@gmail.com*

**Piyush Gupta** MD, FAMS
Professor
Department of Pediatrics
University College of Medical Sciences
New Delhi
Email: *prof.piyush.gupta@gmail.com*

**Praveen Kumar** MD
Professor
Department of Pediatrics
Lady Hardinge Medical College and
Kalawati Saran Children's Hospital
New Delhi
Email: *pkpaed@gmail.com*

**Preeti Singh** MD
Assistant Professor
Department of Pediatrics
Lady Hardinge Medical College and
Kalawati Saran Children's Hospital
New Delhi
Email: *drpreetisingh3@gmail.com*

**Puneet Kaur Sahi** MD
Senior Resident
Department of Pediatrics
Lady Hardinge Medical College and
Kalawati Saran Children's Hospital
New Delhi
Email: *puneetksahi@gmail.com*

**S Aneja** MD
Director–Professor
Department of Pediatrics
Lady Hardinge Medical College and
Kalawati Saran Children's Hospital
New Delhi
Email:*drsaneja@gmail.com*

**S Manazir Ali** MD, DNB, MNAMS, FIAP
Professor and Head
Department of Pediatrics
Jawaharlal Nehru Medical College
Aligarh Muslim University
Aligarh, UP
Email: *manazir1958@yahoo.com*

**Shivani Rohatgi** MSc
Consultant NRC
UNICEF Project (PPMU)
Kalawati Saran Children's Hospital
New Delhi
Email: *rohatgishivani.20@gmail.com*

**Srikanta Basu** MD, MAMS
Professor
Department of Pediatrics
Lady Hardinge Medical College and
Kalawati Saran Children's Hospital
New Delhi
Email: *srikantabasu@gmail.com*

**Subodh Sharan Gupta** MD DNB (MCH)
DNB (SPM)
Professor (Social Pediatrics)
Dr Sushila Nayar School of Public Health
Department of Community Medicine
Mahatma Gandhi Institute of Medical
Sciences, Sewagram
Wardha, Maharashtra
Email: *subodhsgupta@gmail.com*

**Umesh Kapil** MD
Professor and Head
Department of Human Nutrition
All India Institute of Medical Sciences
New Delhi
Email: *umeshkapil@gmail.com*

# Contents

# Burden of Undernutrition

Piyush Gupta, Nidhi Bedi

Nutrition has a powerful impact on maintaining health and preventing disease. Nutritional status of the children of any country is a good window to peep into its development. Nutrition is, therefore, an issue of survival, health, and development for current and succeeding generations.

Nutritional deficiencies of mother and children affect more than half of their global population.[1] Maternal undernutrition results in chronic energy deficiency, anemia, and iodine deficiency in the pregnant women; intrauterine growth restriction in their fetuses; and low birth weight in the offspring. Protein energy malnutrition (including severe acute malnutrition and chronic energy deprivation), underweight, stunting, wasting, and deficiencies of iron, vitamin A, iodine, and zinc are the major public health issues in the developing world in children.[2]

## Macronutrients vs Micronutrients

Carbohydrates, fats, and proteins are the chief sources of energy, and therefore, are also known as **macronutrients** or *proximate principles*. Children require energy for deposition of tissues for growth, whereas pregnant and lactating mothers need additional food supplements for the growth of fetus and maintaining milk secretion, respectively. When an individual is in a state of complete rest, energy is expended for basal metabolism.[3] *Micronutrients* or *protective principles* are nutrients required in tiny amounts, may be a few micrograms per day, and include various minerals and vitamins.[3] Severe acute malnutrition is caused by an acute (or acute on chronic) combined deficiency of macronutrients and micronutrients.

## 1.1 BURDEN OF UNDERNUTRITION

### A. Undernutrition and Child Mortality

Undernutrition (including intrauterine growth restriction (IUGR), protein energy malnutrition (PEM), stunting, wasting, and various micronutrient deficiencies) contributes to 45% of total deaths in children, globally.[3] As per the study conducted by Maternal and Child Undernutrition Study Group, maternal and child undernutrition attributes to 35% of the disease burden in under-five children and 11% of total global disability adjusted life years (DALY).[4] The causes of global under-five mortality are depicted in **Fig. 1.1**. About 35% of deaths in children have one or more of the three underlying risk factors: underweight, micronutrient deficiency, and inadequate breastfeeding.[5] Severe acute malnutrition is the most severe and life threatening form of undernutrition in children.

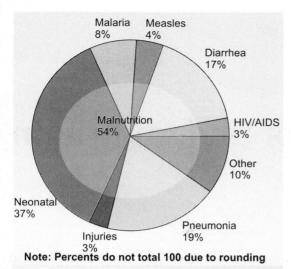

Malaria 8%
Measles 4%
Diarrhea 17%
Malnutrition 54%
HIV/AIDS 3%
Other 10%
Neonatal 37%
Pneumonia 19%
Injuries 3%

**Note: Percents do not total 100 due to rounding**

*Source: CHERG-WHO methods and data sources for child cause of death 2000-2013 (Global Health Estimates Technical Paper)*

**Fig. 1.1** Causes of deaths in children under-5 years (2013)

Majority of under-5 deaths in India are attributed to 4 major diseases—respiratory infections, diarrhea, other infections, and parasitic diseases and malaria. Undernutrition is the major risk factors contributing to these deaths. In India, 54 million children under the age of 5 years are underweight that constitute 37% of total underweight children in the world. Twenty five million under-5 children are wasted and 61 million are stunted in India, which constitute 31% and 28% of wasted and stunted in the world, respectively.[6]

Another category of children with high mortality rates are the low birth weight (LBW) babies i.e; those weighing less than 2500 g at birth. These children have 2–10 times higher risk of death compared to infants with normal birth weight. Low birth weight and early life undernutrition are now also recognized as risk factors for chronic diseases in later life.

## B. Global Prevalence of Undernutrition

In 2014, world had 667 million under-five children. Of these, 159 (23.8%) million were stunted, 90 million (13.5%) underweight, and 50 million (7.5%) wasted.[7] Among the wasted, nearly one-third were severely wasted. Asia alone has 34.3 million wasted children of which more than half are sheltered in South Asia, India being one of the most affected country. Within South Asia, 30% of under-five children are underweight, 37% stunted, and 15% wasted. This percentage is even higher in India. Almost 48% under-five children in India are stunted, 43% are underweight and 20% are wasted.[8] The situation is worse in rural areas, uneducated mothers, and children belonging to schedule caste, schedule tribe, and backward classes.

**Figures 1.2** and **1.3** depict the global prevalence of underweight and stunting in children below 5 years of age, respectively. The Asian data on prevalence of under-nutrition is summarized in **Table 1.1**.

## C. Burden of Undernutrition in India

As per National Family Health Survey (NFHS)-3 (2005-6), approximately 43% of underfive children were underweight, 48% were stunted, and 20% were wasted. Prevalence of severe underweight (<–3SD weight-for-age <–3SD), severe stunting (height-for-age <–3SD), and severe wasting (weight-for-height <–3SD) was 16%, 24%, and 6%, respectively. WHO growth standard median was taken as normal reference value. **Figure 1.4** depicts the trends of nutritional status of children in India from 1993 to 2014. The average annual reduction rate of stunting is 2.6% between NHFS-2 to NFHS-3. It is below the target rate of 3.7%. Wasting has also declined. In 2014, Ministry of Health and Family Welfare, Government of India conducted a rapid survey of children (RSoC) and collected national and state level data. **Table 1.2** and **Fig. 1.5** compare the statistics of NFHS surveys with that of RSoC. NFHS-4 data has been released only for few states and hence a comparative study could not be done.

In a state-wise assessment, as per NFHS-3, undernutrition was most pronounced in

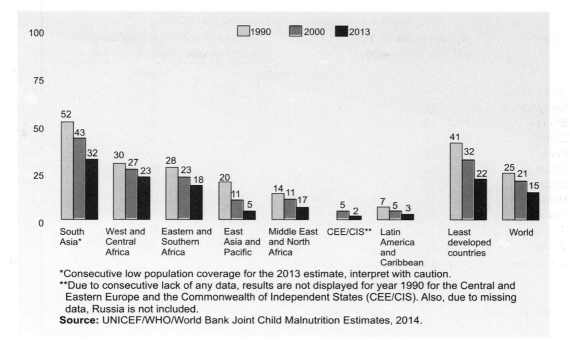

*Consecutive low population coverage for the 2013 estimate, interpret with caution.
**Due to consecutive lack of any data, results are not displayed for year 1990 for the Central and Eastern Europe and the Commonwealth of Independent States (CEE/CIS). Also, due to missing data, Russia is not included.
**Source:** UNICEF/WHO/World Bank Joint Child Malnutrition Estimates, 2014.

**Fig. 1.2** Percentage of children under-5 who areunderweight, by region, 1990 to 2013

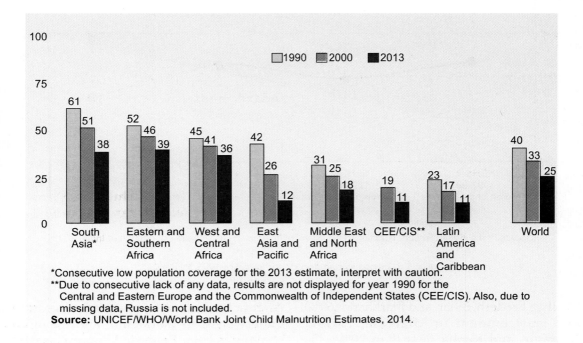

*Consecutive low population coverage for the 2013 estimate, interpret with caution.
**Due to consecutive lack of any data, results are not displayed for year 1990 for the Central and Eastern Europe and the Commonwealth of Independent States (CEE/CIS). Also, due to missing data, Russia is not included.
**Source:** UNICEF/WHO/World Bank Joint Child Malnutrition Estimates, 2014.

**Fig. 1.3** Percentage of children under-5 who are stunted, by region, 1990 to 2013

| Country | Percent of infants born with low birthweight | Percent of under-fives suffering from moderate and severe malnutrition | | |
|---|---|---|---|---|
| | | Underweight | Wasting | Stunting |
| Afghanistan | – | 33 | 9 | 59 |
| Bangladesh | 22 | 37 | 16 | 41 |
| Bhutan | 10 | 13 | 6 | 34 |
| China | – | 3 | 2 | 9 |
| India | 28 | 44 | 20 | 48 |
| Maldives | 11 | 18 | 10 | 20 |
| Myanmar | 9 | 23 | 8 | 35 |
| Nepal | 18 | 29 | 11 | 41 |
| Pakistan | 32 | 32 | 11 | 45 |
| Sri Lanka | 17 | 26 | 21 | 15 |
| World | 16 | 15 | 8 | 25 |

**Table 1.1** Prevalence of Childhood Malnutrition

*Source:* UNICEF, State of the World's Children 2009-2013.

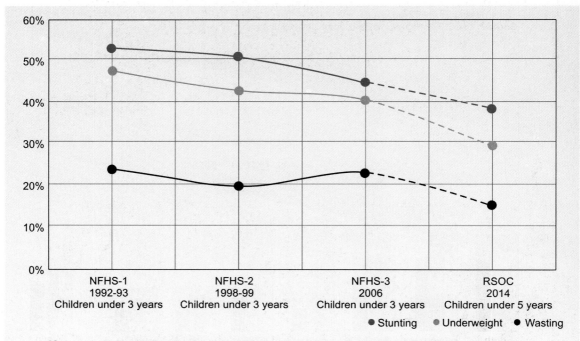

(*Source:* India Health Report: Nutrition 2015. New Delhi, India: Public Health Foundation of India; 2015).

**Fig. 1.4** Trends in nutrition status in India, 1993 to 2014.

Madhya Pradesh, Bihar, and Jharkhand (60%); and least evident in Mizoram, Sikkim, Manipur, and Kerala (less than 20%). The RSoC data has shown maximum wasting in Andhra Pradesh and Tamil Nadu, maximum underweight in Jharkhand, and maximum stunting in Uttar Pradesh. Minimum wasting was recorded in Sikkim, minimum under-

**Table 1.2** Comparison of Prevalence of Undernutrition from two National Surveys

| Indicator | NFHS 3 (2005-6) | RSoC (2014) |
| --- | --- | --- |
| Stunting | 47.9% | 38.8% |
| Wasting | 20.0% | 15.1% |
| Underweight | 43.0% | 29.4% |
| Severe Stunting | 23.7% | 17.3% |
| Severe Wasting | 6.4% | 4.6% |
| Severe Underweight | 15.8% | 9.4% |

NFHS-3: National Family Health Survey (2005-2006)
*RSoC: Rapid Survey of Children (2014)*

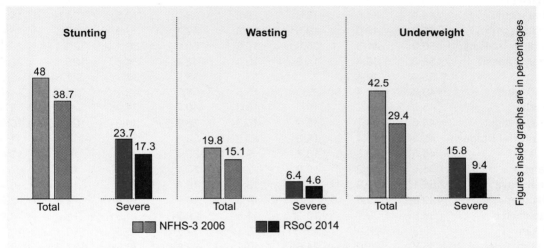

(*Source:* India Health Report: Nutrition 2015. New Delhi, India: Public Health Foundation of India; 2015).

**Fig. 1.5** Comparison of prevalence of undernutrition from two national surveys

weight in Mizoram, and minimum stunting in Kerala (**Table 1.3**). If we analyze the data based on severity (less than –3Z-score), latest figures show maximum severe stunting in Meghalaya, maximum severe wasting in Arunachal Pradesh and Tripura, and maximum severe underweight in Tripura followed by Jharkhand (**Table 1.4**).

## D. Micronutrient Malnutrition

Iron deficiency, vitamin A deficiency, and iodine deficiency are the three most common forms of micronutrient deficiency affecting at least one third of the population (2000 million) worldwide, mostly belonging to developing countries. Iron deficiency anaemia is the most prevalent micronutrient deficiency. It is estimated that just over 2 billion people are anemic, just under 2 billion have inadequate iodine nutrition, and 254 million preschool-aged children are vitamin A deicient. WHO has estimated that 1.5% (0.8 million) of total deaths can be attributed individually to iron deficiency and vitamin A deficiency. In terms of the loss of healthy life, expressed in disability-adjusted life years (DALYs), iron deciency anemia results in 47 million DALYs lost (or 4.7% of the global total), vitamin A deciency in 10 million DALYs lost (or 1% of the global total) and iodine deciency in 4 million DALYs lost (or 0.4% of the global total).[3]

**Table 1.3** Prevalence of Stunting, Wasting, Underweight, and Low-birth weight in Indian States: Comparison of Two National Surveys

| States | Stunting | | Wasting | | Underweight | | Low Birth Weight | |
|---|---|---|---|---|---|---|---|---|
| | NFHS–3 (2005-6) | RSoC (2014) | NFHS–3 (2005-6) | RSoC (2014) | NFHS–3 (2005-6) | RSoC (2014) | NFHS–3 (<5 yrs) | RSoC (<3yrs) |
| India | 48.0 | 38.7 | 19.8 | 15.1 | 42.5 | 29.4 | 21.5 | 18.6 |
| Delhi | 42.2 | 29.1 | 15.4 | 14.3 | 26.1 | 19.4 | 26.5 | 21.9 |
| Haryana | 45.7 | 36.4 | 19.1 | 8.8 | 39.6 | 22.7 | 32.7 | 20.9 |
| Himachal Pradesh | 38.6 | 34.2 | 19.3 | 10.8 | 36.5 | 19.5 | 24.8 | 17.7 |
| Jammu Kashmir | 35.0 | 31.7 | 14.8 | 7.1 | 25.6 | 15.6 | 19.4 | 16.2 |
| Punjab | 36.7 | 30.5 | 9.2 | 8.7 | 24.9 | 16.1 | 27.7 | 20.7 |
| Rajasthan | 43.7 | 36.5 | 20.4 | 14.1 | 39.9 | 31.5 | 27.5 | 23.2 |
| Uttaranchal | 44.4 | 34.0 | 18.8 | 9.3 | 38.0 | 20.5 | 24.6 | 14.2 |
| Chhattisgarh | 52.9 | 43.0 | 19.5 | 12.9 | 47.1 | 33.9 | 17.5 | 16.9 |
| MadhyaPradesh | 50.0 | 41.5 | 35.0 | 17.5 | 60.0 | 36.1 | 23.4 | 23.1 |
| Uttar Pradesh | 56.8 | 50.4 | 14.8 | 10.0 | 42.4 | 34.5 | 25.1 | 22.5 |
| Bihar | 55.6 | 49.4 | 27.1 | 13.1 | 55.9 | 37.1 | 27.6 | 15.0 |
| Jharkhand | 49.8 | 47.4 | 32.3 | 15.6 | 56.5 | 42.1 | 19.1 | 14.7 |
| Odisha | 45.0 | 38.2 | 19.5 | 18.3 | 40.7 | 34.4 | 20.6 | 18.9 |
| West Bengal | 44.6 | 34.7 | 16.9 | 15.3 | 38.7 | 30.0 | 22.9 | 16.9 |
| Arunachal Pradesh | 43.3 | 28.4 | 15.3 | 17.0 | 32.5 | 24.6 | 14.1 | 11.5 |
| Assam | 46.5 | 40.6 | 13.7 | 9.7 | 36.4 | 22.2 | 19.4 | 13.6 |
| Manipur | 35.6 | 33.2 | 9.0 | 7.1 | 22.1 | 14.1 | 13.1 | 7.3 |
| Meghalaya | 55.1 | 42.9 | 30.7 | 13.1 | 48.8 | 30.9 | 18.0 | 10.4 |
| Mizoram | 39.8 | 29.6 | 9.0 | 14.3 | 19.9 | 14.8 | 7.6 | 2.2 |
| Nagaland | 38.8 | 29.1 | 13.3 | 11.8 | 25.2 | 19.5 | 11.0 | 18.9 |
| Sikkim | 38.3 | 28.4 | 9.7 | 5.1 | 19.7 | 15.8 | 10.3 | 10.0 |
| Tripura | 35.7 | 31.0 | 24.6 | 17.1 | 39.6 | 30.5 | 27.3 | 18.5 |
| Goa | 25.6 | 21.3 | 14.1 | 15.4 | 25.0 | 16.2 | 22.2 | 16.7 |
| Gujarat | 51.7 | 41.6 | 18.7 | 18.7 | 44.6 | 33.5 | 22.0 | 19.5 |
| Maharashtra | 46.3 | 35.4 | 16.5 | 18.6 | 37.0 | 25.2 | 22.1 | 20.6 |
| Andhra Pradesh | 42.7 | 35.4 | 12.2 | 19.0 | 32.5 | 22.3 | 19.4 | 18.4 |
| Karnataka | 43.7 | 34.2 | 17.6 | 17.0 | 37.6 | 29.0 | 18.7 | 17.2 |
| Kerala | 24.5 | 19.4 | 15.9 | 15.5 | 22.9 | 18.5 | 16.1 | 16.7 |
| Tamil Nadu | 30.9 | 23.3 | 22.2 | 19.0 | 29.8 | 23.3 | 17.2 | 13.0 |

NFHS-3: National Family Health Survey (2005-2006)
*RSoC: Rapid Survey of Children (2014)*

The intake of iron rich foods is much lower when compared to vitamin A rich foods. As per NFHS-3 data, only 15% children eat foods rich in iron as compared to 50% children (6–35 months) consuming food rich in vitamin A. Only 50% children of 6–35 months live in households using adequately iodized salt. The percentage is much higher in urban areas (68%) than in rural areas (40%).

## 1.2 BURDEN OF SEVERE ACUTE MALNUTRITION

Severe acute malnutrition (SAM) is defined as weight-for-height (or weight-for-length for those less than 2 years age) below –3 Z-score of the median WHO child growth standards, a mid-upper arm circumference (MUAC) < 115 mm, or presence of pedal edema.[9] Worldwide, 26 million under-five children are

**Table 1.4** Prevalence of Severe Undernutrition in Indian States: Comparison of Two National Surveys

| States | Severe stunting | | Severe wasting | | Severe underweight | |
|---|---|---|---|---|---|---|
| | NFHS-3 (2005-6) | RSoC (2014) | NFHS-3 (2005-6) | RSoC (2014) | NFHS-3 (2005-6) | RSoC (2014) |
| India | 23.7 | 17.3 | 6.4 | 4.6 | 15.8 | 9.4 |
| Delhi | 20.4 | 14.1 | 7.0 | 4.6 | 8.7 | 4.9 |
| Haryana | 19.4 | 19.3 | 5.0 | 2.7 | 14.2 | 7.5 |
| Himachal Pradesh | 16.0 | 16.2 | 5.5 | 3.9 | 11.4 | 5.5 |
| Jammu Kashmir | 14.9 | 12.6 | 4.4 | 2.5 | 8.2 | 5.2 |
| Punjab | 17.3 | 13.1 | 2.1 | 3.2 | 8.0 | 4.3 |
| Rajasthan | 22.7 | 17.3 | 7.3 | 2.9 | 15.3 | 11.2 |
| Uttaranchal | 23.1 | 13.9 | 5.3 | 2.6 | 15.7 | 5.9 |
| Chhattisgarh | 24.8 | 16.4 | 5.6 | 2.4 | 16.4 | 9.9 |
| Madhya Pradesh | 26.3 | 18.5 | 12.6 | 5.4 | 27.3 | 12.0 |
| Uttar Pradesh | 32.4 | 28.4 | 5.1 | 2.9 | 16.4 | 12.9 |
| Bihar | 29.1 | 26.1 | 8.3 | 3.9 | 24.1 | 14.7 |
| Jharkhand | 26.6 | 23.7 | 11.8 | 3.7 | 26.1 | 16.1 |
| Odisha | 19.6 | 15.5 | 5.2 | 4.9 | 13.4 | 11.0 |
| Arunachal Pradesh | 21.7 | 19.6 | 6.1 | 7.1 | 11.1 | 13.3 |
| Assam | 20.9 | 21.0 | 4.0 | 2.7 | 11.4 | 7.0 |
| Manipur | 13.1 | 12.6 | 2.1 | 2.4 | 4.7 | 3.5 |
| Meghalaya | 29.8 | 29.4 | 19.9 | 5.2 | 27.7 | 16.0 |
| Mizoram | 17.7 | 15.3 | 3.5 | 6.2 | 5.4 | 6.1 |
| Nagaland | 19.3 | 15.8 | 5.2 | 4.8 | 7.1 | 7.9 |
| Sikkim | 17.9 | 11.0 | 3.3 | 1.4 | 4.9 | 6.5 |
| Tripura | 14.7 | 15.0 | 8.6 | 7.0 | 15.7 | 16.8 |
| Goa | 10.2 | 6.6 | 5.6 | 4.9 | 6.7 | 2.0 |
| Gujarat | 25.5 | 18.3 | 5.8 | 6.7 | 16.3 | 10.1 |
| Maharashtra | 19.1 | 10.0 | 5.2 | 6.3 | 11.9 | 5.7 |
| Andhra Pradesh | 18.7 | 12.0 | 3.5 | 6.0 | 9.9 | 4.7 |
| Karnataka | 20.5 | 15.1 | 5.9 | 6.3 | 12.8 | 9.8 |
| Kerala | 6.5 | 8.0 | 4.1 | 5.4 | 4.7 | 5.7 |
| Tamil Nadu | 10.9 | 9.3 | 8.9 | 6.3 | 6.4 | 6.1 |

NFHS-3: National Family Health Survey (2005-2006)
*RSoC: Rapid Survey of Children (2014)*

suffering from severe acute malnutrition; majority of whom belong to South Asia and Sub-Saharan Africa. Nearly 31% of the total severely wasted children live in India. SAM accounts for nearly 1 million deaths every year in under-five children. Children with SAM have 9 times higher risk of mortality than those in well-nourished children.[9] Mortality rates are highest in children having diarrhea, pneumonia, or measles.

According to the National Family Health Survey-3 (2005-2006),[8] 6.4% of children below 60 months of age are suffering from SAM in India. With the current estimated total population of India as 1100 million, it is expected that there would be about 132 million "under five children" (about 12% of the total population in the country) in India. Of these, it is expected that 6–7%, i.e. 8–9 million children, will be suffering from SAM.

Recently, severe acute malnutrition in infants below 6 months has emerged as a significant cause of infant deaths. The mortality in these children is much higher than those having SAM in older children. Since the main etiology is failure of adequate breastfeeding, treatment is challenging. The defining criteria are also different since MUAC is not considered an age independent criteria in children below 6 months of age. It has been estimated that approximately 4.79 million infants under 6 months of age are severely malnourished, and 5.45 million infants under 6 months of age are moderately malnourished in developing countries (out of a total of 55.8 million infants under 6 months of age in developing countries).[10] In India alone, about 32% of infants under 6 months of age are estimated to be wasted.

Previously, case fatality rates of treatment of SAM in resource poor health facilities were as high as 50–60% but with introduction of WHO management protocol, the fatality rates have come down to nearly half of before.

## 1.3 ECONOMIC BURDEN OF UNDERNUTRITION

Malnutrition still remains a major health problem in Asia and Africa. It is estimated that upto 11% of total productivity in these countries is lost to malnutrition.[11] The annual GDP from low weight, poor child growth, and micronutrient deficiencies averages 11% in Asia and Africa. In global analysis, it is estimated that a 10% increase in GDP can lead to 6% decrease in stunting. Also, economic progression alone is not enough for improvement in nutrition. From 1998-99 to 2005-06, GDP per capita in India expanded by 40% but stunting declined by only 6.1%. Besides, no consistent statistical association between agricultural growth and changes in child undernutrition was noted.[12]

Micronutrient malnutrition has many adverse effects on human health, not all of which are clinically evident. Even moderate levels of deficiency (which can be detected by biochemical or clinical measurements) can have serious detrimental effects on human function. Thus, in addition to the obvious and direct health effects, micronutrient malnutrition has profound implications for economic development and productivity, particularly in terms of the potentially huge public health costs and the loss of human capital formation.

## 1.4 NUTRITION AND HUMAN DEVELOPMENT

In 2015, countries assembled at the United Nations to adopt a new nutrition target as part of the Sustainable Development Goals to end all forms of malnutrition by 2030. In 2016, the United Nations General Assembly declared a decade of Action of Nutrition from 2016 to 2025, which shall translate the commitments into coherent and coordinated actions and initiatives by all national governments.

The rate of reduction in stunting since 2006-2014 in India was 2.3% per year which means India is approaching the rate of decline in other countries with similar level of stunting but still not enough. At this rate, India will reach the current stunting rate of China (10%) by 2055 only. India being a member state of World Health Organization has also endorsed the Sustainable Developmental Goals.

It is clear that human development is not possible without tackling the menace of childhood undernutrition. **Figure 1.6** shows the prevalence of under-5 stunting and level of economic development in selected countries. There is an urgent need of direct nutritional interventions and policy initiatives at the highest level, both for short-term and long term control. Identification and management of children with severe acute malnutrition, the subset of undernourished children reflecting the tip of the iceberg, should be the first priority.

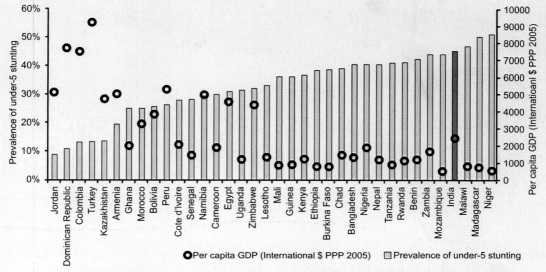

(*Source:* India Health Report: Nutrition 2015. New Delhi, India: Public Health Foundation of India; 2015)

Fig. 1.6 Prevalence of under-5 stunting and level of economic development by selected countries

# References

1. Ahmed T, Hussain M, Sainik KI. Global burden of Maternal and child undernutrition and micronutrient deficiencies. Ann Nutr Metab. 2012;6:8–17.

2. Black RE, Victoria CG, Walker SP, Bhutta ZA, Christian P, de Onis M, *et al.* Maternal and Child Nutrition Study Group. Maternal and child undernutrition and overweight in low income and middle income countries. Lancet. 2013;382: 427–51.

3. Gupta P, Khan AM. Textbook of Community Medicine. New Delhi: CBS; 2016.

4. Bhutta ZA, Das JK, Rizvi A, Gaffey MF, Walker N, Horton S, *et al.* Lancet Nutrition Interventions Review Group. Maternal and Child Nutrition Study Group. Evidence based interventions for improvement of maternal and child nutrition: what can be done and at what cost. Lancet. 2013;382:452–77.

5. World Health Organization. CHERG-WHO methods and data sources for child causes of death 2000-2013. Department of Health Statistics and Information Systems and WHO-UNICEF Child Health Epidemiology Reference Group (CHERG). Geneva: WHO;2014.

6. United Nation Childrens Fund. Improving Child Nutrition: The achievable imperative for global progress: New Delhi: Unicef; 2013.

7. International Food Policy Research Institute. Global Nutrition Report. From Promise to Impact: Ending Malnutrition by 2030. Washington DC: International Food Policy Research Institute; 2016.

8. International Institute for Population Sciences (IIPS). National Family Health Survey (NFHS-3), 2005-06: Mumbai, India: International Institute of Population Sciences; 2007.

9. WHO Child Growth Standards and the Identification of Severe Acute Malnutrition in Infants and Children. A Joint Statement from World Health Organization and United Nations Children's Fund, 2009. Available from:*http://www.who.int/nutrition/publications/severemalnutrition/9789241598163eng.pdf.* Accessed on 12 August 2016.

10. Grijalva-Eternod C, Kerac M, Blencowe H, McGrath M, Shoham J, Seal A. Malnutrition in <6 months old infants: Disease burden in developing countries and implications of WHO Child Growth Standards. Preliminary findings of the MAMI (management of acute malnutrition in Infants) Project presented at the MSF Scientific Day, London. 10th June 2009.

11. Taylor A, Dangour AD, Reddy KS. Only collective action will end undernutrition. Lancet. 2013; 382:490–1.

12. Raykar N, Majumder M, Laxminarayan R, Menon P. India Health Report: Nutrition 2015. New Delhi, India: Public Health Foundation of India; 2015.

# 2

# Epidemiology and Predisposing Factors for Undernutrition

Subodh S Gupta, Abhishek V Raut

Undernutrition is not merely lack of food. It is multifactorial in nature and results as combination of inadequate food intake, recurrent infections, poor quality care, faulty feeding practices, inadequate health services, and unsafe water and sanitation. It is a serious violation of the basic rights of a child to survive and its consequences often are not immediately seen until later stage.[1,2] Child undernutrition is globally recognized as an important public health problem. This led to target childhood undernutrition as one of the Millennium Development Goals (MDGs). The specific target among children younger than 5 years was to reduce by 50% the prevalence of being underweight between 1990 and 2015.[3] The post-MDG global health agenda also continues to lay special emphasis on the need for good nutrition for sustainable development. Goal 2 of the 2015 Sustainable Development Goals (SDGs) aims to "*end hunger, achieve food security and improved nutrition, and promote sustainable agriculture*".[4]

The effects, of child undernutrition on their health, performance, and survival are well established. The initial years of a child's life are absolutely crucial for developing cognitive capacity and physical growth. Lack of adequate nutrition in the initial years has profound, long-lasting, irreversible consequences across the life cycle. The deleterious effects include but may not be limited to stunting, impaired brain development, poorer health status, poor academic performance, and compromised economic productivity. Nearly half (45%) of all under-five deaths are attributed to undernutrition.[5-9]

Children who are well nourished remain healthy, are immune to disease and show better performance in school. Such healthy children, through their life, are better able to contribute to the development of the communities they live in. The rewards of adequate nutrition spill over from one generation to other and help in the development of healthy communities and nations.[2,10]

In this chapter, we focus on delineating burden of child undernutrition and compare its levels in different regions of the world. We will primarily focus on macronutrient deficiency with just a passing reference to problem of micronutrient deficiency just to highlight the need to focus on and address micronutrient deficiency as well. In addition, we will also discuss a causal framework for child undernutrition so that it may facilitate identification of various significant predictors in the causal framework for planning appropriate public health interventions.

## 2.1 INDICATORS FOR CHILD UNDERNUTRITION

Child undernutrition covers a range of disorders including protein-energy malnutrition (PEM) or impaired growth and micronutrient deficiencies. The most basic kind of undernutrition is called protein energy malnutrition (PEM). It is caused as a result of deficiencies in any or all nutrients that include macronutrients, as well as micronutrients. The diet usually is lacking in energy and protein and is deficient in all major macronutrients, such as carbohydrates, fats and proteins. Three indicators based on age, weight and length/height measurements—weight for age (W/A), height for age (H/A), and weight for height (W/H) are used to measure the burden of child undernutrition. For each of these three indicators, a value below –2 Z-score for the growth reference/standards used is considered a measure of undernutrition. This is further classified as moderate undernutrition, if the value is between –2 Z-score and –3 Z-score and severe, if the value is below –3 Z-score for the child growth reference/standards used **(Table 2.1)**.[11]

Currently, the child growth standard commonly used is the WHO Child Growth Standards developed using data collected in the WHO Multicentre Growth Reference Study and first released in 2006.[12,13] India adopted the WHO Child Growth Standards in year 2009 and the Mother and Child Protection Card were developed based on these child growth standards.[14,15] Indian Academy of Pediatrics (IAP) also recommends the new growth standards.[16]

### A. Stunting

**Length/height** is a very stable measure that reflects the total increase in size of the child up to the moment that it is determined, and therefore its total previous health history; however, it changes too slowly to be used in growth monitoring in community-based programs. Furthermore, length or height does not decrease and therefore cannot indicate deterioration in health.

**Stunting** (low height for age) reflects the cumulative effects of undernutrition and infections since and even before birth. The impact of stunting on child growth and development is irreversible and has far reaching consequences, from reduced learning and educational performance, to diminished future earnings.[17]

### B. Wasting

By relating the weight of a child to his/her height or length, an objective measure of the child's degree of thinness can be obtained. Weight for height is more specific in this respect than the measurement of weight alone, which does not distinguish between a tall, thin child and a short, fat child.

**Wasting** refers to a child who is too thin for his or her height. Wasting, or acute malnutrition, is due to recent rapid weight loss or the failure to gain weight. A child who is moderately or severely wasted has an increased risk of death, but treatment is possible. Severe wasting (W/H <–3SD) is also referred to as Severe acute malnutrition (SAM).[17]

### C. Underweight

The relative change of weight with age is more rapid than that of height and is much more sensitive to any deterioration or improvement in the health of the child. Significant changes can be observed over periods of few days to

| Table 2.1 Interpretation of Indicators for Undernutrition | | | |
|---|---|---|---|
| *Indicator* | *< –2 Z-score* | *–2 Z-score to –3 Z-score* | *< –3 Z-score* |
| Height for age (H/A) | Stunting | Moderate stunting | Severe stunting |
| Weight for height (W/H) | Wasting | Moderate wasting | Severe wasting |
| Weight for age (W/A) | Underweight | Moderate underweight | Severe underweight |

few weeks. Weight for age will be low in both acute and chronic malnutrition, and therefore, underweight does not differentiate between acute and chronic malnutrition.

## 2.2 GLOBAL TARGETS FOR UNDERNUTRITION

### A. Millennium Development Goals and Achievements

Reducing underweight was one of the specific targets of MDGs — reduce by 50% the prevalence of being underweight among children younger than 5 years between 1990 and 2015. Between 1990 and 2015, globally the proportion of under-five children who were underweight declined by 11% — from (25% to 14%). Africa experienced the smallest relative decline in underweight prevalence from 23% in 1990 to 16% in 2015; it declined in Asia from 32% to 17% and in Latin America and the Caribbean from 8% to 3%. Although Asia overall almost met the child under-nutrition target of MDG, of halving the 1990 rate of underweight, rates continue to be high in Southern Asia (27%). The underweight rate combined with large population, means that more than half of the world's underweight children live in Southern Asia (49 million out of the global estimate of 93 million in 2015).[18]

### B. Sustainable Development Goals

With sustainable development goals, attention has now shifted from childhood underweight to more specific measures of chronic and acute malnutrition; viz. stunting and wasting. Target 2.2 of the SDG includes, 'By 2030, end all forms of malnutrition, including achieving, by 2025, the internationally agreed targets on stunting and wasting in children under 5 years of age, and address the nutritional needs of adolescent girls, pregnant and lactating women, and older persons'.[19] Global nutrition targets are listed in **Table 2.2**.

• Stunting, which summarizes past nutritional experiences of a child, is a well-established risk marker of poor child development. Childhood stunting predicts poorer cognitive and educational outcomes in later childhood and adolescence and has significant educational and economic consequences at the individual, household and community levels.[20]

• Addressing wasting, the indicator of childhood acute malnutrition is of critical importance because of the increased risk of disease and death. It will gradually become difficult to continue improving child survival rates without reductions in the proportion of children wasted and without adequate provisions for timely and appropriate life-saving treatment for wasted children.[21]

## 2.3 BURDEN OF UNDERNUTRITION, REGIONAL VARIATIONS AND TRENDS

### A. Global Burden

WHO global database on child growth provides adjusted, comparable data for different countries.[22] In 2014, globally 159 million (23.8%) of under-5 children were stunted, 50 million (8%) were wasted and 90

**Table 2.2** Global Nutrition Targets 2025[16]

| Indicators | Targets |
|---|---|
| Childhood stunting | 40% reduction in the number of children under-5 who are stunted |
| Anemia in women of reproductive age | 50% reduction of anemia in women of reproductive age |
| Low birth weight | 30% reduction in low birth weight |
| Childhood overweight | No increase in childhood overweight |
| Breastfeeding | Increase the rate of exclusive breastfeeding in the first 6 months up to at least 50% |
| Childhood wasting | Reduce and maintain childhood wasting to less than 5% |

million (14%) were underweight.[23,24] Amongst the wasted children, nearly a third were severely wasted, global prevalence of severe wasting being around 2.4%. African and Asian countries bear the brunt of problem of undernutrition **(Table 2.3)**. For all developing countries, around one-third of under-5 children were stunted and around one fifth were underweight.[17,25]

Thirty six countries (21 in Africa, 13 in Asia and 1 each in Latin America and Oceania) accounted for 90% of all stunted children worldwide. In absolute terms, south-central Asia was the home to the largest number of stunted children (74 million). Almost all (96%) wasted children under-5 lived in Asia and Africa with the majority (68%) of children under-5 suffering from wasting living in Asia.[17,25]

**Figure 2.1** depicts the global trend in the prevalence of underweight, stunting, and wasting from 1990 to 2014 based on the data available from the WHO global database. Although the prevalence of stunting and underweight shows an overall declining trend when compared to the baseline rates in 1990,

the rate of change is rather slow and variable across countries. Wasting, however, showed only a marginal decline during the same period.

**Figures 2.2** to **2.4** show the global distribution of undernutrition among under-5 children (wasting, stunting, and underweight, respectively) in 2014.

## B. Undernutrition in India

The magnitude of child undernutrition in India is one of the highest in the world. Improvement in nutritional status of under-5 children is rather slow and does not reflect the substantial economic growth and progress which India has made. Almost around two-fifths of the world's stunted children live in India. In India, the burden of undernutrition is available at national and state level through the National Family Health Surveys (NFHS 1, 2 and 3 conducted in 1992-93, 1997-98 and 2005-06, respectively). National report for NFHS-4 conducted in 2014-15 was not available at the time of writing this chapter. The latest figures for undernutrition in India are available from Rapid Survey on Children (RSoC 2013-14) conducted by UNICEF for

**Table 2.3** Prevalence of Childhood Stunting, Wasting, Severe Wasting, and Underweight

| Region | Stunting (HAZ<−2) % (95% CI) | Wasting (WHZ<−2) % (95% CI) | Severe wasting (WHZ<−3) % (95% CI) | Underweight (WAZ<−2) % (95% CI) |
|---|---|---|---|---|
| Africa | 35.6% (33.3–38) | 8.5% (7.4–9.6) | 3.5% (2.9–4.1) | 17.7% (15.7–19.7) |
| Asia | 26.8% (23.2-30.5) | 10.1% (7.9–12.3) | 3.6% (2.4–4.8) | 19.3% (14.6–24.1) |
| Latin America and Caribbean | 13.4% (9.4–17.7) | 1.4% (0.9–1.9) | 0.3% (0.2–0.4) | 3.4% (2.3–4.5) |
| Oceania | 35.5% (16–61.4) | 4.3% (3.0–6.2) | 0.7% (0.5–1.1) | 14% (8.0–23.2) |
| Low & Middle income countries | 28% (25.6–30.4) | 8.8% (7.4–10.4) | 3.3% (2.5–4.0) | 17.4% (14.3–20.4) |
| High income countries | 7.2% (4.1–12.6) | 1.7% (0.8–3.5) | 0.3% (0.0–1.3) | 2.4% (1.7–3.4) |
| Global | 25.7% (23.5–27.9) | 8.0% (6.8–9.3) | 2.9% (2.2–3.6) | 15.7% (13.0–18.4) |

HAZ: Height-for-age Z score; WHZ: weight-for-age Z-score; WAZ: weight-for-age Z-score; CI: confidence interval
(*Adopted from Black, et al Lancet 2013*)[20]

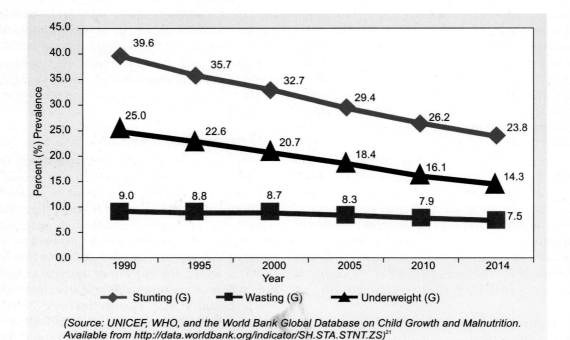

(Source: UNICEF, WHO, and the World Bank Global Database on Child Growth and Malnutrition. Available from http://data.worldbank.org/indicator/SH.STA.STNT.ZS)[21]

**Fig. 2.1** Global trend in prevalence of underweight, wasting and stunting

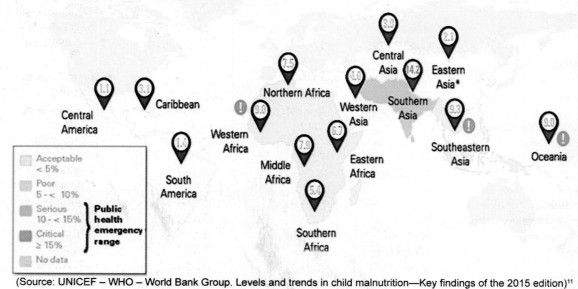

(Source: UNICEF – WHO – World Bank Group. Levels and trends in child malnutrition—Key findings of the 2015 edition)[11]

**Fig. 2.2** Percentage of children under-5 wasted, by United Nations sub-region in 2014

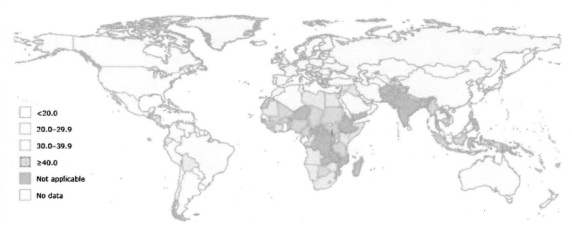

(Source: Prepared using data available from Global Health Observatory data repository)[24]

Fig. 2.3 Percentage of children under-5 stunted, by United Nations sub-region in 2014

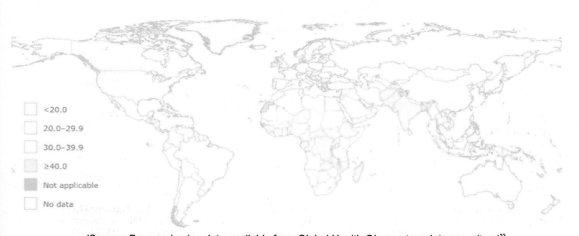

(Source: Prepared using data available from Global Health Observatory data repository)[23]

Fig. 2.4 Percentage of children under-5 underweight, by United Nations sub-region in 2014

Ministry of Women and Child Development (MoWCD) in 2013-14.

**Figure 2.5** shows the proportion of children who were stunted, wasted, and underweight in India based on RSoC 2013-14. Around 39% of under-5 children in India were stunted, 15% wasted, and 29% underweight. More worrisome, 17% of under-5 children were severely stunted, 10% severely underweight,

and 5% severely wasted. This amounts to every sixth child in India being severely stunted, 1 in 10 child being severely underweight, and 1 in 20 being severely wasted.[30]

**Figure 2.6** shows the trend in change in nutritional indicators for India over the last four decades. All the three indicators of stunting, wasting, and underweight have

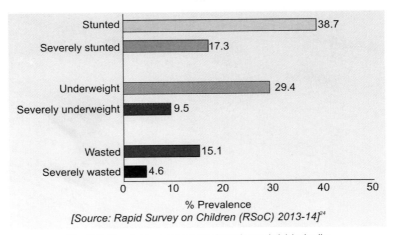

**Fig. 2.5** Stunted, wasted and underweight in India

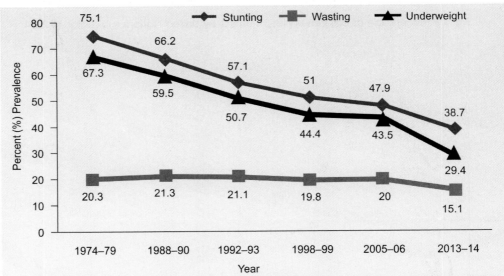

Data sources: 1974-79 - National Nutrition Monitoring Bureau survey; 1988-90 - National Nutrition Monitoring Bureau survey; 1992-93 National family health survey (NFHS-1); 1998-99 - National family health survey (NFHS-2); 2005-06 National family health survey (NFHS-3);2013-14 - Rapid survey on children (conducted by UNICEF for MoWCD)

*[Source: WHO Global Health Observatory data repository & RSOC 2013-14]* [22-24,28]

**Fig. 2.6** Trend in prevalence of underweight, wasting and stunting

improved over time albeit the pace of improvement is slow. Most improvement is seen in reduction in underweight followed by stunting. The improvement in wasting which may present an immediate threat to survival of children is proportionately much less. The rate of decline, that had almost flattened out in the decade between 1996 and 2006 shows improvement after the National Family Health Survey 3 conducted in 2005-06. In the same period, wasting has reduced at a rate of 0.7 percentage points per year while underweight and stunting declined at 2% and 1.3% points per year, respectively. [30-32]

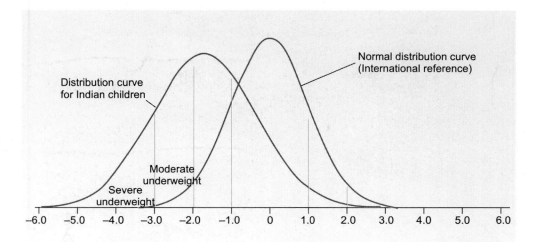

**Fig. 2.7** Comparison of weight-for-age distribution curve of Indian under-3 children with the global reference population[27]

A comparison of the distribution curves for the indicators (H/A, W/H, or W/A) for India with WHO standard normal distribution shows that the entire distribution curve is shifted to the left. The mean of the Indian curve for W/A is closer to –2 Z-score of the global reference population **(Fig. 2.7)**.[33]

Almost every state in India has its own share of nutritional problems and the nutritional status of under-5 children varies substantially across different states. **Figures 2.8 to 2.10** depict the state-wise prevalence of stunting, wasting, and underweight, respectively among under-5 children.

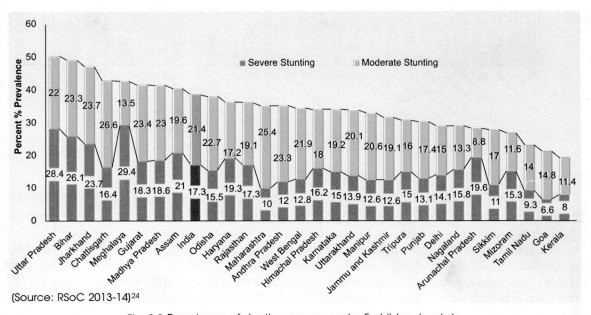

(Source: RSoC 2013-14)[24]

**Fig. 2.8** Prevalence of stunting among under-5 children by state

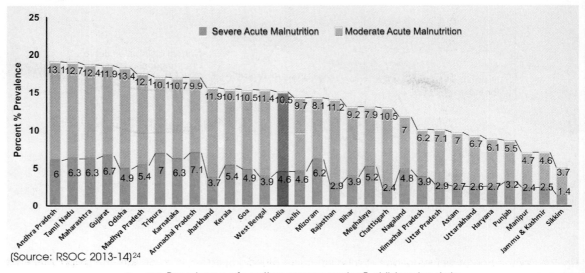

(Source: RSOC 2013-14)[24]

**Fig. 2.9** Prevalence of wasting among under-5 children by state

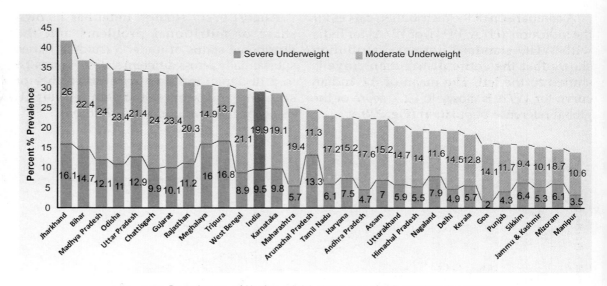

**Fig. 2.10** Prevalence of Underweight among under-5 children by state

## C. Factors in Childhood Undernutrition

Analysis of childhood undernutrition in the demographic surveys points to the role of immediate and underlying drivers of poor nutrition. Infant and young child feeding (IYCF) practices continue to remain poor in the country. According to the recent RSoC data, 65% of 0–5 months children were exclusively breastfed. Only approximately half of children aged 6–8 months were given complementary food and only 20% children age 6–23 months met minimum dietary diversity. **Figure 2.11** shows the level of undernutrition at different age as per NFHS-3. The proportion of children stunted and underweight increases with age till 2 years of

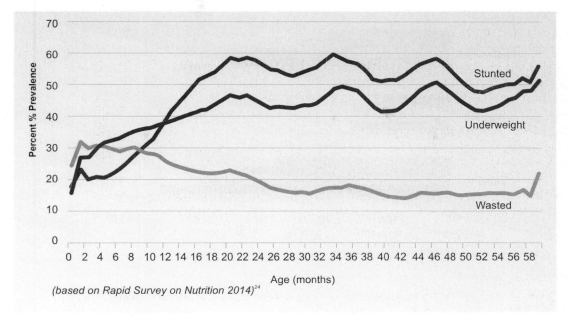

(based on Rapid Survey on Nutrition 2014)[24]

**Fig. 2.11** Undernutrition among under-five children by age

age, thereafter it remains almost at the same level with some fluctuation. This emphasizes on the role, complementary feeding practices plays in causation of undernutrition in India.[35]

The association between poverty and undernutrition is clearly evident from all demographic surveys conducted in India. Stunting, wasting, and underweight show an increasing trend as we move from highest to the lowest quintile of wealth **(Fig. 2.12)**. Other important drivers include maternal nutritional and health status, maternal education and their empowerment, water and sanitation, and issues related to food security.[35]

## 2.4 MAPPING THE MICRONUTRIENT DEFICIENCIES

Around 11% of the under-five deaths each year are attributed to micronutrient deficiencies. Along with child underweight, deficiencies of vitamin A, zinc, and iron are among the 19 leading risk factors to which cause of death is attributed.[26,36–37]

Micronutrient deficiencies are often called as 'hidden hunger' as they may exist even

when the macronutrient needs of an individual are being met. These can be classified as either Type 1 or Type 2.

- *Type 1 micronutrient deficiencies* lead to specific deficiency diseases, need not necessarily always affect growth, but will affect metabolism and immune resistance before signs are clinically apparent. Vitamins, folic acid, iron, iodine, calcium, copper, and selenium are included in this category.

- *Type 2 micronutrient deficiencies* do not present with specific clinical signs. They also affect metabolic processes however result in growth faltering, wasting, and lowered immunity. Sodium, potassium, magnesium, zinc, sulphur, phosphorus, essential amino acids, and nitrogen are grouped in this category.[38]

### A. Vitamin A Deficiency

Vitamin A is compromising the immunity of around 2/5th of the under-five children in developing countries and is attributed for causing early deaths of around one million

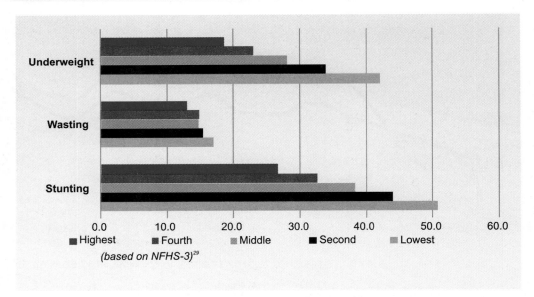

Fig. 2.12 Association between wealth index and undernutrition

under-5 children every year.[39,40] Vitamin A deficiency (VAD) is the commonest cause of preventable blindness among children. World Health Organization (WHO) includes VAD as a priority public health problem. In 2013, VAD affected around one third (29%) of children in 6 to 59 months, globally. VAD rates in sub-Saharan Africa and South Asia are 48% and 44%, respectively and are highest in the world.

Vitamin A supplementation apart from preventing blindness among children complements to maintain strong immune resistance, reduce the absolute risk of diarrhea and measles, and prevents hearing loss. Vitamin A supplementation may help to reduce the all-cause mortality among under-5 children by 12 to 24 percent. The benefits of vitamin A supplementation are strongest in high-risk populations as compared to the low or moderate risk populations.[41, 42]

Despite the proven benefits of Vitamin A supplementation, only a little over two-third of children (69%) were reached in 2014. The rates of supplementation were highest in East Asia and Pacific (86%) and West and Central Africa (83%). In Africa and South Asia where the problem of VAD is highest in terms of absolute numbers as well as rate, the coverage of Vitamin A supplementation was only 62%, far from satisfactory.[43]

## B. Iron Deficiency

Iron deficiency hampers cognitive development of around half of children aged 6–24 months in developing countries.[39,40] Gretchen, *et al.* analyzed demographic and health survey data of 107 countries worldwide from 257 population-representative data sources between 1995-2011 to determine trends and prevalence of anemia in children and pregnant and non-pregnant women. Global mean hemoglobin showed minimal improvement from 10.9 g/dL (10.7–11.1) to 11.1 g/dL (11.0–11.3) in children. Prevalence of anemia decreased from 47% (43–51) to 43% (38–47) in children. In 2011, 273 million (242–304 million) children were anemic globally. South Asia and Central and West Africa had lowest mean hemoglobin concentrations and highest prevalence of anemia. Improvement in anemia was only by 0.2–0.3 percentage points per year over the last two decades that was much lesser than improvement in child underweight for the same period (0.6 percentage points per year).[44,45]

## C. Iodine Deficiency

Iodine deficiency can present in the form of wide variety of health conditions known as iodine deficiency disorders (IDDs). Iodine deficiency has most impact in first trimester of pregnancy and in early childhood. IDDs may lead to cretinism, stillbirth, and miscarriage and can cause serious learning disability.

Although Iodine deficiency has been halved through provision of iodized salt to around 2/3rd of world's household it still continues to remain an important public health problem. Iodine deficiency during pregnancy is the commonest cause of mental impairment in 20 million babies born every year.[39,40]

### Universal Salt Iodization

It has been the most preferred strategy to control and eliminate IDDs over the last three decades. The target is to make iodized salt available for consumption in more than 90% of households, globally. However, in 2013, only around three-fourth of all households consumed iodized salt. East Asia and the Pacific region have the maximum consumption (86%) of iodized salt at household level. In comparison, the rates of consumption of iodized salt in South Asia, Sub-Saharan Africa and Least Developed Countries was 69%, 59%, and 50%, respectively. Out of the birth cohort of 138 million in 2013, 35 million (14 million in Sub-Saharan Africa and 11 million in South Asia) were at risk of iodine deficiency disorders.[46]

## D. Zinc Deficiency

Zinc deficiency contributes to growth failure and compromised immunity in early years of life. It is attributed with increased risk of diarrhea and pneumonia.[39,40]

## 2.5 MICRONUTRIENT DEFICIENCIES BURDEN IN INDIA

### A. Vitamin A Deficiency

VAD has reduced dramatically over the last few decades. There is decline in prevalence of keratomalacia and Bitot's spots. Although the prevalence of Bitot's spot is more than WHO cut-off (to define VAD as a public health problem) of 0.5 percent in some specific pockets and districts of the country especially those areas where there is extreme poverty and little socio-economic development.[46-51]

Because of the dramatic decline in prevalence of Bitot's spot, it is now recommended that the subclinical deficiency of Vitamin A, as assessed by serum retinol (SR) should be used as an indicator for determining the magnitude of VAD. According to WHO, 62% of the Indian population had serum retinol <0.70 μmol/L. The national vitamin A supplementation (VAS) coverage is variable across the country. In 2012, VAS coverage was above 80% in Bihar, Gujarat, Madhya Pradesh, Odisha, Rajasthan, and Tamil Nadu. In comparison, Andhra Pradesh, Kerala, and West Bengal had less than 20% coverage of VAS.[50-53]

Also, there is substantial controversy as regards to universal supplementation of Vitamin A. There is a school of thought that supports targeted supplementation of Vitamin A as against the universal supplementation. [50,54-58]

### B. Iron Deficiency Anemia

WHO classifies the level of public health significance of problem of anemia in India as severe.[59] As per the NFHS-3 data, seven of every 10 children in the age group of 6–59 months were anemic in India. Three percent were severely anemic (less than 7.0 g/dL), 40 percent had moderate anemia (7.0–9.9 g/dL) while 26 percent had mild anemia (10.0–10.9 g/dL).[35]

### C. Iodine Deficiency

India has the largest cohort of vulnerable infants born for likelihood of iodine deficiency disorders (IDD).[60] As mentioned in the National Iodine Deficiency Disorders Control Program (NIDDCP) for India, the goal was to reduce the prevalence of IDD to less than 10 percent by 2012. As per the Government of India report, 263 districts were endemic for IDD with the prevalence of IDD being above 10 percent.The prevalence of goiter was highest in Maharashtra (11.9%) and West Bengal (9%).[51,61,62]

### D. Status of Vitamin A, Iodine, and Iron and Folic Acid Supplementation

As per the RSoC 2013-14, with reference to the 6 months preceding the survey, the percentage of children who had received Vitamin A supplementation and Iron and folic acid supplementation was 45.2% and 13.4%, respectively, which reflects the poor implementation of the available effective public health interventions. The national average for household level consumption of adequately iodized salt (≥15 ppm) was 71% (range 8.2 percent in Tamil Nadu to 91.9 percent in Goa).[30,63]

This emphasizes that due focus should also be given for addressing the 'hidden hunger' in form of micronutrient deficiencies to complement the gains achieved in improving the rates of underweight, wasting, and stunting.

### 2.6 CAUSAL FRAMEWORK FOR CHILD UNDERNUTRITION

Undernutrition is not exclusively related to food and is a complex issue to decipher, with no single apparent cause or one simple solution. An interplay of multiple, interrelated factors is involved in developing undernutrition. It is important to develop a thorough understanding of the multiple complex and subtle causes of undernutrition to gauge the gravity and magnitude of the problem.

**Figure 2.13** depicts the conceptual framework developed by UNICEF to identify the basic and underlying causes of undernutrition that include environmental, social, economic and political factors. This conceptual framework was developed in 1990 as part of the UNICEF nutrition strategy. The framework illustrates that causes of undernutrition are multi-sectoral, including food, health, and child care practices. All causes of undernutrition both directly or indirectly act on the individual and may lead to undernutrition. Direct causes, *e.g.* inadequate dietary intake, diseases are considered as proximal causes and have direct effect in causing undernutrition. Indirect causes *e.g.* poverty, food security, unsafe water and poor sanitation, inadequate health services are the distal causes that act through a longer causal pathway as reflected in this framework. The causes may also be classified as immediate (individual level), underlying (household or family level), and basic (community/societal level), whereby factors at one level influence other levels.[64-66]

- *Immediate causes* These come into picture when there is a gap between the amount of nutrients required and available to the body. Such an imbalance may be due to too little intake of food or some underlying disease that compromises food absorption or a combination of both.

- *Underlying causes* Household food insecurity, inappropriate child caring practices, and inadequate health systems constitute the underlying causes of undernutrition.

- *Basic causes* Poverty, socio-political situation, prevailing cultural customs may prevail over the efforts of households to maintain adequate nutrition and therefore are described as basic causes of under-nutrition.

The conceptual model highlights the complexity of the multiple inter-related elements that may influence nutritional status at either the immediate, underlying, and basic level. More often than not, undernutrition cannot be classified as being only a food issue, or health problem, or care issue. It needs a comprehensive understanding of various factors affecting the nutritional status to look beyond just the food needs of a population.[64-66]

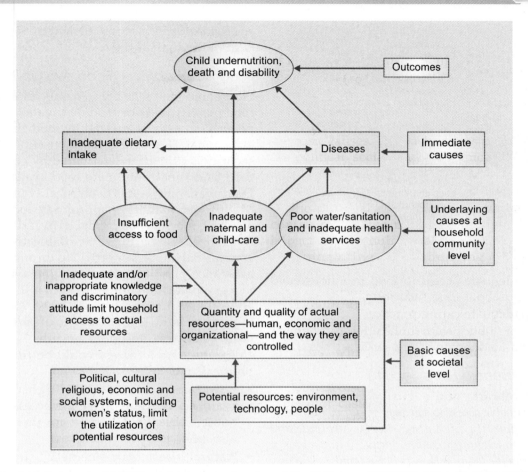

Fig. 2.13 Conceptual framework for causes of undernutrition[58] (*Source:* UNICEF Nutrition Strategy 1990)

## A. Immediate Causes

The immediate causes for undernutrition may be lack of dietary intake, or disease, or both. This may be due to the lesser amount of nutrients absorbed from food as compared to the nutrients required by the body. The cause for this may be consumption of too less food or having some infection that increases body's requirements or reduces appetite or affects the absorption capacity from the gut.

Undernutrition increases the likelihood to get an infection or increase its duration and/or severity. Usually undernutrition and infection co-occur with one increasing the risk for other in the form of a vicious cycle. **Figure 2.14** illustrates the infection-malnutrition vicious cycle—a malnourished child, whose immunity is poor, falls sick and becomes further malnourished that in turn reduces his/her capacity to fight against disease. This vicious cycle needs to be broken by timely and appropriate treatment for infection/s and improved dietary intake.[64-66]

## B. Underlying Causes

Inadequate dietary intake of nutrients or the risk of infection in a child is dependent on some factors operating at the individual household and community/societal level. In the UNICEF framework, these factors are classified as underlying causes. These underlying factors are described as 'food', 'care' and 'health' factors and can be grouped into three broad categories:

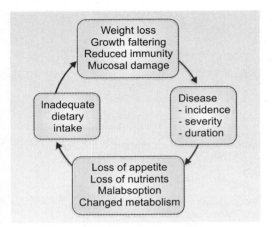

**Fig. 2.14** Infection-undernutrition cycle[58]

1. Inadequate access to food in a household (household food security)
2. Inadequate caring practices
3. Poor public health (unhealthy environment and inadequate health services)

## 1. Household Food Security

Household food security is defined as, *'sustainable access to safe food of sufficient quality and quantity including energy, protein, and micronutrients to ensure adequate intake and a healthy life for all members of the family'*. The key essence of the definition of food security is availability and accessibility of food 'at all times' and to all members in a given household. It is important to understand that in any given community, food security will vary from one season to another and may not be the same for every member of that household.[64-66]

It is important to understand the subtle difference between food shortage, food poverty, and food deprivation as it will help to identify the exact level at which problem lies. Also each of these food security issues requires different types of interventions.

- *Food shortage* is inadequate availability of food due to shortfalls in production or import of food on a national/regional level.
- *Food poverty* is inadequate access of food to a given household.

- *Food deprivation* is insufficient availability at individual level.[67]

## Food Accessibility vs Food Availability

Household food security is mainly an issue of food poverty and/ or food deprivation. Food poverty, in turn, is affected by food shortage at national/ regional level. Household food security is primarily determined by access to food as distinct from mere food availability. Food availability refers to physical availability of sufficient quantity of appropriate food. The available food may be produced by individual household, or be made available through commercial imports or provided through food assistance programs. Food may be available in a given area or community but will not be accessible to those who do not either have the minimum land to cultivate it or adequate money to buy it.

The barriers to access could be financial, physical, and social.

- Low family income and high cost of available food may make it inaccessible to poorer households rendering them food insecure.
- Natural disasters or emergency situations may make the food physically inaccessible for the households.
- Social norms prevalent in that community and unawareness related to dietary needs of people may make adequate food inaccessible to the sub-groups of population, *e.g.* women/girls in a household.

Although the food availability may not be an issue for a given household, the intra-household distribution of food may make some specific members of a household food deprived.[64-66]

## 2. Inadequate Caring Practices

Caring practices such as breastfeeding, timely initiation and appropriate complementary feeding, safe water, sanitation and hygiene, and health seeking behaviors complement good dietary practices.

## 3. *Poor Public Health*

The health status of a child is affected by access to safe water and sanitation, and personal and environmental hygiene in the immediate surroundings. Vector breeding sites, availability and quality of home/shelter, and exposure to extremes of temperatures, air pollution, overcrowding etc. adversely affect the health of a child and thereby his/her nutritional status. Access to basic health services determines the prevention and/or treatment of infection or various disease conditions. Often all these underlying factors also show a seasonal variation.

- Food may not be available in adequate quantities throughout the year and may be ample only in the months following the harvest.
- Floods during monsoon especially so in areas with difficult terrain may make the health facilities inaccessible for those 3 or 4 months of monsoon.

A sick child is dependent on his/her father and/or mother for visiting a health facility for treatment. Mother/father may not be able to spare time to take their sick child to health facility if they fear of losing out on their daily wages or if they have to finish off the farm work before the upcoming sowing season or harvest. In such a case, the time needed to access the health facility become a key determinant for inadequate health care.[64-66]

There is a significant interaction and overlap in the three underlying factors and these do not act in isolation. It is not always easy to determine the attributable fractions for each of the underlying factors for causing undernutrition. The relative contribution of the various underlying causes may vary from one region to another and from one under-nourished child to another. A thorough assessment may help to prioritize which underlying causes we need to address in a given community.

## C. Basic Causes

In the conceptual framework, the third level of factors that can be thought of as the actual reasons (poverty, education, governmental policies etc.) behind the underlying factors contributing to undernutrition and having impact in general on society are referred to as the basic causes. The basic causes usually are the political, social, and economic context as well as the natural physical environment in which the communities live in.

The physical environment in which the communities live may have a significant impact on their nutritional status. Communities inhabiting in challenging physical environment (such as frequent droughts, unreliable rainfall, extremes of temperatures, etc.) or in areas chronically affected by emergencies or conflicts show high prevalence of undernutrition as compared to communities or areas, which do not have to face such adversities.

Political discrimination by virtue of religion or race or caste can lead to marginalization and exclusion from food, livelihood opportunities and other basic services in form of health, education, shelter etc. and is one of the basic causes of undernutrition.[64-66]

## 2.7 EVIDENCE FOR RISK FACTORS OF UNDERNUTRITION

Various studies conducted across the globe support the concept of multi-factorial causation for undernutrition among children as described in the UNICEF framework. Some of these factors act directly (immediate cause) while some of the other factors mediate the effect indirectly through other factors (underlying and basic causes). Following evidence from different studies across the world have identified different risk factors ranging from presence of illness, food insecurity, lack of dietary diversity, maternal nutritional status and education, household income, to lack of access to safe water and sanitation emphasise the need for a multipronged systems approach for tackling the problem of undernutrition. Merely nutritional or food supplementation programs will not help to solve the problem of undernutrition unless the underlying factors are also addressed in a systematic manner.

## Association between Early Childhood Nutrition and Economic Growth

Vollmer S, et al[68] analyzed data from 121 Demographic and Health Surveys from 36 countries to study the association between economic growth (per-head gross domestic product (GDP) as the main independent variable) with stunting, underweight, and wasting in children aged 0–35 months as the outcome variables. Overall magnitude of undernutrition and adjusted odds among children aged 0–35 months are given in **Table 2.4**. The authors concluded that a very small to null association was seen between per-head GDP and early childhood undernutrition, emphasizing the need for direct health investments to improve the nutritional status of children in low-income and middle-income countries.[68]

## Under-5 Undernutrition in China

Zhang, et al[69] in their study on around 84000 under-5 children from different rural areas of China found that the prevalence of underweight, stunting, and wasting was 7.2%, 14.6% and 3.1%, respectively. Stunting and underweight set in mostly before two years of age. Low birth weight, multiparity, preterm birth, multiple birth, maternal illiteracy, low provincial GDP, and low household income have a significant association with stunting. Parity did not show significant relationship with underweight while wasting was not associated with either preterm or multiple births.[69]

## Risk Factors for Chronic Undernutrition in India

Corsi DJ, et al[70] studied the simultaneous contribution of 15 known risk factors for causing chronic undernutrition among children in India. They analyzed data of around 27000 children from National Family Health survey data set. Risk factors studied for probable association with undernutrition were vitamin A supplementation, immunization, usage of iodized salt, indoor air pollution, improved sanitation, safe drinking water, presence of any disease, breastfeed initiation, dietary diversity, maternal BMI, maternal height, maternal education, maternal age at marriage, and socio-economic status. After adjusting for other covariates, the five significant predictors of stunting/underweight were short maternal stature, mother with no education, poorest households, lack of dietary diversity, and maternal underweight. These five factors had a cumulative population attributable risk (PAR) of 67.2% for

**Table 2.4** Association between Indicators of Undernutrition and Per Capita GDP

| Indicator | Sample size | Prevalence % (95% CI) | Range Minimum | Maximum | Adjusted Odds ratio (95% CI) |
|---|---|---|---|---|---|
| Stunting | 462,854 | 35·6 (35·4–35·9) | 8·7% [7·6–9·7] in Jordan | 51·1% [49·1–53·1] in Niger | 0·996 (0·993–1·000) |
| Underweight | 485,152 | 22·7 (22·5–22·9) | 1·8% [1·3–2·3] in Jordan | 41·7% [41·1–42·3] in India | 0·989 (0·985–0·992) |
| Wasting | 459,538 | 12·8 (12·6–12·9) | 1·2% [0·6–1·8] in Peru | 28·8% [27·5–30·0] in Burkina Faso | 0·983 (0·979–0·986) |

*Source:* Vollmer S, et al

stunting and 69.7% for underweight. The other factors contributed with a combined PAR of 11.7% and 15.1% for stunting and underweight, respectively.[70]

## Child Stunting in India

Fenske, et al[71] have conducted secondary analysis of NFHS-3 data for India for children aged 0–24 months to identify the determinants for stunting. After extensive literature search they had identified many potential risk factors for stunting and clubbed them in 16 main groups that could be classified as immediate, underlying, and basic determinants for child stunting as described in the UNICEF conceptual framework of undernutrition. They found that of the 16 main groups, at least one variable within each of 11 groups of determinants was significantly associated with height-for-age. Age and sex of child, household wealth, maternal education, and maternal BMI showed the largest effects. The findings of this study confirm the role of multiple factors in causing child stunting and emphasizes the need to pursue a systems-based approach for tackling stunting among children.[71]

## Undernutrition in Sri Lanka

Rannan-Eliya, et al[72] analyzed data from four Demographic and Health Surveys (DHS) between 1987 to 2006-07 and the 2009 Nutrition and Food Security Survey (NFSS) in Sri Lanka to investigate trends and determinants of child undernutrition in Sri Lanka. They concluded that maternal height, household wealth, length of breastfeeding, and altitude were significant determinants of stunting, but differences in child feeding practices and other factors were not. Of these, maternal height and household wealth had the most influence.[72]

## Determinants of Stunting in Cambodia

Ikeda, et al[73] analyzed data of 10,366 children younger than 5 years available from different national surveys in Cambodia. They found

that child stunting was associated with the child's sex and age, type of birth, maternal height, maternal body mass index, previous birth intervals, family size, household wealth, access to improved sanitation facilities, presence of diarrhea, parental education, maternal tobacco use, and mother's birth during famine. The reduction in the prevalence of stunting during the past decade was attributable to improvements in household wealth, sanitation, parental education, birth spacing, and maternal tobacco use.[73]

Similar results have also been found in studies from Tanzania, Ethiopia, Bangladesh, Vietnam, and other studies from India where literacy and nutritional status of mothers, household wealth index, morbidities, low birth weight, food-insecurity and lack of access to safe water and sanitation were the most significant predictors of stunting and poor linear growth in children under 2 years.[74-78]

## References

1. IFPRI. 2016 Global Nutrition Report - From Promise to Impact: Ending Malnutrition by 2030. Available from: http://ebrary.ifpri.org/utils/getfile/collection/p15738coll2/id/130354/filename/130565.pdf. Accessed 20 Aug 2016.
2. Unicef. The faces of malnutrition. Available from: http://www2.unicef.org:60090/nutrition/index_faces-of-malnutrition.html. Accessed 20 Aug 2016.
3. Unicef Millennium Development Goals (MDG) monitoring: Statistics and Monitoring. Available from: http://www.unicef.org/statistics/index_24304.html. Accessed 20 Aug 2016.
4. United nations System - Standing Committee On Nutrition. Nutrition and the post-2015 sustainable development goals. Available from: http://www.unscn.org/files/Publications/Nutrition__The_New_Post_2015_Sustainable_development_Goals.pdf. Accessed 20 Aug 2016.
5. Caulfield LE, de Onis M, Blössner M, Black RE. Undernutrition as an underlying cause of child deaths associated with diarrhea, pneumonia, malaria, and measles. Am J Clin Nutr. 2004;80:193–8.
6. Chang SM, Walker SP, Grantham-McGregor S, Powell CA. Early childhood stunting and later

behaviour and school achievement. J Child Psychol Psychiatry. 2002;43:775–83.

7. Walker SP, Grantham-Mcgregor SM, Powell CA, Chang SM. Effects of growth restriction in early childhood on growth, IQ, and cognition at age 11 to 12 years and the benefits of nutritional supplementation and psychosocial stimulation. J Pediatr. 2000;137:36–41.

8. World Health Organization. Children: Reducing Mortality. Geneva: WHO;2016. Available from: http://www.who.int/mediacentre/factsheets/fs178/en/. Accessed 20 Aug 2016.

9. Save the Children. Nutrition in the First 1,000 Days. State of the World's Mothers 2012. Available from: http://www.savethechildren.org/atf/cf/{9def2ebe-10ae-432c-9bd0-df91d2eba74a}/State-of-the-Worlds-Mothers-Report-2012-Final.pdf.Accessed 20 Aug 2016.

10. World Bank. Education and learning depend on good nutrition and health. Available from: http://siteresources.worldbank.org/Nutrition/Resources/Tool10-FullReport.pdf.Accessed 20 Aug 2016.

11. World Health Organization. Physical Status: The Use and Interpretation of Anthropometry. Report of a WHO Expert Committee. WHO Technical Report Series No. 854. Geneva: World Health Organization; 1995.

12. World Health Organization [Online]. The WHO Multicentre Growth Reference Study (MGRS). Available from URL: http://www. who.int/childgrowth/mgrs/en/. Accessed 24 Oct 2016.

13. World Health Organization [Online]. WHO Child Growth Standards: length/height-for-age, weight-for-age, weight-for-length, weight-forheightand body mass index-for-age :methods and developments. Available from URL: http://www.who.int/childgrowth/standards/Technical_report.pdf. Accessed 24 Oct 2016.

14. UNICEF, India [Online]. Indian adopts new child growth standards. Available from URL: http://unicef.in/PressReleases/250/India-adopts-new-child-growth-standards. Accessed 24 Oct 2016.

15. Ministry of Women and Child Development [Online]. Mother and Child Protection Card Under ICDS and NHRM. Available from URL: http://icds-wcd.nic.in/icds/mccard.aspx. Accessed 24 Oct 2016.

16. Indian Academy of Pediatrics [Online]. Revised IAP Growth Charts 2015. 2016. Available from URL: http://iapindia.org /Revised-IAP-Growth-Charts-2015.php. Accessed 24 Oct 2016.

17. Unicef/WHO/World Bank Group. Levels and Trends in Child Malnutrition. Unicef/WHO/World Bank Group Joint Child Malnutrition Estimates. Key findings of the 2016 edition. Available from: http://www.who.int/nutgrowthdb/jme_brochure2016.pdf.Accessed 26 Aug 2016.

18. World Health Organization. Underweight in children. Global Health Observatory (GHO) data. Geneva: WHO; 2015. Available from: http://www.who.int/gho/mdg/poverty_hunger/underweight_text/en/.Accessed 26 Aug 2016.

19. United Nations. Sustainable Development Goal 2. Sustainable Development Knowledge Platform 2016. Available from: https://sustainable development.un.org/sdg2. Accessed 10 Oct 2016.

20. World Health Organization. Global Nutrition Targets 2025. Stunting Policy Brief 2014. Available from: http://apps.who.int/iris/bitstream/10665/149019/1/WHO_NMH_NHD_14.3_eng.pdf?ua=1. Accessed 13 Oct 2016.

21. World Health Organization. Global Nutrition Targets 2025. Wasting Policy Brief 2014. (WHO/NMH/NHD/14.8). Available from: http://apps.who.int/iris/bitstream/10665/149023/1/WHO_NMH_NHD_14.8_eng.pdf.Accessed 13 Oct 2016.

22. World Health Organization. Global Targets 2025. Geneva: WHO; 2015. Available from: http://www.who.int/nutrition/global-target-2025/en/. Accessed 13 Oct 2016.

23. World Health Organization. WHO Global Database on Child Growth and Malnutrition. Geneva: WHO; 2015. Available from: http://www.who.int/nutgrowthdb/en/.Accessed 26 Aug 2016.

24. Unicef. Improving Child Nutrition. The achievable imperative for global progress 2013. Available from: http://www.unicef.org/gambia/Improving_Child_Nutrition_the_achievable_imperative_for_global_progress.pdf. Accessed 26 Aug 2016.

25. Black RE, Allen LH, Bhutta ZA, Caulfield LE, de Onis M, Ezzati M, et al. Maternal and child undernutrition: global and regional exposures and health consequences. Lancet. 2008;371(9608):243–60.

26. Black RE, Victora CG, Walker SP, Bhutta ZA, Christian P, de Onis M, et al. Maternal and child undernutrition and overweight in low-income and middle-income countries. Lancet. 2013;382(9890):427-51.

27. The World Bank. Prevalence of wasting, weight for height (% of children under 5) data. Available from: http://data.worldbank.org/indicator/SH.STA.WAST.ZS?end=2014&start=1990&view=chart&year=1990.Accessed 26 Aug 2016.

28. World Health Organization. Children aged <5 years stunted data by country. Global Health Observatory data repository. Geneva: WHO; 2016. Available from: http://apps.who.int/gho/data/node.main.1097?lang=en.Accessed 26 Aug 2016.

29. World Health Organization. Children aged <5 years underweight data by country. Global Health Observatory data repository. Geneva: WHO; 2016. Available from: http://apps.who.int/gho/data/node.main.522?lang=en.Accessed 26 Aug 2016.

30. Government of India. Ministry of Women and Child Development. Rapid Survey On Children 2013-14 National Report; 2014. Available from: http://wcd.nic.in/sites/default/files/RSOC National Report 2013-14 Final.pdf.Accessed 10 Oct 2016.

31. Unicef-WHO-World Bank. Levels and Trends in Child Malnutrition. UNICEF - WHO - World Bank Group joint child malnutrition estimates. Key findings of the 2015 edition. 2015. Available from: http://www.unicef.org/media/files/JME_2015_edition_Sept_2015.pdf.Accessed 10 Oct 2016.

32. United Nations System Standing Committee, (UNSCN) on Nutrition. Progress in Nutrition. Sixth report on the world nutrition situation. 2010. Available from: http://www.unscn.org/files/Publications/RWNS6/html/index.html. Accessed 10 Oct 2016.

33. Gragnolati M, Shekar M, Das Gupta M, Bredenkamp C, Lee Y-K. India's Undernourished Children: A Call for Reform and Action;2005. Available from: http://siteresources.worldbank.org/SOUTHASIAEXT/Resources/223546-1147272668285/IndiaUndernourishedChildren Final.pdf.Accessed 10 Oct 2016.

34. World Health Organization. Children aged <5 years wasted Data by country. Global Health Observatory data repository. Geneva: WHO; 2015. Available from: http://apps.who.int/gho/data/node.main.1099?lang=en.Accessed 26 Aug 2016.

35. Arnold F, Parasuraman S, Arokiasamy P, Kothari M. Nutrition in India. National Family Health Survey (NFHS-3) India 2005-06. Mumbai: International Institute for Population Sciences; 2009.

36. Phelps L. Understanding Malnutrition (Module 3). The Harmonised Training Package (HTP): Resource Material for Training on Nutrition in Emergencies. Version 2. In: Walters T. NutritionWorks. Oxford, UK: Emergency Nutrition Network, Global Nutrition Cluster; 2011. Available from: http://www.unscn.org/en/gnc_htp/htp_documents_pdf.php.Accessed 26 Aug 2016.

37. World Health Organization. Global Patterns of Health Risk. Annexure A 2.1 Geneva: WHO; 2004.

38. Seal A, Timmer A, de R LM. Micronutrient Malnutrition (Module 4). The Harmonised Training Package (HTP): Resource Material for Training on Nutrition in Emergencies. Version 2. In: Dolan C. NutritionWorks. Oxford, UK: Emergency Nutrition Network, Global Nutrition Cluster; 2011.

39. Unicef. Vitamin and Mineral Deficiency. A Global Progress Report. 2004. Available from: http://www.unicef.org/media/files/vmd.pdf.Accessed 26 Aug 2016.

40. Unicef. Vitamin and Mineral Deficiency. A Global Damage Assessment Report; 2004. Available from: http://www.unicef.org/media/files/davos_micronutrient.pdf.Accessed 26 Aug 2016.

41. Francis DK. Vitamin Asupplementation for preventing death and illness in children 6 months to 5 years of age. Cochrane Database Syst Rev. 2011: CD000016.

42. Imdad A, Herzer K, Mayo-Wilson E, Yakoob MY, Bhutta ZA. Vitamin A supplementation for preventing morbidity and mortality in children from 6 months to 5 years of age. Cochrane Database Syst Rev. 2010:CD008524.

43. Vitamin A Deficiency. Current status + Progress. Available from: https://data.unicef.org/topic/nutrition/vitamin-a-deficiency/.Accessed 9 Oct 2016.

44. Stevens GA, Finucane MM, De-Regil LM, Paciorek CJ, Flaxman SR, Branca F, et al. Global, regional, and national trends in haemoglobin concentration and prevalence of total and severe anaemia in children and pregnant and non-pregnant women for 1995-2011: a systematic analysis of population-representative data. Lancet Glob Health. 2013;1(1):e16–25.

45. Mason J, Martorell R, Saldanha L, Shrimpton R, Stevens G, Finucane M, et al. Reduction of anaemia. Lancet Glob Health. 2013;1:e4–6.

46. Unicef. Iodine Deficiency. Available from: https://data.unicef.org/topic/nutrition/iodine-deficiency/. Asscessed 9 Oct 2016.

47. National Nutrition Monitoring Bureau. Prevalence of vitamin A Deficiency among Pre-school children in rural areas. 2006. Available from: http://nnmbindia.org/vad-report-final-21feb07.pdf. Accessed 13 Oct 2016.

48. Ministry of Women and Child Development. Government of India. Report of the Working Group on Nutrition. For the 12th Five Year Plan (2012–2017); 2011. Available from: http://planningcommission.gov.in/aboutus/committee/wrkgrp12/wcd/wgrep_nutition.pdf. Accessed 13 Oct 2016.

49. Akhtar S, Ahmed A, Randhawa MA, Atukorala S, Arlappa N, Ismail T, et al. Prevalence of vitamin A deficiency in South Asia: causes, outcomes, and possible remedies. J Health Popul Nutr. 2013;31(4):413–23.

50. Kapil U, Sachdev HPS. Massive dose vitamin A programme in India-need for a targeted approach. Indian J Med Res. 2013;38(3):411–7.

51. National Nutrition Monitoring Bureau. Prevalence of Micronutrient Deficiencies. NNMB Technical Report No. 22; 2003. Available from: http://nnmbindia.org/NNMB MND REPORT 2004-Web.pdf.Accessed 26 Aug 2016. Accessed 13 Oct 2016.

52. World Health Organization. Global Prevalence of Vitamin A Deficiency in Populations at Risk 1995-2005. WHO Global Database on Vitamin A Deficiency; 2009. Available from: http://apps.who.int/iris/bitstream/10665/44110/1/9789241598019_eng.pdf?ua=1.Accessed 13 Oct 2009.

53. Arlappa N, Balakrishna N, Laxmaiah A, Nair KM, Brahmam GN. Prevalence of clinical and sub-clinical vitamin A deficiency among rural preschool children of West Bengal, India. Indian Pediatr. 2011;48(1):47–9.

54. Kapil U. Ethical issues in vitamin A supplementation in India. Indian Journalfor the Practising Doctor; 2009. Available from: http://www.indmedica.comjournals.php?journalid=3&issueid=132 &articleid=1745&action=article.Accessed 10 Oct 2016.

55. Garner P, Taylor-Robinson D, Sachdev HPS. DEVTA: results from the biggest clinical trial ever. Lancet. 2013;381:1439–41.

56. Benn CS, Fisker AB, Aaby P, Awasthi S, Peto R, Read S, et al. Vitamin A supplementation in Indian children. Lancet. 2013;382(9892):593.

57. Awasthi S, Peto R, Read S, Clark S, Pande V, Bundy D, et al. Vitamin A supplementation every 6 months with retinol in 1 million pre-school children in north India: DEVTA, a cluster-randomised trial. Lancet. 2013;381(9876):1469–77.

58. Chen H, Zhuo Q, Yuan W, Wang J, Wu T. Vitamin A for preventing acute lower respiratory tract infections in children up to seven years of age. In: Wu T, editor. Cochrane Database Syst Rev. 2008;CD006090:20.

59. World Health Organization. The Global Prevalence of Anaemia in 2011. Available from: www.who.int/about/licensing/copyright_form/en/index.html.Accessed 13 Oct 2016.

60. Iodine Global Network. Global Iodine Nutrition Scorecard 2015. Available from: http://www.ign.org/cm_data/Scorecard_2015_August_26_new_1.pdf. Accessed 13 Oct 2016.

61. Pandav CS, Yadav K, Srivastava R, Pandav R, Karmarkar MG. Iodine deficiency disorders (IDD) control in India. Indian J Med Res.2013;138(3):418–33.

62. Annual Report 2010-11. Ministry of Health and Family Welfare. Government of India; 2011. Available from: http://www.mohfw.nic.in/showfile.php?lid=767. Accessed 13 Oct 2016.

63. Unicef. Iodized Salt Consumption SOWC; 2008. Available from: http://data.unicef.org/topic/nutrition/iodine-deficiency/.Accessed 13 Oct 2016.

64. Unicef. The State of the World's Children;1998. Available from: http://www.unicef.org/sowc98/sowc98.pdf.Accessed 26 Aug 2016.

65. Unicef. Response to nutrition in emergencies. Available from: http://www.unicef.org/nutrition/training/2.6/1.html.Accessed 26 Aug 2016.

66. Maxwell S. Causes of Malnutrition (Module 5). The Harmonised Training Package (HTP): Resource Material for Training on Nutrition in Emergencies. Version 2. Walters T.(editor). Nutrition Works. Oxford. UK: Emergency Nutrition Network, Global Nutrition Cluster; 2011.

67. de RoseL, Messer E,Millman S. Who's hungry? And how do we know? Food shortage, poverty, and deprivation. Hongkong; 1998. Available from: https://collections.unu.edu/eserv/UNU:2380/nLib9280809857.pdf.Accessed 7 Oct 2016.

68. Vollmer S, Harttgen K, Subramanyam MA, Finlay J, Klasen S, Subramanian SV. Association between

economic growth and early childhood undernutrition: evidence from 121 Demographic and Health Surveys from 36 low-income and middle-income countries. Lancet Glob Heal. 2014;2(4):e225–34.

69. Zhang J, Shi J, Himes JH, Du Y, Yang S, Shi S, *et al*. Undernutrition status of children under 5 years in Chinese rural areas - data from the National Rural Children Growth Standard Survey, 2006. Asia Pac J Clin Nutr. 2011;20(4):584–92.

70. Corsi DJ, Mejía-Guevara I, Subramanian SV. Risk factors for chronic undernutrition among children in India: Estimating relative importance, population attributable risk and fractions. Soc Sci Med. 2016;157:165–85.

71. Fenske N, Burns J, Hothorn T, Rehfuess EA. Understanding child stunting in India: a comprehensive analysis of socio-economic, nutritional and environmental determinants using additive quantile regression. PLoS One. 2013;8(11):e78692.

72. Rannan-Eliya RP, Hossain SMM, Anuranga C, Wickramasinghe R, Jayatissa R, Abeykoon ATPL. Trends and determinants of childhood stunting and underweight in Sri Lanka. Ceylon Med J. 2013;58(1):10–8.

73. Ikeda N, Irie Y, Shibuya K. Determinants of reduced child stunting in Cambodia: analysis of pooled data from three demographic and health surveys. Bull World Health Organ. 2013;91:341–9.

74. Meshram II, Arlappa N, Balakrishna N, Mallikharjuna Rao K, Laxmaiah A, Brahmam GNV. Trends in the prevalence of undernutrition, nutrient and food intake and predictors of undernutrition among under five year tribal children in India. Asia Pac J Clin Nutr. 2012;21:568–76.

75. Medhin G, Hanlon C, Dewey M, Alem A, Tesfaye F, Worku B, *et al*. Prevalence and predictors of undernutrition among infants aged six and twelve months in Butajira, Ethiopia: the P-MaMiE Birth Cohort. BMC Public Health. 2010;10:27.

76. Ali D, Saha KK, Nguyen PH, Diressie MT, Ruel MT, Menon P, *et al*. Household food insecurity is associated with higher child undernutrition in Bangladesh, Ethiopia, and Vietnam, but the effect is not mediated by child dietary diversity. J Nutr. 2013;143:2015–21.

77. Chirande L, Charwe D, Mbwana H, Victor R, Kimboka S, Issaka AI, *et al*. Determinants of stunting and severe stunting among under-fives in Tanzania: evidence from the 2010 cross-sectional household survey. BMC Pediatr. 2015;15:165.

78. Aguayo VM, Nair R, Badgaiyan N, Krishna V. Determinants of stunting and poor linear growth in children under 2 years of age in India: an in-depth analysis of Maharashtra's comprehensive nutrition survey. Matern Child Nutr. 2016;12 Suppl 1:121–40.

# Identification and Classification of Severe Acute Malnutrition

S Aneja, Preeti Singh

## 3.1 INTRODUCTION

Anthropometry is the universally accepted gold standard tool for assessing the nutritional status in children. It helps to define growth, well-being and predicts overall health and survival. Anthropometric interpretations are influenced by the genetic and environmental factors and among the populations. Anthropometric assessment and regular monitoring helps in early detection of growth faltering. This facilitates timely intervention that prevents children from progressing through severe grades of undernutrition and death. In those who manage to survive, it averts the irreversible consequences of impaired physical, psychosocial, and cognitive development.

Deficits in the individual anthropometric indicators that define childhood stunting and wasting are associated with increased morbidity and mortality.[1,2] The risk of mortality is amplified in the presence of multiple anthropometric deficits as reported in a recent meta-analysis.[3] Hence it becomes important to use valid and reliable tools for early identification of children with undernutrition to prevent motor, cognitive, developmental disability; and mortality.

The anthropometric assessment at the community level helps to estimate the burden and severity of malnutrition, which is instrumental in formulation of public health and nutritional policies. This mandates the precise selection of anthropometric tools that helps to identify the most vulnerable group in a community/population, and target the health and nutritional interventions to improve their health outcomes.

## 3.2 ASSESSMENT OF NUTRITIONAL STATUS

Nutritional status is defined as the inherent state of health of an individual that harmonizes with assimilation of nutrients at the molecular level. This state cannot be measured directly, so a series of indicators (alone or in combination) are used to define it. It encompasses the anthropometric measurements and indices, along with clinical and biochemical indicators which are briefly discussed below.

### A. Anthropometric Assessment

Anthropometric assessment involves measuring the physical dimensions like child's weight, length or height, and mid-upper arm circumference. The measurements taken should be accurate and precise using standardized protocols and well calibrated instruments. All possible precautions are taken to minimize intraobserver and interobserver variations in recording the measurements.

## 1. *Weight*

An electronic/mechanical sliding beam balance type scale is used to measure the weight of children. Infant scales usually have a graduation of 10 grams, while the scale for older children has graduations of 50–100 g.

### *Technique of weighing*

- Weighing scale should be calibrated for zero error.
- Child should be in minimal clothing.
- Infant is placed in the center on the scale tray.
- Children > 2 years are made to stand in the middle of the scale, feet slightly apart, and asked to remain still until the weight appears on the display.
- Weigh infant to the nearest 10 g and older child to nearest 100 g.

If a separate infant weighing scale is not available, the infant can be weighed on the adult scale using 'tared weighing." Tared weighing is also useful for weighing agitated infants who will not remain calm when placed on the infant weighing scale.

## 2. *Length and Height*

Recumbent length is measured using an infantometer for children below 2 years of age. After 2 years, height is measured. Height is measured in light underclothing and without shoes. At least two persons are needed to correctly record a child's length.

### *Technique of recording length*

- Place the child on his back in the center of infantometer placed on a flat, stable surface such as a table, lying straight with his shoulders and buttocks flat against the measuring surface and eyes looking straight up.
- The second helper holds the head along the head piece.
- Align the trunk and legs, extend both legs, and apply gentle pressure to the knees with one hand to straighten the legs without causing injury.

- Bring the movable foot-piece to press firmly against the heels. The toes should be pointing upward with feet flat against the foot-piece.
- Record the length to nearest 0.1 cm.

### *Technique of recording height*

For a child > 2 years, measure standing height unless the child is unable to stand. Use a height board (or a stadiometer) mounted at a right angle between a level floor and against a straight, vertical surface such as a wall or pillar to measure height.

- Ensure shoes, socks, and hair ornaments have been removed.
- The child stands with back of his head, shoulder blades, buttocks, and heal touching the wall, looking straight ahead with lower border of the eye socket in the same horizontal plane as external auditory meatus.
- To keep the head in this position, hold the bridge between your thumb and forefinger over the child's chin.
- A right angled block slides down the scale till it touches the head and compresses the hair.
- Height is recorded to the nearest 0.1 cm.

Note that there is usually a difference of 0.7 cm in the length and height of a child. In case length is recorded for a child > 2 years of age, subtract 0.7 cm from this length to get a true assessment of the height.

## 3. *Mid-upper Arm Circumference*

Mid-upper arm circumference (MUAC) is an age independent criterion for assessment of nutritional status in children >6 months of age. It is especially useful for screening under-nutrition in children when weight and stature cannot be measured.

### *Technique of recording MUAC*

- MUAC is measured in the left arm at a point midway between the acromion process at shoulder and the olecranon process of the ulna.

- With the elbow flexed to 90°, the midpoint is determined by measuring the distance between the two landmarks using a tape measure. Mark the midpoint on the lateral side of arm with a visible marker (chalk, pen) and take the MUAC using a measuring tape keeping the arm hanging loosely by the side.
- Record the MUAC to the nearest 0.1 cm.

## B. Clinical Signs

Visible severe wasting and bipedal edema are important clinical signs that define severe acute malnutrition (SAM). The use of these clinical signs in the identification of cases with SAM requires training and expertise. Although they lack objectivity, still they are valuable tools to identify the most vulnerable group of children during emergency settings and in case of unavailability of anthropometric equipment.

### 1. Visible Severe Wasting

A child with visible severe wasting is extremely thin, has no subcutaneous fat and looks like skin and bones. To assess visible severe wasting, remove the child's clothes and look for muscle wasting of the shoulder, arms, buttocks, and legs. On viewing the side profile, the loose skin folds at the buttocks and thigh are visible those resemble wearing a baggy pant.

### 2. Edema

To identify bilateral pitting pedal edema, normal thumb pressure is applied at the dorsum of both feet simultaneously for 10 seconds. In presence of edema, the impression/pit remains for some time on both feet when the thumb is lifted, at places where the fluid has been displaced out of the tissue. Nutritional edema always starts from feet and extends upwards to other parts of the body. The presence of bilateral pitting pedal edema of nutritional origin is recommended as an independent criteria to screen children with SAM in both community and facility based management. The severity of edema can be graded as follows:

- No edema: 0
- Edema below the ankles: +
- Edema in both feet, legs, and below the knees: ++
- Edema on both feet, legs, arms, sacral pad, and eyelids: +++

## C. Biochemical Parameters

This involves analysis of the components of the metabolic pathways that require sophisticated laboratory facilities *e.g.* serum albumin, serum retinol, serum 25OHD levels. The need for costly equipment, reagents, and skilled and qualified health personnel to collect specimen and conduct and interpret the test results makes biochemical indicators inapt for the community assessment of the nutritional status. They are of use only for facility based care and research purposes.

## 3.3 MEASUREMENTS, INDICES, AND INDICATORS

Let us understand the terms measurements, indices, and indicators, before we apply them to practice in assessment of anthropometry.[4]

### A. Measurements

Measurements refer to baseline anthropometric variables like weight, length/height, and mid upper arm circumference. These anthropometric measurements, by themselves, do not provide any significant information about the nutritional status of the individual.

### B. Indices

The indices are derived from the composite use of measurements. In isolation, weight will not provide any meaningful information unless it is expressed in relation to a stable variable like age or height *e.g.* weight-for-age, or weight-for-height. Therefore, to interpret measurements, they are expressed as indices. The anthropometric indices that are commonly used in pediatric age group include weight-for-age, length/height-for-age, and weight-for-length/height.

Anthropometric indices are expressed with respect to reference/standard growth curves using three different ways:

   i. *Percentile* Position of the observed measurement within a centile distribution of the reference;

  ii. *Percentage of the reference median* Ratio of a measured or observed value in the individual to the median value of the reference data for the same sex and age or height; and as

 iii. Z-score *or standard deviation (SD score)* The difference between the value for an individual and the median value of the reference population for the same age or height, divided by the standard deviation of the reference population.

The preferred and most important means of expression of anthropometric indices is Z-score. The advantage of Z-score is its utility as a summary statistic like computing mean and standard deviation which is not possible with the percentile method. The percentile system will not be able to reflect the absolute changes in the measurement (height or weight) at the extreme ends. The percent of median system cannot compare the deficits across the different anthropometric parameters like weight and height. In addition, the cut-off for median will be different for all three indices (weight-for-age, height-for-age, and weight-for-height) at a particular Z-score. For example; a Z-score of less than –2 corresponds to a cut-off point (percentage of median) of 90% for height-for-age and 80% for weight-for-height.

## C. Indicators

The application of indices to a larger perspective necessitates the need of indicators. These are derived from indices. The indicators used in public health are objective tools that define the state of health for a larger group like population/community and help to quantify and monitor the outcome of the interventions. The anthropometric indicators used for screening children with malnutrition in a community should be able to identify and differentiate those with aberrant anthropometry associated with poor health outcome from the ones who diverge as part of normal variation in the population.

The indicators are defined by cut-off points for indices to make interpretations at population/community level; e.g. weight-for-age <–2 Z-score defines the proportion of children (of defined age and sex) with weight <–2 Z-score below the median of a reference distribution for that age and sex. Some indices such as infant mortality rate can be used as indicators to define the state of public health.

## 3.4 BIOLOGICAL SIGNIFICANCE OF THE INDICES

The deficits in the anthropometric indices are an indicator towards undernutrition and provide clue to its duration and outcome. A well child will have his nutritional parameters (weight-for-age, length-for-age, weight for length/ BMI) within ± 2 Z-scores (standard deviations) of the median expected for the age and sex. Late in the nineteenth century, the terms wasting and stunting were proposed to describe the pathological deficits in weight-for-height and height-for-age, respectively.[5] If the child's WFA, LFA, or WFH/L is less than –2 Z-score, it indicates presence of underweight, stunting, or wasting, respectively. Each of these indices represents different course of malnutrition. The assessment of the nutritional status based on the anthropometric indicators is illustrated in **Table 3.1**.

## 1. Height-for-Age (HFA)

It is a measure of linear growth of an individual, which is interpreted in relation to the age of the child. Stunting signifies deceleration in linear growth and is defined as low height-for-age (<–2 Z-score). It

**Table 3.1** Assessment of the Nutritional Status based on Anthropometric Indicators

| SD (Z) score | Indicators | | |
|---|---|---|---|
| | Weight-for-age | Height-for-age | Weight-for-length/height |
| Median to –1 | Normal | Normal | Normal |
| Below–2 | Moderately underweight | Stunted | Wasted |
| | | | Moderate acute malnutrition (MAM) |
| Below –3 | Severely underweight | Severely stunted | Severely wasted |
| | | | Severe acute malnutrition (SAM) |

characterizes failure to reach the linear growth potential.

## Etiopathogenesis of Stunting

Stunting evolves over a period of time due to chronic suboptimal food intake, recurrent infections and has a strong association with poor socioeconomic conditions. It represents a longstanding or chronic phase of malnutrition/suboptimal health. It is important to understand that linear growth is a slow process and an individual can fail to gain height but will never lose it. In the preschool age, stunting indicates failure to grow while in later phase reflects that the child had failed to grow. The catch up in length/height may or may not occur depending on the time line at which intervention is initiated. Linear growth is usually not used as an indicator to monitor the response to interventions.

## 2. Weight-for-Height (WFH)

It is the measure of weight with respect to the height and does not account for the age of the individual. Wasting is defined as low WFH (<–2 Z-score) as it signifies the loss of fat mass and tissue that occurs in comparison with a normal child of the same length or height. It indicates present state of undernutrition, regardless of the age.

## Etiopathogenesis of Wasting

Wasting develops as a result of severe and acute weight loss or when there is failure to gain weight, which can occur with acute illness, inadequate dietary intake, or in a natural disaster. In case the underlying cause continues for long period, it would affect the linear growth also and lead to stunting. Severe wasting indicates a high risk of morbidity and mortality. An important attribute of wasting is its rapid development and renewal once the underlying cause is treated.[6]

## 3. Weight-for-Age (WFA)

It is an indicator of body weight with respect to the chronological age. It is a composite measure of both height-for-age as well as weight-for-height making its interpretation difficult. Low weight-for-age (<–2 Z-score) can reflect either low weight-for-height or low height-for-age or both thereby encompassing both acute and chronic malnutrition.

Under the ICDS scheme, growth monitoring of children attending the Anganwadi Center (AWC) is done using growth charts (based on World Health Organization growth standards) based on weight-for-age for boys and girls. It has three color coded categories: green for normal, yellow for under-weight (WFA between –2 Z-score to –3 Z-score) and red for severely underweight (WFA <–3 Z-score) child. The limitation of WFA assessment is its inability to differentiate between acute and chronic malnutrition.

## 4. Mid-Upper Arm Circumference (MUAC)

Mid-upper arm circumference (MUAC) is a measure of the diameter of the upper arm that encompasses both fat reserves and muscle mass. In areas where weight and height measurements are not possible especially in field/community set up, MUAC is an extremely useful tool to assess the nutritional status. **Low MUAC indicates wasting**.

MUAC and MUAC for height (MUAC/H) are age independent indicators of malnutrition as there is very small variation in the reference median (approximately 17 mm) over 1–5 years of age.[7,8] The predictive power of mortality of MUAC is also independent of age even in children below 1 year of age.[9,10] In both community and hospital settings, MUAC is superior to WFH in predicting childhood mortality.[11,12]

- *Shakir's tape:* Shakir's tape is a tool used by the peripheral health workers for measuring MUAC. MUAC is read in three visual Zones – red < 12.5 cm (signifies malnutrition), yellow between 12.5–13.5 cm (borderline) and green > 13.5 cm (normal).
- *New WHO tape:* In 2009, WHO and UNICEF issued a joint statement for identification of children with SAM and to translate it, a new MUAC tape was introduced. This tape also displayed three color zones but with different cut-offs (red–0 to 11.5 cm, yellow–11.5 to 12.5 cm, and green >12.5 cm).
- *Bangle test:* Another alternative to assess MUAC is the Bangle test. A bangle is passed above the elbow, whose internal diameter is 4 cm (circumference about 12.5 cm). If the bangle can be passed above the elbow it indicates that the child has severe malnutrition.

Other age independent indices of anthropometry are given in **Table 3.2**.

## 5. Body Mass Index (BMI)

BMI is defined as the weight in kilos divided by the square of height in meters. The index varies with age for children and adolescents, and must therefore be interpreted in relation to BMI-for-age reference charts. BMI is an important tool to measure undernutrition or thinness. Currently WHO classifies undernutrition as "thinness" and "severe thinness" using cut-offs at –2 Z-score and –3 Z-score of BMI for age, respectively. This classification is used for children > 5 years of age.

## 3.5 SELECTION OF AN INDICATOR AND CUT-OFF POINTS

The best anthropometric indicator to define the nutritional status of an individual may not be the most suited tool for the community assessment program or facility based care. This is because the community based programs primarily focus on preventing mortality and hence they use indices that define the most vulnerable group (highest risk of dying) that would presumably show prompt response to nutritional interventions.

Sackett and Holland[13] devised a scoring system to assess the appropriateness of the anthropometric tools used for identification of cases (screening) in various settings. They defined the essential attributes which a case

| Name of index | Calculation | Normal value | Value in malnutrition |
|---|---|---|---|
| Kanawati and McLaren index | Mid-upper arm circumference/ head circumference (cm) | 0.32–0.33 | Severely malnourished: <0.25 |
| Rao and Singh index | (Weight (kg)/height² (cm)) × 100 | 0.14 | 0.12–0.14 |
| Dugdale index | (Weight (kg)/height 1.6 (cm)) × 1 | 0.88–0.97 | <0.79 |
| Quacker arm circumference measuring stick (Quac stick) | Mid-upper arm circumference that would be expected for a given height | | 75–85%-malnourished <75%- severely malnourished |
| Jeliffe's ratio | Head circumference/chest circumference | | Ratio <1 in a child >1 year: malnourished |

**Table 3.2** Age-Independent Anthropometric Indices

defining indicator should have i.e. simplicity, acceptability, low cost, accuracy (closeness to the true measurement), precision (degree of reproducibility), and reasonable degree of sensitivity/specificity/predictive value that varies across the clinical/epidemiological settings. In usual circumstances, the indicator used for nutritional surveillance and screening should be highly specific with a reasonable degree of sensitivity.

For a community based screening, Beaton and Bengoa[14] suggested that the indicator used should be objective and quantitative in addition to the above enumerated properties. The concept of age independent criteria was proposed by Jelliffe and Jelliffe[15] as in community based settings it is often difficult and unfeasible to ascertain the age accurately.

The selection of an indicator also depends upon the skill and knowledge of the people who would apply the indicator. The conventional cut-off points (–2 Z-score) are applicable where resources are adequate. When the resources are limited, the cut-offs are determined by the finances and capacity available to screen and treat rather than the need to treat. In such cases, the cut-off points are lowered to take care of the most vulnerable group at highest risk of morbidity and mortality. This will automatically increase the specificity of the indicator at the expense of low sensitivity. Multiple screening indices can be utilized for screening large numbers and with meagre resources.

Different anthropometric indicators have varied applications and interpretation across the populations and settings. The selection of an appropriate anthropometric indicator to identify the cases of interest depends upon the setting in which the case detection is being done. The most important application is to identify individuals or populations at risk of poor health outcome i.e. morbidity or mortality. The indicator selected for this purpose should reflect the present/past risk or predict the future risk of adverse health outcome. The second important application of an anthropometric indicator is to assess the effectiveness of an intervention/therapeutic program. The indicator used for this purpose should be able to predict the benefit or the response.

## Facility Based Inpatient Care

WHO and UNICEF recommend the WFH cut-off <–3 Z-score (WHO 2006 Growth standards) to identify children under 5 years of age with Severe acute malnutrition (SAM). This cut-off –3 Z-score for WFH has a high specificity of 99% and the proportion identified carry a 9 fold high risk of mortality as compared to those with WFH >–1 Z-score.[16] Other reasons for selecting this as cut-off are as follows:

i. Children identified as SAM using this cut-off demonstrate a higher weight gain and recovery when put on therapeutic diets;

ii. Virtual absence of healthy population below –3 Z-score (<1%); and

iii. No risks identified in application of therapeutic protocols to this subgroup.

This classification is designed for clinical settings/facility care and intended to be used by skilled clinical staff. The cost and complexity of the above classification has precluded its use by the community volunteers.

Stunting or low HFA (<–2 Z-score) indicates long standing undernutrition in early childhood (past risk) and increased risk of mortality (present risk) but it loses its reliability to predict future risk with advancing age. HFA does not show prompt response to nutritional rehabilitation.

## Community-based Therapeutic Care

For community based programs, the use of multi-component indicators (i.e. WFA, HFA, WFH,) defies the properties of simplicity and acceptability since it involves the use of multi-dimensional tables/growth charts and familiarity with arithmetic concepts.[17] Moreover, the unskilled staff employed in community based screening programs will be unable to use them with accuracy and precision. Indicators with age component (i.e. HFA, WFA) are subject to random errors in age estimation.[18,19]

MUAC in comparison with the above indicators is a simple and low cost tool that can be utilized for door to door screening in community.[20] MUAC has an operational advantage of not needing any reference charts for interpretation. A single cut-off can be applied to screen children (6–59 months of age) with wasting, irrespective of age, sex, and height.[21] MUAC is a fairly accurate and reproducible/precise tool when put to use in field settings.[22,23] The median for MUAC shows very little variation with age[8] and its predictive power for mortality is again age independent.[24,25]

The introduction of color banded cards by Shakir and Morley[26] has further simplified the technique to be used by minimally trained paramedical staffs in the field setting. WFH also displays age independent properties between 1 and 5 years[27] but the predictive power (i.e. mortality) of WFH may change with age.[28] In most studies across developing countries to assess the sensitivity of indicators for predicting mortality at a high specificity, MUAC is reported superior to HFA and WFA while WFH was observed as least effective predictor.[11,29] Even in emergency/disaster conditions,MUAC is a reasonably good indicator to screen children (6 months -5 years) with acute malnutrition.

The current WHO classification of malnutrition defines the cut-off of MUAC <115 mm to classify SAM as it increases the risk of dying in the same proportion as defined by WFH <–3 Z-score.[30]

## Edematous Malnutrition

The WFH or MUAC in isolation cannot definitively identify both the spectra of malnutrition i.e. marasmus and kwashiorkor (edematous malnutrition). WFH will not be able to reliably identify the subgroup of edematous SAM, as the retained fluid will mask the otherwise low WFH. Therefore, the presence of bilateral bipedal edema is used as an independent adjunctive tool to detect cases of edematous SAM in children in both facility as well as community assessment. Since edema has a strong association with mortality, it is employed for screening and surveillance purposes to designate children with SAM independent of other anthropometric parameters.

However, in a study from Malawi, MUAC was reported to be more sensitive and specific than WFA and WFH used in isolation to identify children with edematous malnutrition.[31] **Table 3.3** summarizes the anthropometric screening tools and their cut-offs to identify children with malnutrition in different clinical settings.

## 3.6 EVOLUTION OF GROWTH CHARTS

### 1. Growth Reference vs Growth Standard

The anthropometric indices obtained for an individual are interpreted by comparing with the population reference or standards using growth charts.The growth charts can be classified as growth reference charts and growth standards that differ in their conceptual design and approach.

- The growth references are the descriptive charts that describe the growth of an individual at a cross-sectional point (time and place) e.g. NCHS or CDC charts.
- On the other hand, the growth standards are the prospective growth charts that describe the growth of the healthy children longitudinally under optimal environment/ nutrition, e.g. WHO (2006) growth charts.

### 2. From NCHS to WHO Growth Charts

In 1977-78, the NCHS (National Center for Health Statistics, USA) developed smoothened percentile curves of weight, height, and head circumference from birth to 18 years using cross-sectional data from US Health examination surveys and longitudinal data

**Table 3.3** Anthropometric Tools and their Cut offs to Identify Malnutrition in Children

| Type of setting | Purpose | Index | Cut offs |
|---|---|---|---|
| Emergency setting | Identify children less than 5 years requiring immediate intervention | 1. Mid upper arm circumference (MUAC)<br>2. Bilateral pitting pedal edema | Depends on resources. Conventional cut offs used when resources adequate; MUAC <12.5 cm. In case of limited resources, cut offs brought down < 11.5 cm. |
| Non-emergency settings for facility based care | Screening children < 5 years for nutrition rehabilitation and/or other health intervention | 1. Weight-for-height/ length (WFL/H)<br>2. Mid-upper arm circumference (MUAC) in 6–59 months<br>3. Bilateral pitting edema of both feet | WFL/H <–3 Z-score * or MUAC <11.5 cm* or B/L pedal edema* |
| Non-emergency settings for community based therapeutic care | Screening for Nutritional surveillance and rehabilitation | 1. Mid-upper arm circumference (MUAC) in 6–59 months<br>2. Bilateral pitting pedal edema of both feet | Conventional cut offs used when resources adequate; MUAC <12.5 cm*<br>In case of limited resources, cut offs brought down to < 11.5 cm. |

*Indications for hospitalization: Age less than 6 months, presence of any emergency signs, hypothermia (axillary temperature < 35°C), poor appetite, persistent vomiting, lethargic and apathetic, diarrhea with dehydration, severe anemia, evidence of systemic infections or complications.

from Fels Research Institute.[32] They were later adapted by Centers for Disease Control and Prevention (CDC, Atlanta), USA. The major limitation of the NCHS curves was the use of two different data sets representing different age groups and in different time frame for compilation. The charts had disjunction in the measurement of length and height during the transition period from 2 to 3 years. Besides, the charts lacked racial and genetic diversity of the population surveyed and the infants included in the data were formula fed predisposing children to obesity by promoting excessive weight gain in infancy. These growth reference curves[33] were recommended and endorsed by WHO for international use as growth reference curves till the introduction of the WHO Growth Standards in 2006.

## 3. WHO Growth Standards 2006

In 2006, the WHO released new Multicentre Growth Reference Standards (MGRS) for assessing the growth and development of children from birth to 5 years of age.[34] The WHO (2006) Growth Standards (WHO-GS) are prescriptive, longitudinal growth standards that represent optimal growth. They are based on international sample of breastfed infants of different ethnic origins from 6 diverse geographical locations (Brazil, Ghana, India, Norway, Oman, and the United States) who were raised in optimal conditions and measured in a standardized way. The WHO-GS validate the fact that the differences in growth of children till 5 years of age across the boundaries are primarily determined by environmental factors and the role of genetic and ethnic factors is very small. Hence they have been adopted as universal standards for growth assessment for under-5 children globally. These new standards have been endorsed by international bodies such as the United Nations Standing Committee on Nutrition,[35] The International Union of

Nutritional Sciences and International Paediatric Association[36] and have been adopted in more than 90 countries.[37] The Centers for Disease Control and Prevention, USA also recommends the use of WHO standards in US population up to 2 years of age.

## 3.7 CLASSIFICATION OF MALNUTRITION

Historically, many classification systems have been proposed to grade the severity of malnutrition. One of the initial classifications was based on weight-for-age, as proposed by Gomez in 1956.[38] Subsequently, Seoane and Latham[39] developed a classification using WFH and HFA to identify wasting and stunting, respectively. The use of Z-scores or Z-score below the cut-off to define underweight (low weight-for-age), stunting (low height-for-age) and wasting (low weight-for-height) was suggested by Waterlow in 1977.[40,41] In 1981, WHO defined 3 clinical variants of protein energy malnutrition as marasmus, kwashiorkor, and a mixed form, marasmic kwashiorkor on the basis of phenotypic features. Subsequently in 1999, WHO came up with classification system of malnutrition for children 6–59 months of age based on Z-score of WFH, HFA, or the presence/absence of bilateral symmetrical pedal edema involving at least the feet (edematous malnutrition) **(Table 3.4)**.[42]

The NCHS (1978) growth reference charts were used as the reference population data to classify malnutrition till 2006. The IMNCI classification of malnutrition was introduced in 2005 based on clinical signs like visible severe wasting (marasmic spectrum) and bipedal edema (kwashiorkar).[43] Under IMNCI, growth monitoring was done using weight-for-age; however, this failed to differentiate between acute and chronic malnutrition. Visible severe wasting had limitations of being subjective and an unreliable indicator to detect severe wasting in the community.[30,31]

### 1. Severe Acute Malnutrition

To address the problem of acute and severe malnutrition, the nomenclature "Severe acute malnutrition" (SAM) was introduced. It was defined as very low weight-for-height (WFH<–3 Z-score), visible severe wasting, or the presence of nutritional bipedal edema. In 2007, the United Nations agencies endorsed a low MUAC<110 mm as an independent diagnostic criterion for SAM, besides a WFH <–3 Z-score or nutritional bipedal edema.[44,45] After the introduction of WHO 2006 GS, WHO and UNICEF recommended similar cut-offs for WFH (<–3Z-score) using WHO-GS, as used earlier by NCHS standards to define SAM. This resulted in a 2–4 fold rise in the proportion of children identified as SAM (using WHO-GS) than by the NCHS reference.

| | Table 3.4 WHO Classification of Malnutrition[42] | |
|---|---|---|
| | *Moderate malnutrition* | *Severe malnutrition* |
| Symmetrical edema | No | Yes **(edematous malnutrition)** |
| Weight-for-height | Between –3 and <– 2 Z-score OR 70–79% of median | Z-score <–3 OR <70% of median **Severe wasting** |
| Height-for-age | Between –3 and <–2 Z-score OR 85–89% of median | Z-score <–3 OR <85% of median **Severe stunting** |

It was of public health importance as the increase in case load would have a substantial impact on the existing resources and had programmatic repercussions. For MUAC using a cut-off <115 mm, the prevalence of wasting and the risk of mortality was reported to be similar to that of WFH <–3 Z-score.[46] This led to an increase in the cut-off of MUAC to <115 mm (from 110 mm) to take care of the increased case burden and was observed to align more closely to WFH <–3 Z-score using 2006 WHO-GS. In 2009, a higher cut-off point of MUAC (115 mm) was recommended in a joint statement by WHO and UNICEF.[46] The cut-off selected to define SAM — WFH (<–3 Z-score) and MUAC (< 115 mm) observed a high specificity (>99%) over the age range 6–60 months.[31]

## 2. What is in Practice Today?

The nutritional status of children 6 months to 5 years of age can be classified as underweight, wasted, and stunted based on the indicators WFA, WFH, and HFA Z-scores, respectively **(Table 3.4)**. The WHO 2006 growth standards are used for comparing the anthropometric indicators.

The current recommendation by WHO for defining severe acute malnutrition in children less than 5 years of age is elaborated in **Table 3.5**.[51] Visible severe wasting is not used as diagnostic criteria for SAM, as there is not enough evidence to support it as an

independent criterion. The discharge criteria used for exit from the nutritional rehabilitation program depends upon the anthropometric criteria used for admission. The cut-offs values recommended for discharge is WFH/L ≥ 2Z-score and MUAC ≥ 125 mm. Children admitted on the basis of bipedal edema are discharged once edema resolves using either of the above anthropometric indicators. Discharge criteria are further discussed in Chapter 10.

## 3. Comparison of WFH and MUAC for Identifying SAM

An important caveat to the use of independent case definitions using WFH and MUAC is that they do not identify same set of children with SAM.[47,48] There is only 40% degree of agreement using both the indicators in detection of cases with SAM, leaving a large proportion of potentially high risk cases as untreated.The probable explanation to it is that children identified by low WFH Z-score and missed by low MUAC are more likely to be males and the incongruence observed increases with advancing age. The community based longitudinal data from Senegal[49] was analyzed to establish the relationship between anthropometric parameters and mortality and to determine the benefit of combination of the WFH and MUAC in identifying children with SAM. They observed no added advantage in using both WFH<–3 Z-score and MUAC

**Table 3.5** WHO Recommended Criteria for Identification of Severe Acute Malnutrition[51]

| Age | Criteria |
|---|---|
| 6 months–5 years | • Weight-for-height/length <–3 Z-score and/or <br>• Mid-upper arm circumference (MUAC) < 11.5 cm and/or <br>• Bilateral pitting edema of both feet* |
| Less than 6 months ** | • Weight-for-height/length <–3 Z-score** and/or <br>• Bilateral pitting edema of both feet* |

*Unilateral edema is not indicator of SAM and there should not be a known cause of edema like nephritic syndrome, congestive heart failure, etc.

** For children with length less than 45 cm, visible severe wasting can be used to identify SAM.

<115 mm for detection of high risk cases, and MUAC alone was observed to be superior to WFH.[50] There has been no RCT to compare the outcomes of children admitted independently on the basis of low WFH versus MUAC.

## 3.8 CHALLENGES OF ANTHROPOMETRIC ASSESSMENT IN YOUNG INFANTS

In young infants (age < 6 months), the application of anthropometric tools is an arduous task that requires resources, equipment, and skill. It is recommended to measure weight using the instrument with a least count of 10 g rather than the conventional 100 g graduated scale and an infantometer is needed to correctly measure the length. Though weight is commonly measured during infancy at every health visit, but WFA does not reliably differentiate between acute and chronic malnutrition. It is influenced by the birth weight and the gestational age of the individual.

Weight-for-length (WFL) is a useful tool to assess acute malnutrition in children less than 5 years but its utilization in young infants depends upon the availability of infantometer, familiarity, ability to use it correctly, and the skill needed for its interpretation. Measurements of length in young infants are subject to errors and unlikely to yield precise results. Studies to compare the interobserver variability in the assessment of MUAC and WFL Z-score in infants <6 months by community health workers, reported higher reliability for MUAC than WFL Z-scores.[52,53] They observed that WFL Z-scores were extremely sensitive to even small variation in the measurements of length. MUAC offers the technical advantage of a simple, inexpensive and easy to use tool in the hands of community health workers, in comparison to WFL Z-score estimation. The validity and accuracy of MUAC Z-score in young infants (< 6 months of age), as tool to identify the most vulnerable group with a highest risk of morbidity and mortality has not been established. It warrants further research to define the age appropriate cut-offs in young infants before its wider application.

Currently according to WHO, severe acute malnutrition(SAM) and moderate acute malnutrition (MAM) in a young infant is defined in the same way as for older children i.e. WFL<–3 Z-score and WFL between –3 Z-score and –2 Z-score respectively.[51] In addition there are no WFL Z-scores available for infants with length <45 cm. This has led to the utilization of the clinical signs like visible severe wasting as a clinical indicator of SAM. Though bilateral pedal edema is not a common finding in young infants with SAM, it continues to be one of the indicators of SAM (< 6 months), as its presence is associated with high risk of mortality.

### Gaps in Knowledge

There is a need to establish thresholds for MUAC for identification of SAM in < 6 months and after 5 years of age. The sensitivity and specificity of MUAC at different age strata across 5 years needs further evaluation. Discharge criteria from nutritional rehabilitation programs, based on MUAC versus WFH Z-score needs validation by evidence based, robust good quality research comparing the impact on treatment outcomes.

### References

1. Black RE, Allen LH, Bhutta ZA, Caulfield LE, de Onis M, EZZati M, Mathers C, Rivera J. Maternal and child undernutrition: global and regional exposures and health consequences. Lancet. 2008;371:243–60.
2. Pelletier DL, Frongillo EA Jr., Schroeder DG, Habicht JP. The effects of malnutrition on child mortality in developing countries. Bull World Health Organ. 1995;4:443–8.
3. McDonald CM, Olofin I, Flaxman S, FawZi WW, Spiegelman D, Caulfield LE, Black RE, EZZati M, Danaei G; et al. Nutrition Impact Model Study.The effect of multiple anthropometric deficits on child mortality: meta-analysis of individual data in 10 prospective studies from developing countries. Am J Clin Nutr. 2013;97: 896–901.

4. WHO. Use and Interpretation of Anthropometric Indicators of Nutritional Status. Report of a WHO Working Group. Bull World Health Organ. 1986;64:929–41.

5. Waterlow JC. Classification and definition of protein-calorie malnutrition. BMJ. 1972;3:566–9.

6. Ashworth A. Growth rates in children recovering from protein-calorie malnutrition. British J Nutr. 1969;23:835–45.

7. Burgess HJ, Burgess AP. The arm circumference as a public health index of protein-calorie malnutrition of early childhood. A modified standard for mid upper arm circumference in young children. J Trop Pediatr. 1969;15:189–93.

8. de Onis M, Yip R, Mei Z. The development of MUAC for- age reference data recommended by a WHO Expert Committee. Bull World Health Organ. 1997;75:11–8.

9. Briend A, Garenne M, Maire B, Fontaine O, Dieng K. Nutritional status, age and survival: the muscle mass hypothesis. Eur J Clin Nutr. 1989;43:715–26.

10. Berkley J, Mwangi I, Griffiths K, Ahmed I, Mithwani S, English M, Newton C, Maitland K. Assessment of severe malnutrition among hospitalized children in rural Kenya: comparison of weight-for-height and mid upper arm circumference. JAMA. 2005;294:591–7.

11. Briend A, Zimicki S. Validation of arm circumference as an indicator of risk of death in one to four year old children. Nutr Res. 1986;6:249–61.

12. Sachdeva S, Dewan P, Shah D, Malhotra RK, Gupta P. Mid-upper arm circumference weight-for-height Z-score for predicting mortality in hospitalized childrenunder 5 years of age. Public Health Nutr. 2016;19:2513–20.

13. Sackett DL, Holland WW. Controversy in the detection of disease. Lancet. 1975;25:357–9.

14. Beaton GH, Bengoa JM. Practical population indicators of health and nutrition. In: Beaton G, Bengoa JM (eds). Nutrition and Preventive Medicine, Monograph Series 62. Geneva: WHO;1976.p.500–19.

15. Jelliffe EFP, Jelliffe DB. The arm circumference as a public health index of protein-calorie malnutrition of early childhood. J Trop Pediatr. 1969;15:179–92.

16. Black RE, Allen LH, Bhutta ZA, Caulfield LE, de Onis M, EZZati M, Mathers C, Rivera J; Maternal and Child Undernutrition Study Group. Maternal and child undernutrition: global and regional exposures and health consequences. Lancet. 2008;371:243–60.

17. Velzeboer MI, Selwyn BJ, Sargent F, Pollitt E, Delgado H. The use of arm circumference in simplified screening for acute malnutrition by minimally trained health workers. J Trop Pediatr. 1983;29:159–66.

18. Hamer C, Kvatum K, Jeffries D, Allen S. Detection of severe protein-energy malnutrition by nurses in The Gambia. Arch Dis Child. 2004;89:181–4.

19. Bairagi R. Effects of bias and random error in anthropometry and in age on estimation of malnutrition. Am J Epidemiol. 1986;123:185–91.

20. Alam N, Wojtyniak B, Rahaman MM. Anthropometric indicators and risk of death. Am J Clin Nutr. 1989;49:884–8.

21. Burgess HJ, Burgess AP.The arm circumference as a public health index of protein-calorie malnutrition of early childhood. J Trop Pediatr. 1969:189.

22. Velzeboer MI, Selwyn BJ, Sargent F, Pollitt E, Delgado H. The use of arm circumference in simplified screening for acute malnutrition by minimally trained health workers. J Trop Pediatr. 1983;29:159–66.

23. Feeney B. Investigation into community volunteers using an admission criteria of middle upper arm circumference of below 110 mm and length equal to or greater than 65 cm for children to a community programme for severely malnourished children in Ethiopia.MSc Thesis. London: London School of Hygiene and Tropical Medicine; 2004.

24. Briend A, Garenne M, Maire B, Fontaine O, Dieng K. Nutritional status, age and survival: The muscle mass hypothesis, Eur J Clin Nutr. 1989;43:715–26.

25. Berkley J, Mwangi I, Griffiths K, Ahmed I, Mithwani S, English M, Newton C, Maitland K, et al. Assessment of severe malnutrition amongst hospitalized children in Rural Kenya: Comparison or weight-for-height and mid upper arm circumference JAMA. 2005;294:591–7.

26. Shakir A. Arm circumference in the surveillance of protein-calorie malnutrition in Baghdad. Am J Clin Nutr. 1975;28:661–5.

27. Ross DA, Taylor N, Hayes R, McClean M. Measuring malnutrition in famines: Are weight-for height and arm circumference interchangeable? Int J Epidemiol. 1990;19:636–45.

28. Katz J, West KP, Tarwotjo I, Sommer A. The importance of age in evaluating anthropometric indices for predicting mortality. Am J Epidemiol. 1989;130:1219–26.

29. Vella V, Tomkins A, Ndiku J, Marshal T, Cortinovis I. Anthropometry as a predictor for mortality among Ugandan children allowing for socio-economic status. Eur J Clin Nutr. 1994; 48:189–97.

30. Myatt M, Khara T, Collins S. A review of methods to detect cases of severely malnourished children in the community for their admission into community-based therapeutic care programs. Food Nutr Bull. 2006; 27(3 Suppl):S7–23.

31. Sandiford P, Paulin FH. Use of mid-upper-arm circumference for nutritional screening of refugees, Lancet. 1995;345:1120.

32. Hamill PV, Drizd TA, Johnson CL, Reed RB, Roche AF, et al. NCHS growth curves for children birth-18 Years: United States. Vital Health Stat. 1977;i-iv:1–74.

33. Centers for Disease Control and Prevention. CDC growth charts: United States: Centers for disease control and Prevention. Available fromwww.cdc. gov/growth charts, 2000. Accessed 20 November, 2016.

34. WHO Multicentre Growth Reference Study Group. WHO child growth standards based on length/height,weight and age. Acta Paediatr. 2006;450:76–85.

35. UN Standing Committee on Nutrition. SCNendorses the New WHO Growth Standards for Infants and Young Children. Available at: http://www.who.int/childgrowth/ endorsement_scn.pdf.Accessed 20 November, 2016.

36. International Union of Nutrition Sciences. Statement of Endorsement of the WHO Child Growth Standards. 2006. Available at: http:// www. who.int/childgrowth/endorsement_ IUNS.Accessed 20 November, 2016.

37. International Pediatric Association Endorsement. The New WHO Growth Standards for Infants and Young Children. 2006. Available at: http://www. who.int/childgrowth/Endorsement_IPA. pdf.Accessed 20 November, 2016.

38. Chavez R, Frenk S, Galvan Rr, Gomez F, Munoz Jc, Vazquez J, et al. Mortality in second- and third-degree malnutrition. J Trop Pediatr. 1956;2:77–83.

39. Seoane N, Latham MC. Nutritional anthropometry in the identification of malnutrition in childhood. J Trop Pediatr Environ Child Health.1971;17:1271-4.

40. Waterlow JC. Classification and definition of protein calorie malnutrition BMJ.1972;3:566–9.

41. Waterlow JC, Buzina R, Keller W, Lane JM, Nichaman MZ, Tanner JM, et al. The presentation and use of height and weight data for comparing the nutritional status of groups of children under the age of 10 years. Bull World Health Organ. 1977;55:489–98.

42. Management of Severe Malnutrition: Amanual for physicians and other senior health workers. Geneva: World Health Organization; 1999. Available from: http://apps.who.int/iris/ bitstream/10665/41999/1/a57361.pdf.Accessed 20 November, 2016.

43. Department of Child and Adolescent Health and Development, WHO. Handbook IMNCI: Integrated Management of Childhood Illness. Geneva: World Health Organization; 2005.

44. WHO, UNICEF, and SCN Informal Consultation on Community-based Management of Severe Malnutrition in Children. SCN Nutrition Policy Paper No. 21. 2006. Available at: http:// www.who. int/child_adolescent_health/ documents/pdfs/ fnb_v27n3_suppl.pdf.Accessed 20 November, 2016.

45. WHO/UNICEF/WFP/SCN Joint Statement. Community-based management of severe acute malnutrition. Geneva, New York, Rome, 2007. Available at: http://www.who.int/child_ adolescent_health/documents/pdfs/ severe_acute_ malnutrition_en.pdf.Accessed 20 November, 2016.

46. A Joint Statement by the World Health Organization and the United Nations Children's Fund. WHO child growth standards and the identification of severe acute malnutrition in infants and children. Geneva: WHO/UNICEF; 2009.

47. Berkley J, Mwangi I, Griffiths K, Ahmed I, Mithwani S, English M, et al. Assessment of severe malnutrition among hospitalized children in rural Kenya: comparison of weight-for-height and mid upper arm circumference. JAMA. 2005;294: 591-7.

48. Luque Fernandez M, Delchevalerie P, Van Herp M. Accuracy of MUAC in the detection of severe wasting with the new WHO growth standards. Pediatrics. 2010;126:e195-e201.

49. Garenne M, Maire B, Fontaine O, Briend A. Distributions of mortality risk attributable to low nutritional status in Niakhar, Senegal. J Nutr. 2006;136:2893–2900.

50. Briend A, Maire B, Fontaine O, Garenne M. Mid-upper arm circumference and weight-for-height

to identify high-risk malnourished under-five children. Matern Child Nutr. 2012;1:130–3.

51. WHO. Guideline: Updates on the Management of Severe Acute Malnutrition in Infants and Children. Geneva: World Health Organization; 2013. Available from http://www.who.int/nutrition/publications/guidelines/updates_management_SAM_infantandchildren/en/.Accessed 20 November, 2016.

52. Mwangome MK, Fegan G, Mbunya R, Prentice AM, Berkley JA. Reliability and accuracy of anthropometry performed by community health workers among infants under 6 months in rural Kenya.Trop Med Int Health. 2012;17:622–9.

53. Mwangome MK, Berkley JA. The reliability of weight for- length/height Z scores in children. Matern Child Nutr. 2014;10:474–80.

# Pathophysiology of Undernutrition

Bhavna Dhingra, Piyush Gupta

Severe acute malnutrition is a clinical syndrome due to an imbalance between demand and supply of calories, proteins and micronutrients, with complex interplay of various pathological mechanisms. An understanding of the pathophysiological processes is required for proper management of these children. Lack of nutrients leads to decrease in the lean body mass and total protein thus hampering normal growth and development. This affects virtually all organ systems of the body thereby leaving the child more vulnerable to infections. Each episode of infection further precipitates malnutrition, thus establishing a vicious cycle. Under-nourished mothers deliver low birth weight babies who due to inappropriate feeding practices, poor hygiene, poverty and illiteracy, land up being undernourished.

## 4.1 REDUCTIVE ADAPTATION

All the bodily functions get affected by undernutrition to varying degrees. The body tries to adapt to this suboptimal state and makes certain changes to combat this chronic deprivation of nutrients. This adjustment is known as *reductive adaptation* and includes reduced physical activity and growth, reduced basal metabolism and attenuated immune and inflammatory responses. The malnourished child is able to survive an ongoing deficit in energy and protein even with increased energy requirements due to associated infections, due to these adaptations in various metabolic pathways.

Various theories have been put forth to explain this phenomenon.

### A. Gopalan Theory of Adaptation

Chronic deficit of calories makes the body adapt over a period of time thereby stimulating the adrenocortical axis. This leads to increased cortisol secretion which causes breakdown of muscle protein. This results in severe muscle wasting (non-edematous malnutrition or marasmus). If this adaptation does not occur or the adaptation breaks down due to an intercurrent illness, it leads to an insufficient increase in plasma cortisol and growth hormone thereby leading to lipolysis and fatty liver (edematous malnutrition or kwashiorkor).[1] **Figure 4.1** describes the pathogenesis of adrenocortical response and development of malnutrition.

### B. Golden Theory of Free Radical Injury

Golden proposed that an excess of free radical formation in the body due to decreased protein intake, reduced synthesis, and recurrent infections leads to excessive oxidative stress and reduced antioxidant capacity. All these factors play a role in the development of edematous malnutrition.[2]

47

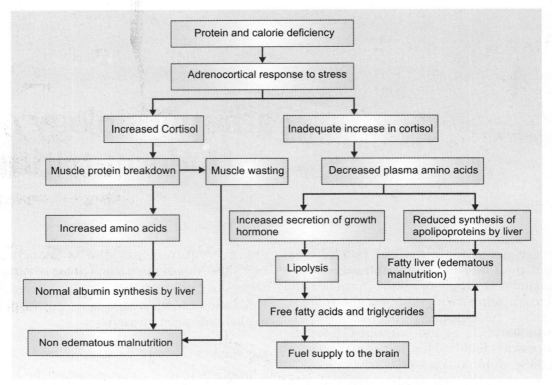

**Fig. 4.1** Adrenocortical response and biochemical changes in undernutrition

## 4.2 BODY FUNCTIONS AND COMPOSITION IN UNDERNUTRITION

### A. Protein and Amino Acid Metabolism

Total body protein and plasma proteins are markedly reduced with the greatest reduction being in albumin, in cases of edematous malnutrition.[3] The most severely affected organs are the muscles and fat while the heart and the brain are relatively spared.[4]

### Albumin and Globulin

Due to decreased intake of protein for prolonged periods, protein synthesis and total protein turnover gets reduced. The catabolic rate and synthesis of albumin are both reduced in severe malnutrition. Globulin metabolism remains largely unaffected and synthesis of gamma globulins may be increased in the presence of infection.[5] Plasma transferrin is markedly reduced.[6]

### Amino Acids

Due to reduced protein intake the body tries to conserve nitrogen and there is a reduction in the proportion of amino acids metabolized to urea thereby decreasing urinary nitrogen excretion. The total plasma amino acids are reduced to about half of the normal value in severe PEM. In edematous malnutrition, most of the essential and branched chain amino acids like threonine and tyrosine are markedly reduced while lysine and phenylalanine are less affected and the non-essential amino acids remain normal or increased.[7] High levels of growth hormone along with raised cortisol in the plasma is postulated to be the cause for marked reduction of branched chain amino acids as these two hormones have antagonistic effects on amino acid metabolism.[8] Therefore the availability of amino acids for protein synthesis in the muscles is markedly reduced.

Redistribution of endogenous amino acids occurs to the visceral organs at the expense of muscles. During rehabilitation phase, provision of adequate good quality protein in the diet is essential for replenishment of these aminoacids to promote endogenous protein synthesis.

## Urea and Creatinine Turnover

Creatinine turnover remains almost constant even in severe malnutrition which may partly be explained by the impairment of renal function in malnutrition and the presence of small bowel bacterial overgrowth which metabolizes creatinine.[9] Plasma urea and urinary urea excretion are greatly diminished in severe malnutrition but ammonia excretion remains largely unaltered. Due to a decrease in the total body potassium, there is inability to secrete hydrogen ions and thus the acid formed from the endogenous protein breakdown and fatty acid metabolism gets secreted in the form of ammonium iron.[10]

When adequate diet is replenished to the malnourished kids, they have a hypermetabolic state with increased protein synthesis, catabolism, and turnover leading to recovery.

## B. Carbohydrate Metabolism

Long term deficit of calories in undernutrition leads to various adaptations in the carbohydrate metabolism in the body. *Undernourished children have lower fasting blood glucose and thus are at risk of potentially life threatening hypoglycemia.* The level of glycogen stores, the rate of its breakdown in liver, the rate of gluconeogenesis and peripheral utilization of glucose are some of the important factors which regulate the blood glucose levels in the malnourished. Increased activity of hepatic glucose-6-phosphatase helps in maintaining the blood glucose levels in malnutrition.

In children with severe malnutrition, liver glycogen stores are reduced, glycogen oxidation is reduced and gets completed earlier than normal. There is efficient recycling of the products of glycolysis which helps to maintain the glucose production and blood glucose levels in the malnourished child.

Brain and red blood cells are dependent on glucose as the energy source and gluconeogenesis from three carbon substrates meets this requirement. In other tissues, after depletion of glycogen stores, fat oxidation becomes the major source of energy.[11]

## C. Lipid Metabolism

In non-edematous malnutrition, plasma concentration of triglyceride, cholesterol, β lipoproteins and free fatty acids are essentially normal. In edematous malnutrition, there is severe fatty infiltration of liver, even in the absence of hepatomegaly. Fasting plasma concentration of β lipoproteins is reduced, while triglycerides may be normal or elevated and fall to normal during recovery. There is reduced synthesis of VLDL apo B-100 lipoprotein. The liver's ability to remove triglyceride gets reduced and it accumulates in the liver thus giving rise to hepatic steatosis (fatty liver).[12]

Deficiency of essential fatty acids can give rise to scaly skin, reduced growth, and increased susceptibility to infections.

## D. Basal Metabolism

The basal metabolic rate (BMR) is decreased in severe undernutrition leading to decreased physical activity, reduced emotional responsiveness, bradycardia, and decreased temperature. The absolute weight of the various organs gets reduced to varying degrees, with muscle and fat bearing the maximum brunt while brain, kidneys, and heart are affected to a lesser extent. The liver becomes heavier in edematous malnutrition due to fat accumulation but weighs less than normal in case of non-edematous malnutrition. The chemical composition of the various tissues also gets altered thereby contributing to a reduced organ metabolic rate.

*Temperature Regulation*

Gross depletion of substrates for energy production puts the child at high risk of developing hypothermia which is usually associated with hypoglycemia and may be life threatening. Children with non-edematous malnutrition are at higher risk of hypothermia due to marked reduction in the subcutaneous fat and total specific thermal insulation as compared to children with edematous malnutrition who have relatively well preserved subcutaneous fat and better thermal insulation. Thermogenesis is reduced due to depletion of brown fat stores in the interscapular region.[13]

Hypothermia occurs more frequently at night as the heat production reduces further due to sleep and physical inactivity coupled with decreased ambient temperature.

## 4.3 BODY FLUIDS AND ELECTROLYTES IN UNDERNUTRITION

### A. Body Fluids

#### 1. Total Body Water

Malnourished children have increased total body water, most of which is accounted for by an increase in the extracellular fluid space. The risk of developing congestive cardiac failure is high in edematous malnutrition with parenteral fluid replacement. Children with non-edematous malnutrition have the highest total body water with marked reduction in adipose tissue and lean body mass. Thus, the risk of developing fluid overload is high and intravenous fluids should be used very judiciously in children with severe malnutrition, irrespective of presence of edema. During early rehabilitation phase, on high energy intake there is a significant increase in total body water.

#### 2. Edema

The development of edema in malnutrition is multifactorial. Hypoproteinemia (hypo-albuminemia) is one of the major contributing factor. It has also been postulated that there is defective inactivation of anti-diuretic hormone (ADH) due to structural and functional changes in the liver. These changes also lead to the presence of ferritin into the plasma which has an anti-diuretic action mediated through the posterior pituitary. Increased aldosterone secretion and reduced total body potassium also play in role in developing edema. Deficiency of vanadium and increased free radicals also contribute to the development of edema. **Figure 4.2** shows the pathogenesis of edema in malnutrition.[14]

## B. Mineral Metabolism

### 1. Sodium and Potassium

Total body sodium is increased in children with undernutrition. Studies have reported higher than normal concentration of sodium in muscles, brain, erythrocytes, and leucocytes of undernourished children.[15-17] Dilutional hyponatremia can occur due to fluid retention or due to acute kidney injury following an episode of diarrhea.

Impaired adenosine triphosphate (ATP) production and utilization leads to failure of the energy dependent sodium pump. For each mol of ATP consumed, the pump transports 3 sodium molecules outwards and 2 molecules of potassium inwards. Thus, a fall in total body potassium is associated with a rise in intracellular sodium.[17]

Undernutrition is associated with total body deficit of potassium. Dietary deficiency and gastrointestinal losses in diarrhea contribute to the body deficit. Once rehabilitation is initiated, potassium levels take several weeks to come back to normal due to slow recovery of the sodium pump.

### 2. Magnesium

There is true magnesium deficit in the muscles of the malnourished kids and the serum levels also may be low. Magnesium is important for cellular metabolism and has membrane stabilizing properties; its deficiency may lead

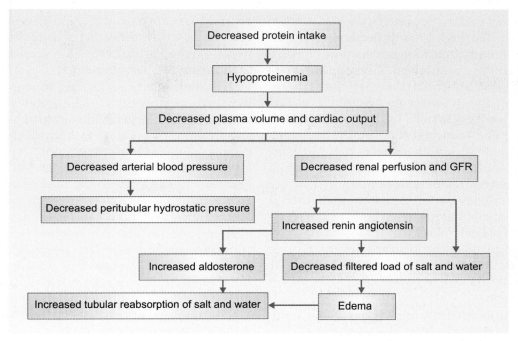

**Fig. 4.2** Pathogenesis of edema formation in malnutrition

to hyperirritability, convulsions, apathy, and cardiovascular morbidity. Coexistent magnesium and potassium deficit require the provision of both ions in order to achieve potassium repletion. Magnesium supplementation has been shown to decrease mortality in malnourished children.

### 3. Phosphate

Malnourished children have low blood phosphate at admission and there is a further decline, reaching a nadir within the first couple of days. This has been shown to be associated with increased mortality. During treatment phase, these children are at risk of refeeding hypophosphatemia.

Refeeding syndrome may be observed in some children during recovery phase and presents with self-limited tremors (*kwashi shake*), encephalitis like picture, increase in liver size, hypertrichosis, gynecomastia, parotid swelling, ascites, splenomegaly, and eosinophilia. The probable pathophysiological mechanisms are excess hormone secretion

during recovery, dysmyelination, vitamin deficiencies, neurotransmitter imbalance, and high solute load on the kidneys.

During refeeding, a shift occurs from fat to carbohydrate metabolism as the body moves from a catabolic to anabolic state. This leads to insulin release and increases cellular uptake of electrolytes, including phosphate. Routine monitoring of electrolytes is therefore required, and if phosphate is not supplemented in diet, hypophosphatemia gets precipitated.

To prevent refeeding syndrome, the WHO guideline on inpatient management of SAM includes a stabilization phase with a low-energy formula (F-75), as well as a gradual transition to F-100 diet.[18]

## 4.4 ENDOCRINE FUNCTIONS IN UNDERNUTRITION

### A. Growth Hormone

In edematous malnutrition, the levels of growth hormone are high at presentation, while in non-edematous malnutrition they have been variably reported to be low, normal, or high. The high growth hormone levels in edematous malnutrition remain unresponsive to arginine stimulation. Growth hormone levels in malnutrition are negatively correlated with the serum albumin level. GH levels are also related to the metabolism of alanine and branched chain amino acids.

Rehabilitation with a protein rich diet helps in normalization of these raised levels. Insulin like growth factor and somatomedins are comparatively low in edematous malnutrition than non-edematous cases. Low insulin levels help in peripheral release of fuel for the brain and high growth hormone level helps to provide substrate in malnourished kids.

## B. Insulin

Edematous malnutrition is associated with low fasting levels of plasma insulin, impaired glucose tolerance, and a reduced response to stimulation by intravenous glucose and glucagon. Glucose tolerance is largely normal in non-edematous malnutrition while it is impaired in edematous malnutrition.

Pancreas exhibits marked structural changes in malnourished children. Damage to β cells leads to poor insulin secretion. Coexistent potassium deficiency and inefficient utilization of glucose by peripheral tissues contributes to glucose intolerance. Pancreatic β cells involvement is variable and thus the levels of glucagon are also variable.

Chromium acts as a glucose tolerance factor and potentiates the peripheral action of insulin. Its deficiency in severe malnutrition contributes to glucose intolerance.

## C. Cortisol

Malnutrition is associated with atrophy of adrenal cortex and medulla, but there is a good functional reserve of cortisol in response to corticotrophin. Plasma cortisol levels are raised in children with non-edematous malnutrition. The diurnal rhythm of cortisol secretion is altered and clearance of exogenous cortisol is impaired.[20] Children with edematous malnutrition have a marked rise in plasma free cortisol, especially if associated with severe hypoalbuminemia.

Recurrent infections leading to stress and hypoglycemia contribute to the elevation in plasma cortisol levels, which in turn leads to suppression of cellular immunity thereby predisposing to development of infections.[21] Hypothermia, hypoglycemia, and acidosis also lead to elevation in the plasma cortisol levels.

Adrenocorticotropin (ACTH) and plasma aldosterone levels are normal in non-edematous malnutrition despite raised cortisol levels. The rate of secretion of aldosterone is increased in cases of non-edematous malnutrition, while it is normal in edematous malnutrition and its reduced hepatic clearance leads to elevated plasma levels.

Once rehabilitation is initiated, these metabolic abnormalities normalize slowly.

## D. Thyroid

Severe malnutrition is associated with depressed thyroid function as the BMR is decreased and there is reduced protein synthesis. Iodine uptake by the thyroid and protein bound iodine are reduced. Edematous malnutrition is associated with iodine malabsorption and negative iodine balance. There is relative hypothyroidism of pituitary origin leading to low serum thyroxine (T4) but variable levels of free T4.[22]

## 4.5 IMMUNE FUNCTIONS IN UNDERNUTRITION

Immunity is depressed in children with severe malnutrition, cell mediated immunity being affected severely as compared to humoral immunity. There is atrophy of lymph nodes, tonsils, and thymus. Synthesis of secretory IgA and complement is reduced. Delayed hypersensitivity in response to purified protein derivative and response to vaccine antigens are impaired. There is marked reduction in phagocytosis. Malnourished children are unable to mount classical response of fever and leukocytosis in case of infections. Compromised skin barrier serves as a good portal of entry for microorganisms.

Free radicals play an important role in immunological response, which induces the increase oxidative stress in severe malnutrition. Increased production of reactive oxygen intermediates such as superoxide anion ($O_2-$), hydroxyl radical (OHo), singlet oxygen, and hydrogen peroxide ($H_2O_2$) within the erythrocytes, and of malondialdehyde (MDA) from lipid peroxidation, contributes to the increased cellular oxidative stress. Superoxide dismutase (SOD) which scavenges free radicals and other reactive oxygen species (ROS), and is the first line of defense against free radical damage, is markedly reduced in severe malnutrition.[23]

Deficiency of trace metals, selenium and zinc, which are critical for the functioning of metalloenzymes, like zinc-superoxide dismutase (SOD), which forms an integral part of the antioxidant defense system, contributes to the depressed immunity.

Vitamin E deficiency is common in the severely malnourished and is implicated as a causative factor in anemia in edematous malnutrition. It adds to the morbidity and mortality of the disease.

## 4.6 GASTROINTESTINAL FUNCTION IN UNDERNUTRITION

### A. Malabsorption

Shortage of nutrients due to inadequate diet can be exaggerated due to coexisting malabsorption which is common in undernutrition. Reduced capacity for digestion and absorption is a physiological adaptation to reduced intake. Breakdown of this adaptation leads to malabsorption of fat, carbohydrates, and fat soluble vitamins. Associated gut infections further compound the malabsorption by reducing the digestive and absorptive capacity of the gut thus increasing the malnutrition. The bacteria in the guts of malnourished children are predominantly pathogenic and therefore lead to persistent gut inflammation, increased permeability, and malabsorption of nutrients. Children with non-edematous malnutrition have lesser gut microbial diversity as compared to those with edematous malnutrition.

### B. Changes in the Gut

Due to a decreased intake of nutrients the gut tries to adapt by making certain changes in its structure and function. There is a reduction in the villous height, protein and DNA content, disaccharidases and dipeptidase content, cell division, and migration rates.

Decreased gut motility, hypochlorhydria, and immunoparesis lead to overgrowth of bacteria in the small bowel, which increases the recycling of urea through the small bowel in malnourished children. This dysbiosis leads to increased deconjugation of bile salts, decreased pool of bile salts with increased turnover, increase in deoxycholate/cholate ratio, increase in glycine/taurine ratio, and reduced ability to form micelles. Bacterial endotoxins affect the cell membrane functions thereby altering leucocyte membrane permeability to sodium and contributing to the electrolyte imbalance and malabsorption.[24]

On rehabilitation, there is a rapid return to normalcy in absorptive functions of the gut, while morphological abnormalities may persist and take longer to recover.

### C. Liver and Pancreas

Malnutrition is associated with lactose intolerance and deficiency of lactase, maltase, and sucrase in the small bowel mucosa. Exocrine pancreatic insufficiency leading to deficiency of amylase and trypsinogen, and biochemical signs of pancreatitis are seen in malnourished children and are more marked in cases of edematous malnutrition. These changes are known to reverse during rehabilitation phase. There is atrophy of the pancreas and reduction in the number of zymogen secreting pancreatic acinar cells.[25]

Liver is infiltrated by fat and there is reduced hepatic protein synthesis and gluconeogenesis. Capacity of the liver to metabolize and inactivate toxins is markedly diminished. Liver has decreased number of peroxisomes and high amount of rough endoplasmic reticulum and mitochondria.

Intestinal flora is responsible for bile acid metabolism, deconjugation and synthesis. Dysbiosis of intestinal flora thus affects bile acid metabolism leading to bile acid malabsorption in malnourished children.[26]

## 4.7 CARDIAC, RENAL AND NEUROLOGICAL CHANGES

### A. Cardiac Function

Severe malnutrition is associated with reduced cardiac output, stroke volume, and peripheral blood flow. There is prolongation of systemic recirculation time and bradycardia. Blood pressure is low. The heart size is reduced and there are nonspecific changes on the electrocardiogram (ECG). Anemia, hypothyroid state, and decreased oxygen consumption due to low BMR also affect cardiac function in severely malnourished.

The chances of developing congestive cardiac failure are high if intravenous fluids are given rapidly to malnourished children, due to sodium and water retention.

It has been postulated that malnutrition in fetal period and early childhood when an individual is developmentally plastic increases the risk of cardiovascular disease in adulthood. Systemic vascular resistance is higher in adulthood in survivors of malnutrition. They also have smaller outflow tracts and cardiac output and are more likely to develop hypertension in later life, especially when exposed to obesity.[27]

### B. Renal Function

Glomerular filtration rate and renal plasma flow are reduced, which may be compromised further during an acute episode of diarrhea. Disturbance of tubular function leads to aminoaciduria and inefficient acid secretion. Sodium and phosphate excretion is reduced. Retention of sodium and water contributes to the development of edema. Changes in the epithelium of the urinary tract predispose the malnourished children to development of urinary tract infections. Serum urea and creatinine levels are within the normal range in the absence of dehydration. If deranged, they normalize quickly after correction of dehydration.

### C. Nervous System

Myelination of neurons, dendritic arborization, and morphology of dendritic spines get affected by malnutrition in early childhood. Cerebral atrophy occurs in malnourished children and affects the higher brain functions and may lead to permanent neuropsychological and cognitive damage which are irreversible even after nutritional rehabilitation. Learning disabilities are frequent in survivors of childhood undernutrition.

## References

1. Gopalan C. Malnutrtion in childhood in the tropics. Br Med J. 1967;4:603–7.
2. Golden MH, Ramdath D. Free radicals in the pathogenesis of Kwashiorkor. Proc Nutr Soc. 1987;46:53–68.
3. Whitehead RG, Alleyne GA. Pathophysiological factors of importance in protein-calorie malnutrition. Br Med Bull. 1972;28:72–9.
4. GarrowJS, Fletcher K, Halliday D. Body composition in severe infantile malnutrition. J Clin Invest.1965;44:417–25.
5. Cohen S, Hansen JD. Metabolism of albumin and gamma-globulin in kwashiorkor. Clin Sci. 1962;23:351–9.
6. Antia AU, McFarlane H, Soothill JF. Serum siderophilin in kwashiorkor. Arch Dis Child. 1968;43:459–62.
7. Holt LE Jr, Snyderman SE, Norton PM, Roitman E, Finch J. The plasma amniogram in kwashiorkor. Lancet. 1963;2:1342–8.
8. Catt KJ. Growth hormone. Lancet. 1970;1:933–9.

9. Jones JD, Brunett PC. Creatinine metabolism and toxicity. Kidney Inst Suppl. 1975;3:294–8.

10. Tannen RL, Wedell E, Moore R. Renal adaptation to a high potassium intake. The role of hydrogen ion. J Clin Invest. 1973;52:2089–101.

11. Alleyne GAO, Hay RW, Picou DI, Stanfield JP, Whitehead RG, editors. Protein-energy Malnutrition. 1st Indian ed. New Delhi: Jaypee Brothers;1989.p.54–92.

12. Waterlow JC, Bras G. Nutritional liver damage in man. Br Med Bull. 1957;13:107–12.

13. Brooke OG. Thermal insulation in malnourished Jamaican children. Arch Dis Child. 1973;48:901–5.

14. Klahr S, Alleyne GA. Effects of chronic protein-calorie malnutrition on kidney. Kidney Int. 1973;3:129–4.

15. Halliday D. Chemical composition of the whole body and individual tissues of two Jamaican children whose death resulted primarily from malnutrition. Clin Sci. 1967;33:365–7.

16. Khalil M, Kabeil A, el-Khateeb S, Aref K, el-Lozy M, Jahin S, et al. Plasma and red cell water and elements in protein-calorie malnutrition. Am J Clin Nutr. 1974;27:260–7.

17. Hilton PJ, Edmondson RP, Thomas RD, Patrick J. The effect of external potassium concentration on leucocyte cation transport in-vitro. Clin Sci Mol Med. 1975;49:385–90.

18. Namusoke H, Hother AL, Rytter MJ, et al. Changes in plasma phosphate during in-patient treatment of children with severe acute malnutrition: an observational study in Uganda. Am J Clin Nutr. 2016;103:551–8.

19. Grant DB, Hambley J, Becker D, Pimstone BL. Reduced sulphation factor in undernourished children. Arch Dis Child. 1973;48:596–600.

20. Alleyne G, Young VH. Adrenocortical function in children with severe protein-calorie malnutrition. Clin Sci. 1967;33:189–200.

21. Schonland MM, Shanley BC, Loening WE, Parent MA, Coovadia HM. Plasma- cortisol and immune suppression in protein-calorie malnutrition. Lancet. 1972;2:435–6.

22. Beas F, Monckeberg F, Horwitz l. The response of the thyroid gland to thyroid stimulating hormone (TSH) in infants with malnutrition. Pediatrics. 1966;38:1003–8.

23. Ghone RA, Suryakar AN, Kulhalli PM, Bhagat SS, Padalkar RK, Karnik AC, et al. A study of oxidative stress biomarkers and effect of oral antioxidant supplementation in severe acute malnutrition. J Clin Diagn Res. 2013;7:2146–8.

24. Kristensen KH, Wiese M, Rytter MJ, Özçam M, Hansen LH, Namusoke H, et al. Gut microbiota in children hospitalized with oedematous and non-oedematous severe acute malnutrition in Uganda. PLoS Negl Trop Dis. 2016;10:e0004369.

25. Bartels RH, Meyer SL, Stehmann TA, Bourdon C, Bandsma RH, Voskuijl WP. Both exocrine pancreatic insufficiency and signs of pancreatic inflammation are prevalent in children with complicated severe acute malnutrition: An observational study. J Pediatr. 2016;174:165–70.

26. Zhang L, Voskuijl W, Mouzaki M, Groen AK, Alexander J, Bourdon C, et al. Impaired bile acid homeostasis in children with severe acute malnutrition. PLoS One. 2016;11:e0155143.

27. Tennant IA, Barnett AT, Thompson DS, Kips J, Boyne MS, Chung EE, et al. Impaired cardio-vascular structure and function in adult survivors of severe acute malnutrition. Hypertension. 2014;64:664–71.

# Clinical Features of Undernutrition

Srikanta Basu, Puneet Kaur Sahi

## 5.1 INDICATORS OF UNDERNUTRITION

Clinical features of undernutrition are diverse and depend on several factors. The common underlying mechanism is the deficiency of energy, proteins, and nutrients in these children relative to their needs. Clinical manifestations of undernutrition in a child will depend upon the magnitude of deficiency and the type of nutrients that are lacking. This in turn is determined by the duration of nutrient inadequacy, the quantity and diversity of foods that are lacking in the diet, the presence of antinutrients such as phytates, individual variations in requirements, number and severity of co-existing infections and their duration. Response to noxious stimuli also leads to increased nutrient utilization and may lead to their deficiency. Thus, the protean manifestations of severe acute malnutrition depends on the heterogeneity of extent and nature of nutrient deficits in affected children.

Malnutrition is broadly divided into underweight, stunting, and wasting based on three indices–weight-for-age, height/length-for-age, and weight-for height/length.

A child is said to be **underweight** if the weight-for-age (WFA) is low as compared to standard for his/her age and sex. It can result from either acute or chronic malnutrition or both and is thus a composite measure of stunting and wasting. It is often used to determine the nutritional status of a population as weight is easy to measure. Underweight can be categorized into 2 groups *viz.* moderately underweight and severely underweight.

**Stunting** is defined as height-for-age (HFA) less than –2 Z-score of the median reference for that age and sex. Stunting is an indicator of linear growth retardation that results from failure to receive adequate nutrition over a long period or because of recurrent infections. It is an indicator of past growth failure. It may result in delayed mental development, reduced intellectual capacity, and poor scholastic performance.

Weight-for-height/length less than –2 Z-score of the median reference for that sex is defined as **wasting**. It results from inadequate food intake, incorrect feeding practices, diseases, infection, or a combination of these factors. *Wasting indicates acute malnutrition* resulting from failure to gain weight or actual weight loss. A wasted child looks weak, thin with gradual loss of fat and muscles.

Acute malnutrition is classified according to the degree of wasting and presence of edema.

- **Moderate acute malnutrition** (MAM) is defined as a weight-for-height/length between –2 Z-score and –3 Z-score for that sex, and/or mid-arm circumference between 115 mm and 125 mm.

- **Severe acute malnutrition** is defined as weight-for-length <-3 Z-score, and/or MUAC <115 mm, and/or bilateral pedal edema of nutritional origin in children 6 months to 5 years. In children < 6 months, all of the above except MUAC are applicable.[1] This definition of severe acute malnutrition distinguishes the wasted/edematous children from those who are simply stunted, as the latter are not a priority for acute clinical care.

The term protein energy malnutrition is not used now as it does not reflect the complex multideficiency etiology of undernutrition.

## 5.2 CLINICAL SYNDROMES

### 1. Visible Severe Wasting

Deprived nutrition initially leads to failure to gain weight, followed by weight loss. Initially, wasting occurs at the site of brown fat, as it is metabolically more active and is important for thermogenesis. Wasting is most visible in the buttocks, thighs, upper arms, ribs, and scapulae where the fat and skeletal muscle mass loss is the greatest. The face retains a relatively normal appearance till very late. However continued lack of nutrition can lead to sunken eyes due to loss of retro-orbital fat. Dry eyes and dry mouth can result from atrophy of the lacrimal and salivary glands. The buccal pad of fat is the last to be lost (as it is metabolically less active) and gives a hollow cheek appearance akin to an "old man". The child should be examined after removing the clothes to look for loss of subcutaneous fat in lower limbs and buttock as presence of buccal pad may be misleading. The skin becomes loose and lacks turgor due to loss of subcutaneous tissues which are used up for providing energy, enhancing the "wrinkled old man" look. Weakened abdominal muscles and gaseous distension of the abdomen due to gut bacterial overgrowth lead to a protruded belly. In cases of severe wasting, folds appear on the buttocks and thighs as if the child is wearing a "baggy pants" **(Fig. 5.1)** and will have a very low weight for height.

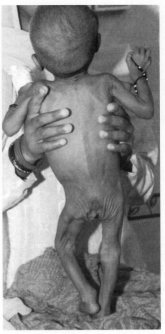

**Fig. 5.1** Baggy pant appearance in severe acute malnutrition

*Another term used for these children who are visibly severely wasted is Marasmus.* Children with marasmus usually are alert and have a good appetite. However, continued dietary deprivation later turns them irritable. As the appetite is maintained in marasmus, their treatment is easier and more effective than kwashiorkor.

Grading of Marasmus is as follows:[2]

*Grade I*     Wasting of axilla and groin
*Grade II*    Wasting of axilla and groin + thigh and buttocks
*Grade III*   Wasting of axilla and groin + thigh and buttocks + chest and abdomen
*Grade IV*    Wasting of axilla and groin + thigh and buttocks + chest and abdomen + buccal fat

### 2. Edema

It appears first in the most dependent part, *i.e.* feet, followed by the legs. Eventually, edema can become generalized involving the face, arms, and hands. The pathogenesis of

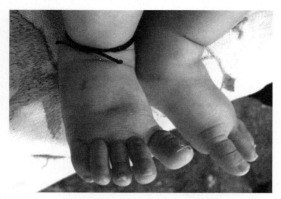

Fig. 5.2 A 7-month-old child with bilateral nutritional edema in the feet

edema is multifactorial. To be considered as a sign of malnutrition, the edema should be present in both the legs (bipedal) and nutritional in origin (cardiac, renal, and hepatic cause are ruled out).

Bilateral pitting pedal edema can be demonstrated by applying firm pressure over the dorsum of bilateral feet for 10 seconds. A dent seen at the site of pressure indicates pitting edema (Fig. 5.2). Edema of malnutrition can be graded in following way:

Mild (+)      Edema confined to both the feet.
Moderate (++)  Edema of both feet plus lower legs, hands or lower arms.
Severe (+++)   Generalized edema including feet, legs, hands, arms, and face.

## Pathophysiology

Low albumin concentration leads to decreased intravascular osmotic pressure, causing fluids to move to third space. This leads to decreased plasma volume, decreased cardiac output, and decreased renal blood flow. These changes activate the renin angiotensin aldosterone system and increase re-absorption of sodium and water. Decreased ADH inactivation by the liver promotes further water retention. Also, due to decreased activity of the Na⁺K⁺ ATP pump, sodium accumulates inside the cells, decreasing its extracellular concentration and hence the filtered load in the kidney. Thus,

more sodium and water is retained by the kidneys leading to edema. Vanadium deficiency, free radicals, and serum ferritin are also known to be causal agents for water retention.

## 3. Kwashiorkor

This entity was first described by Prof Cicely Williams in 1933 and thought to be caused by predominant protein deficiency. The term "sugar baby" has also been used to stress the dietary origin of the disease. Children 1 to 4 years of age are usually affected and main sign is pitting edema. Due to prominent cheeks (moon facies) and edema, child may appear well fed and healthy to the parents. A classic case of kwashiorkor is an apathetic, miserable child with edema, stunting, hepatomegaly, anemia, skin and hair changes. The characteristic pigmentary changes of hair have earned the alternate name "red boy" for kwashiorkor. **Essential triad of kwashiorkor includes edema, growth retardation, and psychomotor changes. Table 5.1** summarizes the important differences between marasmus and kwashiorkor.

## 4. Other Clinical Syndromes

Apart from the above, undernutrition can also present with the following clinical syndromes:

*Marasmic kwashiorkor* When edema develops in a marasmic child, the term marasmic kwashiorkor is used.

*Prekwashiorkor* The deficient children have some features of kwashiorkor like hepatomegaly, moon face, skin and hair changes, but no edema.

*Nutritional dwarfing* Prolonged nutritional deficiency early in life which does not manifest as severe forms of undernutrition like marasmus or kwashiorkor, may present later with nutritional dwarfing. These children are stunted but not wasted. They are also known as *bonsai children* or *pocket editions*. Micronutrient deficiency is now thought to cause such dwarfing.

| Feature | Marasmus | Kwashiorkor |
|---|---|---|
| Cause | Occurs due to deficiency of both carbohydrates and proteins | Mainly due to deficiency of proteins, other factors are implicated as well |
| Prevalence | More common | Less common |
| Age group | <1 year | 1–5 years |
| Appearance | Old man like face | Moon face |
| | Severe visible generalized wasting | Dependent edema which masks the muscle wasting |
| Weight for age | <60% | 60–80% |
| Growth retardation | ++ | + |
| Edema | Absent | Present (Pitting) |
| Activity | Alert | Apathetic |
| Skin changes | Nil/Mild | Present |
| Hair changes | Nil/Mild | Present |
| Anemia | Less common | More common |
| Appetite | Present but less | Poor |
| Hepatomegaly | Absent | Present |
| Infections | Less prone | More prone |
| Life threatening complications | Less common | More common |
| Recovery | Good | Poor |
| Pattern of recovery after initiating treatment | Steady weight gain | Initial weight loss due to loss of edema fluid followed by weight gain (Tick sign) |
| Mortality | Less than kwashiorkor | High in early stage |
| Proteins and albumin | Low | Very low |
| Carrier protein | Low | Very low |
| Anabolism | Decreased | Very decreased |
| Catabolism | Very increased | Increased |

**Table 5.1** Differences between Marasmus and Kwashiorkor[2]

*Invisible PEM:* These children do not have overt wasting or stunting, however when their growth is plotted on the growth chart a flat or downward curve is observed. Children between the ages of 6–24 months, who show breast addiction, often develop invisible PEM. They receive only 60% of their caloric requirement and have decreased resistance to infection, no outward signs of hunger except for a frequent desire to breastfeed.

## 5.3 PATHOPHYSIOLOGY OF SAM: REDUCTIVE ADAPTATION

The basic pathophysiological changes in severe malnutrition arise due to imbalance between the demand and supply of major nutrients and micronutrients. When the child's intake is compromised, the metabolic and physiological changes take place to conserve energy and prolong life. This process of slowing down is called **reductive adaptation**.[3] Initially, the fat stores are mobilized to meet the demand. With ongoing imbalance, protein is also mobilized from various organs like muscles, skin, and GIT. The body tries to conserve energy by limiting the growth, physical activity, basal metabolic rate, immune and inflammatory response, and functional reserve of the various organs. Finally, these physiological and metabolic derangements lead to various consequences and are responsible for clinical features and complications seen in children with SAM:

- Most children with severe acute malnutrition have asymptomatic infections because their immune system fails to respond with chemotaxis, opsonization, and phago-cytosis of bacteria, viruses, or fungi. The typical sign of inflammation *i.e.* fever is less commonly seen as the inflammatory system is depressed.

- There is fatty degeneration of liver and metabolic function of liver is compromised. The liver makes less amount of glucose which may lead to hypoglycemia. Various transport proteins, albumin, and transferrin are produced in inadequate amount. Furthermore, liver is unable to deal with excess dietary proteins and toxins.
- The kidneys are not able to excrete excess fluid and sodium effectively which may lead to fluid overload and electrolyte imbalance.
- Due to fatty degeneration, the cardiac size and output are reduced and cardiac function is further compromised specially in presence of edema. If not recognized, this leads to iatrogenic fluid and sodium overload leading to cardiac failure and death.
- The sodium-potassium pump often functions sub-optimally leading to accumulation of sodium, fluid retention, and edema. Similarly due to pump failure, potassium leaks out of the cells and is excreted in urine, leading to hypokalemia.
- Digestion and absorption is impaired, as the gut produces less gastric juice and enzymes. Motility is reduced, and bacteria colonize the stomach and small intestine, and damage the mucosa.
- Malnourished children become dehydrated, hypothermic and hypoglycemic more quickly and severely than others due to loss of subcutaneous fat, which markedly reduces the body's capacity for temperature regulation and water storage.
- Muscle protein is also lost along with losses and deficiency of magnesium, zinc, copper, and potassium.
- Severe malnutrition is furthermore associated with chronic hypovolemia, which leads to secondary hyperaldosteronism, and further complicates fluid and electrolyte balance.

## 5.4 GENERAL SIGNS OF UNDERNUTRITION

### 1. Skin Changes

The term "nutritional dermatosis" is used to describe the skin changes associated with malnutrition. It usually indicates severe degree of malnutrition. The skin becomes loose and wrinkled due to loss of subcutaneous fat whereas in kwashiorkor, it becomes shiny and edematous due to water retention. Skin may become hypopigmented, hyperpigmented, erythematous, or black in color.

- *Flaky paint dermatosis* is pathognomonic of kwashiorkor and is characterized by patches of hyperpigmented skin which peel off to reveal raw areas. It involves the extremities more often than the trunk especially the buttocks, perineum, and the thighs.
- *Crazy pavement dermatosis* refers to cracked skin lesions in flexures, joints, and buttocks which get ulcerated and infected. Pathogenesis of these skin lesions is attributed to the deficiencies of tyrosine, niacin, zinc and vitamins.

Apart from skin color changes and easy ulceration, nutritional dermatosis is also marked by poor wound healing and increased risk of secondary infections. Sometimes skin changes can be attributed to vitamins or other micronutrient deficiencies which often co exist in children with SAM **(Table 5.2)**.[4]

### 2. Mucosal Changes

Glossitis **(Fig. 5.3)** (swollen tongue), stomatitis (inflammation of the mouth) and cheilitis (inflamed lips) occur due to deficiency of vitamin $B_2$, vitamin $B_3$, and folic acid. A bald and smooth tongue occurs due to atrophy of the papillae in vitamin $B_{12}$ deficiency. Spongy bleeding gums can be a manifestation of vitamin C deficiency.

**Table 5.2** Summary of the Skin Findings in Various Nutritional Deficiencies[4]

| Nutrient deficiency | Skin changes |
|---|---|
| Vitamin A | • Dry and scaly skin (generalized xerosis)<br>• Follicular hyperkeratosis especially in arms, shoulders, legs, buttocks |
| Riboflavin (vitamin $B_2$) | • Seborrheic dermatitis-like eruptions |
| Niacin (vitamin $B_3$) | • Scaly, symmetrical, well demarcated dermatitis on areas exposed to irritants like sunlight, heat, friction or pressure. Skin lesions resemble sunburn and subside leaving a dusky, brown-red color.<br>• Lesions on the face resemble a butterfly eruption<br>• Lesions on hands and feet resemble the glove and stocking pattern<br>• Lesions on the front of the neck resemble a Casall's necklace<br>• Vesicles and bullae can also develop |
| Pyridoxine ($B_6$) | • Seborrheic dermatitis-like eruptions |
| Cyanocobalamin (vitamin $B_{12}$) | • Hyperpigmentation of knuckles and palms |
| Biotin (vitamin H) | • Scaly periorifical dermatitis, seborrheic dermatitis like eruptions |
| Vitamin C | • Hyperkeratosis of hair follicles, poor wound healing, hemorrhagic manifestations like petechiae, ecchymosis and purpura at pressure points, perfollicular hemorrhages |
| Vitamin E | • Hemorrhagic skin manifestations |
| Zinc | • Eczematous eruptions of hands, feet, and anogenital regions.<br>• Fingers, flexural creases and palms show characteristic flat, grayish bullous lesions surrounded by red-brown erythema.<br>• In chronic cases, the lesions are seen on areas subject to repeated pressure and trauma, such as elbows, knees, and knuckles. They are well demarcated, thickened, and brownish, and may later develop lichenification and scaling. |
| Copper | • Depigmentation of skin |

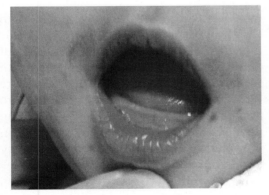

**Fig. 5.3** One and half year severely malnourished child with glossitis and oral ulcers

occur. Change in hair color may be due to deficiency of substrate (e.g., tyrosine) and coenzymes. During periods of improved nutrition, hair regain their pigmentation. Thus, distinct bands consisting of hypopigmented hair tips alternating with normally pigmented hair roots develop, this appearance is called as the **flag sign**. Eyelashes become thin and long and are called as *broom stick eyelashes*. Alopecia occurs due to deficiency of vitamin A, biotin and zinc, apart from protein deficiency. Decreased copper in diet can produce depigmented hair and skin.

## 3. Hair Changes

Hair become dull, sparse, thinner, straighter, brittle, and easily pluckable. Hypopigmentation of hair (hypochromotrichia) may

## 4. Nail Changes

• *Onycholysis* (separation of the nail from the nail bed) can occur in iron deficiency and Vitamin $B_3$ (niacin) deficiency.

- *Leuconychia* (white lines on nails) occur in hypoalbuminemia, calcium, vitamin B$_3$, and zinc deficiency.
- *Platynychia* (flattening of nails) followed by koilonychia (spooning of nails) is characteristically seen in iron deficiency anemia.
- *Koilonychia* occurs secondary to growth of the nail plate over a relatively low set distal matrix compared to the proximal matrix.
- *Haplonychia* or soft nails can occur in deficiencies of vitamin A, vitamin B$_6$, vitamin C, vitamin D, and calcium.
- *Beau's lines* are transverse depressions or grooves on the nail plate and occur in protein and vitamin B$_3$ deficiency.[5]

## 5. Teeth

Delayed tooth eruption can occur in vitamin D deficiency. Deficient vitamin A can lead to defective tooth enamel. Dental caries occur in fluoride deficiency.

## 6. Eye Changes

Eyes can be involved in children with SAM mostly due to infection or vitamin A deficiency. Eye lesions **(Fig. 5.4)** are the most characteristic and specific findings of co-existing vitamin A deficiency, the spectrum of which has been named as xerophthalmia

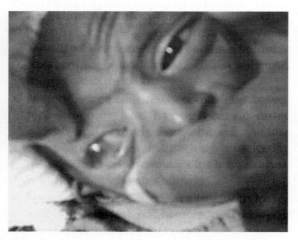

**Fig. 5.4** A 6-month-old child with xeropthalmia (keratomalacia)

**Table 5.3** WHO Staging of Xerophthalmia (Vitamin A Deficiency)

| Stage | Clinical feature |
| --- | --- |
| XN | Night blindness |
| IA | Conjunctival xerosis |
| IB | Bitot's spot |
| II | Corneal xerosis |
| III A | Corneal ulcer <1/3 of corneal area |
| III B | Corneal ulcer > 1/3 of corneal area/ keratomalacia |
| XS | Corneal scar |
| XF | Xerophthalmic fundus |

(literally meaning dry eye) **(Table 5.3)**. These signs usually develop insidiously and rarely occur before the age of 2 years.

- A delayed adaptation to the dark is the earliest manifestation (due to decreased rhodopsin) which progresses to night blindness or nyctalopia (due to complete absence of rhodopsin).
- Lack of vitamin A causes loss of mucus secreting cells leading to conjunctival xerosis and hyperkeratinization of the conjunctiva leading to Bitot spots. These are triangular white, foamy lesions usually seen in the temporal paralimbal areas of eyes.
- Corneal dryness and ulceration can occur which may progress to keratomalacia in which more than 1/3rd of the cornea is ulcerated. The ulcers can be punched out or fluffy and are commonly associated with secondary infection and are signs of severe vitamin A deficiency and may lead to blindness if left untreated. The underlying pathology involves corneal edema, thickening, and collagen necrosis secondary to vitamin A deficiency.
- Ocular abnormalities associated with beriberi include central scotomas and external ophthalmoplegia particularly affecting the third and sixth cranial nerves.
- Vitamin B$_2$ deficiency can cause conjunctivitis, keratitis, corneal vascularization, lacrimation, and photophobia. Corneal neovascularization is of special concern to

the ophthalmologists because it is one of the earliest signs of vitamin $B_2$ deficiency.

- Conjunctivitis can be produced by a biotin deficient state.
- Vitamin C deficiency may cause sub-conjunctival hemorrhages, and in advanced case hyphemas and retinal hemorrhages have been observed.[6]

## 7. Glands

Bilateral parotid gland enlargement occurs in chronic malnutrition especially in young children. Atrophy of the lacrimal and salivary glands occurs leading to dry eyes and mouth.

## 5.5 SYSTEMIC MANIFESTATIONS OF UNDERNUTRITION

### 1. Central Nervous System

The period from mid-conception up to the third year of postnatal life is the critical time when the brain grows at an unmatched pace. Although the number of neurons becomes complete by mid-gestation, the neuronal migration, glial proliferation, synaptic connections, dendritic arborization, myelination and cerebellar growth continue up to 3 years of life. Any insult during this phase is bound to affect the above processes and impair brain growth and development affecting central as well as peripheral nervous system.[2,5]

- Severe malnutrition results in decreased brain growth, reduced neurotransmitter production and synaptic connections, resulting in decreased cognitive abilities.
- Impaired myelination results in decreased conduction velocity of the peripheral nerves.
- In the spinal cord, anterior horn cells are reduced in number and size and degenerative changes occur. This has been termed as "*Kwashiorkor myelopathy*".
- Overall, reduction in head circumference, development quotient, motor nerve conduction velocity, brain stem auditory evoked potential, CSF cholesterol and

phospholipid content have been found in severe malnutrition.

- Irritability and apathy are common. Brain edema, electrolyte imbalance, hypokalemia and hypomagnesemia are the proposed causes. Alteration of neurotransmitter synthesis and release is also known to occur. Playfulness is decreased as is environmental and familial interaction.
- Tremors are usually seen during treatment. They occur due to deficiency of vitamin $B_{12}$, electrolyte imbalance, imbalance in the production of GABA, and dysmyelination. Blinking frequently, tremulous cry due to vocal cord tremor, and tremors of the body are seen and designated as "*Kwashi shake*". Most of these changes are relatively more common in babies in Kwashiorkor, which is seen far less in Indian population.

### Long-term Effects on Intelligence

Deficits in motor coordination tasks have been demonstrated due to cerebellar involvement. General reasoning, perceptual abilities, and sensory integration are most severely affected; followed by deficits in short term memory and learning skill. Language ability is the last to be affected.[3]

### 2. Hematological Changes

The most common hematologic change in the children with severe malnutrition is anemia and major cause of anemia is iron deficiency. Bone marrow of most patients with severe acute malnutrition has normal cellularity with dysplastic changes due to the inadequate and imbalanced intake of protein and energy.[8] Purpura or bleeding can occur due to deficiency of vitamin C or vitamin K; and in Gram negative septicemia and disseminated intravascular coagulation.

### 3. Gastrointestinal Changes

Mucosal atrophy, delayed mucosal repair, and disaccharidase deficiency occurs. Cholangitis and ascending pancreatitis may occur due to bacterial overgrowth in the upper gut and duodenum. Hepatomegaly occurs due to fatty infiltration of the liver. Ascites may be present.

## 4. Immune Function

Worldwide, acute malnutrition is probably the leading cause of immunodeficiency in children. The immune responses of the body are produced by cells arising in the lymphoreticular organs (the thymus, lymph nodes and spleen) which develop rapidly in the first two years of life.

- In severe malnutrition the thymus, tonsils, spleen, and other lymphoid tissues are atrophied. These changes are accompanied by delayed or absent tuberculin response and other skin hypersensitivity reactions; reduced complement activity in the serum, especially the C3 component; and reduced numbers of thymus dependent lymphocytes (T-cells) in the blood.

- Protein deficiency is the primary cause for the above changes though a lack of zinc, folate and other nutrients also contribute to the immunodeficient state.

- Total circulating lymphocytes are reduced in number. T-lymphocytes have a poor response to in vitromitogenic stimulator. Vitamin A deficiency produces reduced CD4/CD8 ratio and total CD4 naive T cells. This immunocompromised status improves with dietary rehabilitation, functional recovery occurs within 2 weeks and the total lymphocyte count recovers within 4 weeks.

- The concentration of B lymphocytes in lymphoid tissues and peripheral blood is normal and the immunoglobulin synthesis is increased as reflected in elevated total circulating IgA, IgM, IgG, IgD, and IgE levels. The concentrations are greater in children with kwashiorkor than those with marasums.

- Malnourished children have reduced secretary IgA (sIgA) levels in nasal washings, duodenal fluids, and tears despite the elevated level of IgA in the serum. The loss of secretory immunity may contribute to an increase in the respiratory and intestinal infections.

- The response of polymorphonuclear (PMN) leukocytes to chemotactic stimulation is normal, but that of the macrophages is reduced.

- All children with severe malnutrition have depressed concentrations of specific complement factors (Ciq, Cis, CZ, Cs, C6, C8, C9 and C3 PA).[9]

## 5. Cardiovascular Changes

Decreased cardiac output, hypotension, bradycardia and rarely small vessel vasculopathy are observed. However, congestive cardiac failure and cardiomyopathy may be seen secondary to anemia, thiamine, and selenium deficiency.[3]

## 6. Musculoskeletal Changes

Muscle wasting occurs due to protein deficiency. In addition, several skeletal changes occur secondary to calcium, vitamin D or vitamin C deficiency. Hypocalcemia can be detected by signs for latent tetany (Trousseau sign or Chvostek sign).

## 7. Mineral and Trace Element Deficiencies

Eleven major elements constitute 99% of the human body. These include hydrogen, carbon, nitrogen, oxygen, sodium, potassium, calcium, magnesium, sulfur, phosphorus, and chlorine. In addition, the body has trace elements which comprise of less than 0.01% of the body weight. These trace elements are chiefly components of metalloenzymes. Children are especially prone to trace element deficiency symptoms as their growth increases demands. Gastrointestinal disorders which increases trace element losses are commoner in children and some organs like the brain are likely to sustain permanent damage due to trace element deficiency in childhood.

## 5.6 COMPLICATIONS OF SEVERE ACUTE MALNUTRITION

### A. Complicated SAM

This term is used to describe children in whom severe acute malnutrition is worsened by co-existence of infection, any metabolic disturbance, edema, anorexia, or poor appetite (fail the appetite test). Conditions which are included in complicated SAM comprise of other comorbid conditions like severe anemia, complicated malaria, other severe infections like severe respiratory infection, meningitis or sepsis, diarrhea with dehydration, lethargy or acute neurological disorders with or without HIV infection, hypoglycemia, temperature instabilities, and dyselectrolytemia.[1,11]

### B. Uncomplicated SAM

This refers to severely malnourished children who are free from the above co-morbidities and retain a good appetite. It is important to differentiate between the two as the former need hospital admission whereas the latter can be managed at home/at community level.

### C. Common Complications

#### 1. *Hypothermia*

Rectal temperature less than $35.5°$ C or an axillary temperature less than $35°$ C indicates hypothermia. Due to low body fat reserves, decreased metabolic rate and poor thermo-regulatory control, severely malnourished children are at increased risk of hypothermia especially those with denuded skin or co-existing infections.

#### 2. *Hypoglycemia*

Children with SAM are at increased risk of hypoglycemia (blood sugar <54 mg/dL) because of decreased glucose synthesis and increased demand. In addition to decreased intake of glucose, synthesis is also decreased due to impaired gluconeogenesis in the liver along with decreased glycogen reserves in the

wasted muscles. Increased demands occur due to increased activity of the immune system to fight the presence of superadded infections.[9]

Hypoglycemia may be symptomatic or asymptomatic. Symptoms may include lethargy, unconsciousness, seizures, hypothermia, and peripheral circulatory failure. Features of sympathetic stimulation like pallor and sweating are rare in malnourished children but may occur.[12]

Malnourished children may arrive at the hospital in the hypoglycemic state if they have been vomiting, if they have been too sick to eat, or if they have undertaken long journey without food. In hospital also they may develop hypoglycemia if they are not fed regularly specially at night time, or have been waiting for admission.

#### 3. *Infections*

Classic signs of infection i.e. fever, tachycardia, tachypnea are often absent in severely malnourished children. There are few localizing signs. Hypothermia, hypoglycemia, and septicemia often coexist in a triad in malnourished children. Thus, the presence of one should prompt the exclusion of the other two. The skin, respiratory, alimentary and urinary tracts are the most common systems infected. Septicemia, acute respiratory tract infection, infective diarrhea, urinary tract infection, tuberculosis, HIV, measles are some of the infective conditions which are known to be commonly associated with SAM in children.[13] Gram negative organisms are the commonest cause of infections in SAM. In addition, TB should be ruled out as it occurs more commonly and has a poorer outcome in children with SAM.[14] Moreover, malaria should be investigated for in endemic areas and CSF done if signs of meningitis are present.

#### 4. *Diarrhea and Dehydration*

Diarrhea in any form complicates SAM. Dehydration, however can be overestimated in children with severe malnutrition. Loss of skin elasticity may be due to loss of subcutaneous fat as well as due to dehydration. Likewise, skin pinch can be slow due to either reason. Therefore the main diagnosis comes from history rather than examination. If there is recent history of significant fluid loss in the form of watery diarrhea and if there is recent change in appearance of the child, the child is presumed to have dehydration. Sometimes, other signs of dehydration *i.e.* dry oral mucosa, excess thirst, hypothermia, weak pulses, and oliguria are better indicators of dehydration.

Since an accurate estimation of dehydration is difficult in malnourished children, it is safe to assume that all malnourished patients with watery diarrhea have *Some dehydration* except when the child presents with shock, which indicates *Severe dehydration* or septic shock.[1]

## 5. *Electrolyte Disturbances*

Total body sodium is elevated in severely malnourished children even though plasma sodium may be low. Thus, sodium intake should be restricted to prevent sodium excess and water retention as this may precipitate congestive cardiac failure. Potassium and magnesium deficiencies are present in all severely malnourished children and take at least two weeks to correct.

## References

1. WHO. Pocket Book of Hospital Care for Children: Guidelines for the Management of Common Childhood Illnesses (2nd ed). Geneva: World Health Organization; 2013.
2. Elizabeth KE. Triple burden of malnutrition. In: Nutrition and Child Development. 4ed. Hyderabad, New Delhi: Paras Medical Publisher; 2010.p.164–260.
3. Müller O, Krawinkel M. Malnutrition and health in developing countries. CMAJ 2005;173:279–86.
4. Oumeish YO, Oumeish I. Nutritional skin problems in children. Clin Dermatol. 2003;21:260–3.
5. Michael W, Cashman BA, Sloan SB. Nutrition and nail disease. Clin Dermatol. 2010;28:420–5.
6. Bloch R. Gastrointestinal and nutritional diseases. In: Duane TD, Jeagear EA (eds). Clinical Ophthalmology. Volume 5. Philadelphia, London: JB Lippincott Company; 1988. p.427.
7. Rodríguez-Salinas LC, Amador C, Medina MT. Malnutrition and Neurologic Disorders: A Global Overview. *In*: Medina MT, Amador C, Hernández-Toranzo R, Hesse H, Holden KR, Morales-Ortíz A, Rodríguez-Salinas LC (eds). Neurologic Consequences of Malnutrition. Volume 6. New York: Demos Medical Publishing; 2008.p.4–6.
8. Özkale M, Sipahi T. Hematologic and bone marrow changes in children with protein-energy malnutrition. Pediatr Hematol Oncol. 2014;31:349–58.
9. Johanne M, Rytter H, Kolte L, Briend A, Friis H, Christensen VB. The immune system in children with malnutrition- A systematic review. PLoS One. 2014;9:e105017.
10. Greenbaum LA. Micronutrient mineral deficiencies. *In*: Kliegman R, Nelson WE, ed. Nelson Textbook of Paediatrics. Vol. 1. 20 ed, Philadelphia PA: Elsevier/Saunders; 2016.p.343–5.
11. WHO. Guideline: Updates on the management of severe acute malnutrition in infants and children. Geneva: World Health Organization; 2013.
12. Bhatnagar S, Lodha R, Choudhury P, Sachdev HPS, Shah N, Narayan S, *et al*. IAP guidelines 2006 on hospital based management of severely malnourished children (adapted from the WHO Guidelines).Indian Pediatr. 2007;44:443-61.
13. Jones KD, Thitiri J, Ngari M, Berkley JA. Childhood malnutrition: Toward an understanding of infections, inflammation, and antimicrobials. Food Nutr Bull. 2014; 35: S64–S70.
14. Chisti MJ, Ahmed T, Pietroni MA, Faruque AS, Ashraf H, Bardhan PK, *et al*. Pulmonary tuberculosis in severely-malnourished or HIV-infected children with pneumonia: a review. J Health Popul Nutr. 2013;31:308–13.

# Principles of Care in Severe Acute Malnutrition

Preeti Singh, S Aneja

## 6.1 INTRODUCTION

Severe acute malnutrition (SAM) is a significant public health problem in India and many developing countries. Globally it is responsible for >50% mortality in children under 5 years of age after the first month of life.[1] Malnutrition is a state of negative balance at the cellular level; the supply of nutrients and energy are inadequate to meet body's demand to ensure growth, maintenance, and specific functions. The physiology of a child with SAM is different from a child who has normal nutritional status and these differences affect the essential components of care in SAM. The course of illness of a child with SAM is often complicated by metabolic and medical complications which may or may not be clinically apparent. Application of the usual protocols of treatment in such children may be detrimental or can result in mortality. Despite the variability in presentation of children with SAM across countries worldwide, the principles of management of these children are largely based on the understanding the pathophysiology in SAM. The factors which precipitate the acute illness vary and the spectrum of infections or infestations which complicate the disease is characteristic of the local geographical area. The management of children with SAM essentially has dual objectives: (a) to decrease the mortality; and (b) to achieve early complete recovery. Multiple socioeconomic factors including food insecurity, poverty, illiteracy, lack of health education, and poor environmental sanitation are involved in causation of malnutrition. Addressing the underlying factors are unequivocally important in holistic management of children with SAM.

## 6.2 NEED FOR EARLY IDENTIFICATION AND TREATMENT

Estimates suggest that the prevalence of severe acute malnutrition (SAM) in children below 5 years of age in India is about 6.4 %, accounting for nearly 8.1 million children.[2] Acute malnutrition predisposes the children to die while the immediate cause of mortality could be diarrhea, pneumonia, measles, or malaria. A severely wasted and stunted child has 9 and 4 times, respectively increased risk of death as compared to children with normal nutritional status.[3]

Children with SAM have increased susceptibility to infections which makes them prone to multiple episodes of illness and longer recovery period. At the same time, infection results in loss of appetite, increased nutrient requirements and/or decreased absorption of nutrients consumed, further perpetuating the vicious cycle of malnutrition.

Prolonged undernutrition in first 2 years of life leads to stunting and irreversible changes in brain growth leading to poor motor skills, social skills, and cognitive decline. This vulnerable group if left untreated enter adolescence in a state of undernutrition, thereby affecting growth potential, schooling, and ultimately unfavorable employment opportunities and poor productivity outcomes.

## Why Children with Severe Acute Malnutrition Need to be Treated Differently?

A child with SAM undergoes several physiological and metabolic changes in the body to allow survival on limited calories called as *reductive adaptation* (Also See Chapter 4). These biochemical changes predispose children with malnutrition to environmental stress and infection. There is a gradual decline in the functioning of the organ systems and the energy reserves are diverted towards basic physiological functions to sustain life.

The complex metabolic, biochemical, and hormonal adaptations are a consequence of limited calorie and protein intake. Inadequate calorie intake leads to glycogenolysis and gluconeogenesis with mobilization of amino acids, pyruvate, and lactate from skeletal tissue. This is followed by a phase of protein conservation and utilization of fat stores through lipolysis and ketogenesis. An important component of reductive adaptation is decrease in number and slow functioning of the glycoside sensitive energy-dependent sodium pump which generates a state of excess sodium and low potassium in the body.[4]

A child with SAM conserves energy mainly by reducing physical activity and growth; reducing basal metabolism by slowing protein turnover; reduced fat, muscle, and visceral mass; and poor inflammatory and immune responses. Reduction in muscle, mass is accompanied by loss of intracellular nutrients and smaller reserves of muscle glycogen. As a consequence of the reductive adaptation, the work and function of each and every organ

system suffers putting the child in a vulnerable state. The effects of reductive adaptation on different organ systems are described in **Table 6.1**.

Median case fatality rate in hospitalized children with SAM is very high *i.e.* approximately 23.5% and it rises to 50% in edematous SAM if these changes are not kept in mind.[5] Reasons for high case fatality are enlisted in **Table 6.2**. The case fatality can be brought down to approximately <10% by standard case management protocol.[6]

## 6.3 UNFOLDING PRINCIPLES OF NUTRITIONAL MANAGEMENT OF SAM

The old prevalent theory of energy and protein deficiency, leading to marasmus and kwashiorkor, respectively, stands disproved. Although the quantity of food available, suboptimal living conditions, poor child care practices, and acute/chronic infection, independently and in combination contribute to malnutrition but they are not the primary cause of it. The weight loss in malnutrition can be explained by the impaired appetite which develops due to consumption of poor quality diets deficient in essential micronutrients.

### A. Type I *vs.* Type II Micronutrients

Essential micronutrients can be divided into two classes as suggested by Golden.[7,8]

*Type I micronutrients* which consists of nutrients (iron, calcium, iodine, vitamin A, thiamine, riboflavin, vitamin $B_{12}$, folate, and selenium) responsible for various biochemical, hormonal, and immunological functions in the body. Deficiency of Type I nutrients would allow the child to grow and consume the body stores with eventual signs and symptoms of deficiency. Their need is determined by the demand for specific functions and the need to replenish the body stores.

*Type II nutrients* (essential amino-acids, potassium, magnesium, zinc, phosphorous) are the essential building blocks which are needed for all biochemical pathways. There

**Table 6.1** Consequences of Reductive Adaptation on Various Organ Systems in Severe Acute Malnutrition

| Organ system | Effects | Clinical implication |
|---|---|---|
| Liver | Unable to synthesize glucose. Impaired ability to excrete excess proteins and detoxify toxins and drugs. | Increased risk of hypoglycemia and hypothermia. Ensure frequent small volume feeds throughout day and night Limit protein intake to avoid stressing the liver. |
| Gastrointestinal system | Reduced gastric acid secretion. Gut mucosa is flattened with villous atrophy and crypt hypoplasia and resultant loss of disaccharidases and other enzymes. There is poor gut motility with bacterial colonization of the small bowel mucosa. Pancreatic atrophy is also seen leading to fat malabsorption. | During stabilization, feeds must be small in amount and the composition should be such as to avoid exceeding the gut's functional capacity. The physical presence of nutrients helps in early repair of the gut mucosa. |
| Cardiovascular system | The heart is small with thinned out myofibrils. Impaired cardiac contractility and reduced output. | Bradycardia and hypotension may be seen. They are susceptible to develop arrhythmias in presence of dyselectrolytemias. The fluid intake should be carefully monitored as any excess fluid in the circulation can cause mortality from heart failure. The composition of the feeds and rehydrating fluid should be low in sodium. |
| Renal system | Decreased glomerular filtration rate and lowered capacity to concentrate the urine and excrete an acid load. | Excess fluid and sodium (from feeds or rehydration fluid) can lead to fluid overload. Feeds should be enteral, never parenteral, to reduce the risk of fluid overload. |
| Hematopoietic system | Red cell mass is reduced, liberating iron. Free iron promotes the growth of pathogens and the production of free radicals which damage cell membranes. | During stabilization phase withhold iron and provide vitamins and minerals to mop up free radicals. |
| Respiratory system | Low minute ventilation as a result of reduced thoracic muscle mass, low metabolic rate, and electrolyte abnormalities (hypokalemia and hypophosphatemia) | Predisposed to hypoxemia because of impaired ventilator response. |
| Immune system | Thymus, lymph nodes, and tonsils undergo atrophy. Impaired cell mediated immunity resulting in loss of delayed hypersensitivity reactions. Impaired phagocytosis, and low secretory IgA. | Increase susceptibility to invasive infections. May or may not manifest clinical signs of sepsis. Presume infections and give broad spectrum antibiotics |
| Endocrine system | Hypofunction of thyroid gland (reduced levels of tri-iodothyronine (T3) due to poor deiodination by liver, decreased | Low metabolic rate Poor physical growth |

*Contd.*

**Table 6.1** Consequences of Reductive Adaptation on Various Organ Systems in Severe Acute Malnutrition (*Contd.*)

| Organ system | Effects | Clinical implication |
|---|---|---|
| | levels of thyroxine-binding prealbumin and globulins are due to decreased synthesis by liver, low plasma T4; TSH levels are normal). Low insulin as it regulates the release of glucose. Low Insulin-like Growth Factor-1 (IGF-1) - poor growth. Elevated levels of growth hormone and cortisol to provide substrate when intake is limited. | |
| Neurological system | Brain growth suffers due to reductions in the number of neurons, synapses, dendritic arborisations, and myelination. | Global developmental delay; neonates and infants are most susceptible as phase of exponential brain growth. Need for early recognition and intervention to prevent permanent neurological sequelae. |

**Table 6.2** Reasons for High Mortality in Severe Acute Malnutrition

1. Hypoglycemia and hypothermia unattended
2. Use of intravenous fluids to manage some dehydration
3. Inappropriate monitoring during rehydration — fluid overload
4. Untreated infection
5. Use of diuretics for edema
6. Use of albumin for edema
7. Inability to distinguish between initial and rehabilitation phases
8. Use of therapeutic diets high in protein and sodium during initial stabilization phase
9. Failure to monitor food intake
10. Use of oral iron in the initial stabilization phase

are no body stores of Type II nutrients except the functional tissues and hence need to be supplemented if lost during a catabolic stress.[9] Deficiency of Type II nutrients leads to growth failure; at the expense to conserve and maintain their normal plasma levels of potassium, magnesium, zinc, and essential amino acids. Indeed in severe deficiency, the body goes into a catabolic state with poor appetite.

## B. Type II Nutrient Deficiency Leads to Reductive Adaptation

It is now understood that the primary reason of wasting and stunting is severe and mild deficiency of Type II nutrients, respectively, leading to state of reductive adaptation.[10] Hence Type II nutrients need to be supplemented in appropriate amounts during stabilization and rehabilitative phase for regeneration of wasted tissues and their functions. Concurrently some children with SAM have deficiency of Type I nutrients predisposing them to oxidative stress thereby compromising their health and wellbeing.[7,8] Deficiency of Type I nutrients does not lead to growth failure so they may not necessarily lose weight or become stunted. During convalescence besides the optimal calories and proteins, unless a diet rich in essential nutrients (Type I and II) is provided, there would be incomplete recovery.

## C. Therapeutic Diets

Conventional old diets provided empty calories for weight gain but failed to regain the functional tissue for physiological, biochemical, and immunological recovery. Such children might become obese due to excess adipose tissue but continue to have malnutrition. The adequacy of the therapeutic diets should not be judged by the potential to gain weight. Growth velocity is a better indicator of nutritional adequacy.[10] Modern therapeutic diets are based on the principles of reductive adaptation.

- The **F-75 starter diet** has been designed with low sodium and protein content and relatively optimal levels of potassium, magnesium, zinc and Type I nutrients which would be easily tolerated by the compromised intestine. This diet is based on the physiological adaptation in children with malnutrition to help regain the enzymatic functions. It helps to tide over the stabilization phase, assists in loosing edema, but would not support weight gain or growth.

- On the other hand, the **F-100 catch up formula** contains the essential nutrients required to regain appetite and promote early and complete recovery to premorbid functional, biochemical, and immuno-logical state. It helps to rebuild the wasted tissues and promotes catch-up growth. However F-100 diet is not suitable for children with edematous SAM and for those admitted with complications during the initial stabilization phase.

## 6.4 CLINICAL ASSESSMENT OF A CHILD WITH SAM

The growth and development in children is a complex process determined by the genetic potential and accompanying health and nutritional status. Assessment of growth provides an indicator to the health and the nutritional status. A complete nutritional assessment in a child with SAM includes a thorough history of the clinical illness and accompanying complications, anthropometric assessment, and a detailed dietary and socioeconomic history to elucidate the underlying factors responsible for

malnutrition. Before going through a detailed history, initial evaluation warrants a quick look for the emergency signs and their appropriate treatment if present. In the absence of emergency signs a detailed evaluation is conducted to determine the cause of malnutrition (primary or secondary), accompanying complications, current state of health and appetite, underlying socio economic factors, the ability of caregiver to deliver the requisite care, and finally decide the platform of management — facility based or community based. Identification of SAM in children under 5 years is done as per WHO criteria.[11] We have already discussed identification of SAM in Chapter 3.

## 6.5 DECIDING THE LEVEL OF CARE

### A. Community-based Care

Evidence shows that children with SAM who have good appetite and are free of medical complications **(Table 6.3)**, can be managed at home under community based program.[12]

- This community based therapeutic care aims to ensure increased access and care to a large number of children with SAM who do not require inpatient care.

- In addition, this strategy prevents the risk of nosocomial sepsis in case of hospitalization.

- It does not disrupt the family, comes out as a cost effective approach for the family as it saves on the patient costs, transport, and loss of wages from work absenteeism.

- It involves active case finding so that many undetected children with SAM are screened and provided appropriate care.

Under a community based therapeutic care program, these children are enrolled at a nearby health facility where they receive locally prepared therapeutic food (Ready to Use Therapeutic Food–RUTF) and medicines (as applicable) for home consumption. RUTF is an energy dense palatable food enriched with vitamins and minerals that has a nutritional profile similar to WHO-

**Table 6.3** Criteria for Hospitalization in Children with Severe Acute Malnutrition[11,14]

| 6–59 months | < 6 months |
|---|---|
| i. Presence of any emergency signs<br>ii. Hypothermia (axillary temperature < 35°C)<br>iii. Edema<br>iv. Persistent vomiting<br>v. Poor appetite, apathetic<br>vi. Fever (axillary temperature > 39°C)<br>vii. Fast breathing, chest indrawing<br>viii. Extensive skin and eye lesions.<br>ix. Diarrhea with dehydration<br>x. Severe anemia<br>xi. Purpura or bleeding tendency<br>xii. Evidence of systemic infections or complications | i. Any clinical condition or medical complication as outlined for infants ≥6 months of age with SAM.<br>ii. Recent weight loss or failure to gain weight<br>iii. Ineffective feeding (attachment, positioning and suckling) directly observed for 15–20 min in a supervised separated area<br>iv. Presence of pitting edema<br>v. Any medical or social issue needing more detailed assessment or intensive support (e.g. disability, depression of the caregiver, or other adverse social circumstances). |

recommended therapeutic diets for inpatient management.[13] They can be easily and safely administered to children > 6 months of age with SAM by the caregiver. The absence of water in RUTF gives them protection against bacterial contamination and the ease of storage at home even without refrigeration.

Mothers should attend health facility/nutritional centers weekly for monitoring the response to treatment and to receive additional supplies of therapeutic food. The community-based program should be linked with the facility-based component, so that children with medical complications, non-responders to community based management can be referred to the facility level, and those stabilized on facility-based management can be transferred in the community for continued care.

## B. Health-facility based Care

Children with SAM who have poor appetite and/or medical complications and/or edema, or are aged < 6 months at outset are managed in a health facility as inpatients preferably at a Nutrition Rehabilitation Center.[14] These children need immediate attention and management otherwise are at a high risk of mortality. The medical complications that mandate hospitalization are given in **Table 6.3**. Other indications for facility based

management are children whose mother/caregiver is unable to deliver requisite care at home, or child not responding/experience weight loss while being managed in a community based program. Successful implementation of the standardized WHO protocol[15] in facility based care has reduced the case fatality rates in Bangladesh and South Africa.[16,17] It is important to realize that the protocols were followed in well-resourced hospitals by skilled and motivated health staff which were the main determinants of their favorable outcome.

The consensus statement by the Indian experts on the management of children with SAM based on the WHO and UNICEF specifications were published in 2006[18] and revised in 2013.[19] The observational studies from Indian subcontinent on the experience and outcome of children with SAM using therapeutic diet in community settings and inpatient care have highlighted promising results.[20,21]

## 6.6 LABORATORY INVESTIGATIONS

All children with SAM admitted to a health facility should undergo appropriate tests to assess the current state of health, confirm apparent diseases, actively screen for occult infections, and explore secondary causes of SAM. At the outset, check blood glucose, serum electrolytes, hemoglobin (along with red cell indices) with peripheral smear. Hypoglycemia, dyselectrolytemia, and severe anemia need immediate attention as they increase the risk of mortality. Investigations to screen and confirm infections include total and differential leukocyte count; blood culture; urine routine and microscopic examination with culture; peripheral smear for malarial parasite; chest X-ray and Mantoux test; and stool examination in case of persistent and chronic diarrhea. If facilities exist, serum electrolytes (sodium, potassium, magnesium, and phosphate) should be monitored closely in the early treatment phase to identify refeeding syndrome. Additional tests may be required depending upon the clinical condition of the child.

## 6.7 ESSENTIAL COMPONENTS OF CARE

The management of children with SAM in a facility/NRC essentially constitutes of 10 steps distributed over initial stabilization and rehabilitative phase.[15] Resources and skilled dedicated staff should be provided for optimal delivery of care to these children. Standardized anthropometric tools should be available to monitor the response to treatment. Initial management steps primarily deal with awareness of common problems (hypoglycemia, hypothermia, infections, and fluid and electrolyte imbalance) and appropriate steps to prevent, identify, and manage them at the earliest. Round the clock meticulous and intensive monitoring is the cornerstone of successful initial stabilization. The rationale behind the steps involved in the management of children with SAM is briefly discussed below.

### 1. Hypoglycemia and Hypothermia

Children with SAM are eminently susceptible to hypoglycemia and hypothermia and this could be a reason of early demise if unattended. Hypothermia develops in a SAM child as less heat is generated when physically inactive and their BMR is low because of reductive adaptation. Moreover they tend to lose more heat than usual due to higher body surface area per kg body weight and lack of subcutaneous fat that provides insulation. Hence suitable arrangements should be made to nurse these children in a warm area (25–30°C), free from draughts. Ensure appropriate clothing to keep them fully covered including head, hands, and feet. Washing should be kept to a minimum, following which they should be dried immediately.

Hypoglycemia is an important metabolic problem faced by children with SAM. There exists problem of poor glucose delivery from the hepatic and muscle stores because of depleted reserves and impaired release while the body has a constant high demand for it. Therefore, early initiation and continuous small frequent feeds is of utmost importance to maintain a regular supply of glucose. Hypoglycemia frequently coexists with hypothermia and infection so immediate attention should be directed to address all the three problems simultaneously.

### 2. Rationale of Antibiotics in Children with SAM

It is clearly evident through literature review that children with SAM have high prevalence of pneumonia, bacteremia, urinary tract infections, otitis media, and other systemic infections. However the clinical signs and symptoms may not be apparent due to impaired immunological response in SAM. They often do not have fever or signs of inflammation even in presence of fulminant sepsis. So, it is prudent to suspect infection in all children with SAM. It is recommended to treat with antibiotics according to the local prevailing antibiotic resistance patterns even without any obvious clinical signs of infection.[12,22]

Children with uncomplicated SAM should receive oral antibiotics while those who need inpatient management are started on broad spectrum parenteral antibiotics while investigating for coexisting infections.[14]

The use of oral antibiotics in children with uncomplicated SAM prevents the development of small bowel bacterial overgrowth and the risk of bacteremia due to translocation of gut microbes. Oral antibiotics are not warranted in any child with undernutrition without SAM unless they harbor clinical sign or symptoms of infections. However the recent research has questioned the role of oral antibiotics in the outpatient management of uncomplicated SAM[23,24] as it failed to demonstrate improvement in nutritional recovery.

## 3. Fluid Management

Children with SAM have altered fluid and electrolyte homeostasis and are extremely vulnerable to rapid changes in the fluid volume and composition. As a result of reductive adaptation, the sodium potassium pumps decrease in number and function sluggishly. Sodium leaks into cells leading to excess body sodium while potassium leaks out of cells and is lost in urine. Besides, physiological adaptive mechanisms result in a small heart with reduced cardiac output and kidneys are unable to excrete excess fluid and sodium. This explains the propensity of children with SAM to retain fluid and develop heart failure when provided with excessive fluids. It becomes practically impossible to get the fluid and excessive sodium out of a child with SAM in such a situation. Hence there is a need to restrict sodium, provide potassium, and follow guarded approach to fluid management in children with SAM. The challenge is even tougher in cases with diarrhea as signs of dehydration are highly unreliable to classify and assess the severity of dehydration in a wasted or edematous SAM child. Wrong assessment of hydration status and overzealous fluid given for its correction is often the cause of mortality in SAM. The use of intravenous fluids is not recommended to correct dehydration unless the child is in altered sensorium or in shock.

## Fluids in Children with SAM and Diarrheal Dehydration

The use of standard WHO ORS for the management of dehydration in children with SAM has raised concern of causing fluid overload and heart failure due to their high sodium content (90 mEq/L). In addition the need for potassium supplementation in them is much more than provided by the standard ORS.

## Which fluid to use?

- **ReSoMal** (Rehydrating Solution for severely malnourished children) was introduced in 1999[15] to manage dehydration in children with SAM as it contained less sodium (45 mEq/L) as compared to the conventional ORS and had added potassium (40 mEq/L) and minerals appropriately suited for these children. ReSoMal continues to be recommended (low quality of evidence) by WHO to manage some and severe dehydration in children with SAM and diarrhea.[14,25]

- Another alternative is to use half strength low osmolarity ORS with added glucose and potassium as ReSoMal is not commercially available. One sachet of standard WHO low-osmolarity oral rehydration solution is dissolved in 2 L water (instead of 1 L). To this add 50 g of sugar and 1 level scoop of commercially available combined minerals and vitamins mix or 40 mL of mineral mix solution.[14]

- A randomized controlled trial from India to compare the safety and efficacy of low-osmolarity ORS vs. modified ReSoMal for treatment of children with SAM and diarrhea observed comparable success rate of rehydration in both the groups.[26] Though the children in modified ReSoMal group achieved early rehydration but a higher proportion (15.4%) developed hyponatremia as compared to 1.9% on low osmolarity ORS. In case of cholera or profuse watery diarrhea, ReSoMal is not desirable and instead standard low osmolarity ORS is used to treat dehydration.[14,25]

## Duration for Correction of Dehydration

To avoid rapid changes in homeostasis in children with SAM, the dehydration correction is done orally (or nasogastric tube) and slowly alternating with feeds (F-75 therapeutic diet) over 10–12 hours with intensive monitoring of vitals. The fluid requirements can change during the course of rehydration depending upon the ongoing losses, ability to drink, vomiting, and appearance of signs of overhydration.

## Monitoring during Correction

Intensive vital monitoring is absolutely imperative in children with SAM during initial 48–72 hrs especially in case of edematous SAM and where rehydration is ongoing along with therapeutic diet F-75. During initial stabilization phase when F-75 diet is initiated, the cell membranes regain their function to pump sodium out of the cells and potassium goes back inside the cell. Children can characteristically develop signs of fluid overload and heart failure if overhydrated and not monitored. Close observation will pick up subtle signs like tachypnea, tachycardia, weight gain, and worsening edema suggestive of fluid overload, and impending heart failure.

## Fluid Management in SAM with Shock

Management of children with SAM who present with shock continues to remain a challenge. Shock can evolve due to fluid losses following diarrhea and dehydration or as part of septic shock or may have both the components. The greatest clinical challenge is to differentiate between hypovolemic and septic shock. The clinical assessment of hydration status is an arduous task as signs of dehydration are quiet unreliable. At the same time these children are susceptible to risk of overhydration, heart failure, pulmonary edema, and clinical deterioration if rapid and large volumes of fluid are used for management of shock.

- The outcome of FEAST (Fluid Expansion as Supportive Therapy) trial conducted in children with febrile illness in resource-poor hospitals in sub-Saharan Africa provided robust evidence that fluid boluses increased 48-hour mortality in critically ill children with impaired perfusion.[27] However, children with severe malnutrition were excluded from this trial.
- Another RCT conducted in Kenyan children with SAM comparing the efficacy of Ringer's lactate isotonic fluid (RL), half-strength Darrow's in 5% dextrose (HSD/5D), and 4.5% human albumin solution (HAS) was prematurely terminated due to high mortality and inadequate correction of shock in all study arms.[28]
- There are no well conducted randomized controlled trials to guide us on the best possible fluid to resuscitate, rate of infusion, and outcome in terms of mortality or recovery in children with malnutrition.

*In presence of shock or lethargy/unconsciousness, WHO recommends half-strength Darrow's solution with 5% dextrose, or Ringer's lactate solution with 5% dextrose or 0.45% saline with 5% dextrose initially @ 15 mL/kg/h with meticulous monitoring of vital parameters to identify signs of overhydration and congestive heart failure.[14,15,25] The clinical response to this bolus will determine the need for further fluid (if shock improves) or inotropes (in case of deterioration).*

Once the shock improves, rest of the fluid rehydration is carried out orally or via nasogastric tube as in case of some dehydration over next 10–12 hours. Feeds are initiated at earliest alternating with oral fluids as the child recovers from shock.

## 4. Management of Dyselectrolytemia

### Treat Hypokalemia

Children with severe acute malnutrition are in a state of excess sodium while potassium stores are depleted due to poor function of sodium potassium pumps. So we need to restrict sodium and give potassium supplements. Potassium is essential to maintain cellular physiology and is needed in substantial amounts for convalescent growth. F-100 diet contains 2400 mg (61 mmol) of potassium/1000 kcal to replete body stores in couple of weeks[29] and support rapid weight gain.

## Treat Hypomagnesemia

Undernutrition leads to tissue magnesium deficit which also needs to be replenished. Magnesium helps potassium to enter the cells and be retained because it is an important co-factor controlling the sodium pump.[30] Magnesium deficiency also contributes to the osteoporosis of malnutrition. To successfully treat hypocalcemia/rickets with calcium and vitamin D supplements, correction of magnesium deficiency must accompany or precede treatment.

## Phosphate Deficiency

Phosphorous is an intracellular anion found in soft tissue, bone, and brain. It is required for many biological functions as all intermediate metabolites are phosphorylated before they are utilized in the metabolic pathways. Phosphorous deficiency in the face of adequate carbohydrate and protein intake can be detrimental or may even cause mortality because of hepatic ATP consumption.[31,32] Phosphate is needed to buffer the acid generated in the body by increasing the excretion of the titratable dihydrogen-phosphate in the urine. The acidosis associated with diarrhea, pneumonia, and malaria does not get corrected when there is relative phosphate deficiency. All children with malnutrition have phosphate deficiency.[33]

The WHO recommended therapeutic diets (F-75 and F-100) contain optimal, accessible soluble phosphorous from cow milk required for stabilization and rehabilitation. Substitution of F-75 with rice porridge during

stabilization in children with diarrhea was associated with a lower rise in phosphorous concentration as compared to F-75 in an observational study from Uganda.[34] Hence there is a need to fortify alternative diets with adequate mineral mix solutions (prepared from local ingredients) and assess their efficacy before utilizing them in the management of children with SAM.

## 5. Management of Severe Anemia in SAM

Severe anemia is a frequent associated comorbidity in children with SAM. Anemia in malnutrition is due to multi-nutrient deficiency (folate, cobalamin, riboflavin, pyridoxine, vitamin C, vitamin E, and copper). It is important to note that iron stores are replete in SAM due to reductive adaptation. It is thus incorrect to give only iron to treat anemia in SAM as it can even increase mortality.[35]

Besides dietary deficiency, malaria, severe sepsis, and hookworm infestations can contribute to anemia in a severely malnourished child. A hospital based study from India reported 25% of 131 children 6–59 months admitted with SAM to have required blood transfusion.[36] Both microcytic hypochromic (38.6%) and megaloblastic (30.5%) anemia were described as causes of nutritional anemia in the children studied. Thus, it is important to supplement vitamin $B_{12}$ along with iron and folic acid.

## Need for Blood Transfusion

A chid with SAM needs blood transfusion if the hemoglobin falls below 4 g/dL or < 6 g/dL if associated with signs of respiratory distress. Severe anemia is known to precipitate heart failure if associated with sepsis. It is recommended to give 10 mL/kg of packed red cells or whole blood 5 mL per kg of body weight slowly over 3 hours.[14] Besides hematinics and nutritional rehabilitation, etiology of anemia should always be looked into and optimally treated.

## 6. Rationale of Therapeutic Diets in the Management of Children with SAM in the Hospital Setting

### A. F-75: The Starter Diet

Children with SAM can survive on limited calories due to various adaptive physiological and metabolic changes in the body. Hence they cannot tolerate usual amounts of protein, fat, and sodium present in normal diet. So they must be initially given a diet that is low in protein and sodium and high in carbohydrates. The Starter diet (F-75) is designed to fulfil these requirements.

F-75 is a low-protein milk-based formula diet which contains 75 kcal and 0.9 g protein per 100 mL. This diet provides the necessary glucose to maintain homeostasis, allows recovery of the gut epithelium and at the same time does not overwhelm the body's systems. Children with SAM cannot tolerate long periods of fasting as they have poor glycogen reserves and impaired gluconeogenesis. Therefore, feeding must be started at the earliest in frequent (2 hourly), small amounts throughout day and night. F-75 diet is continued with gradually increasing interval (in the same amount) for next 3–7 days until the child is stabilized. After the initial stabilization when the child's appetite improves and there are no medical complications, "catch-up" formula (F-100) diet is started during rehabilitation phase to regenerate from the debilitated state.[14,15]

### B. F-100: The Catch-up Diet

Catch-up diet (F-100) contains more calories and protein: 100 kcal and 2.9 g protein per 100 mL. This will allow repair and remodelling of the body tissues. The transition of diet from F-75 to F-100 should occur gradually over a period of 2–3 days. During this phase an equal amount of F-75 is replaced by F-100 and child is carefully monitored for any signs of feed intolerance.[14] Subsequently, the amount of F-100 is slowly increased till child is allowed to take *ad libitum*. There is substantial evidence that there is risk of refeeding syndrome and osmotic diarrhea in children fed large amounts of F-100 diet in rehabilitative phase without this transition.[37,38] The recommended energy intake during this transition phase is 100–135 kcal/kg/day.

### C. Transition to RUTF

The transition of F-75 diet to ready to use therapeutic food (RUTF) should also follow the same principles as F-100 but it is individualized depending on the availability and skill of the supervisory staff. Children doing well and gaining weight on F-100 diet in rehabilitative phase should be changed to RUTF before discharge and transfer to the outpatient program. Daily weight records are maintained to monitor and assess the response to therapeutic diets and investigate the reasons of failure in non-responders.

### D. Refeeding Syndrome

It develops as a result of the electrolyte and hormonal changes that take place on rapid reintroduction of feeds in children with SAM.[30,31] During periods of starvation the body uses fat and proteins over glucose and basal metabolic rate falls by 20–25%. As feeding begins, the body shifts back to carbohydrate metabolism from protein and fat catabolism, and glucose becomes the primary source of energy once again. The increased glucose load leads to a corresponding increase in insulin secretion that stimulates glycogen, fat, and protein synthesis. This process requires cellular influx of potassium, magnesium, and phosphate, and cofactors such as thiamine. The shift of electrolytes back into the cell causes hypokalemia, hypomagnesemia, and hypophosphatemia. A functional deficit of these electrolytes and a sudden rise in the basal metabolic rate are responsible for clinical effects of refeeding syndrome. A fall in serum phosphorous levels can affect virtually every physiological and metabolic function of the body. Hypokalemia and hypomagnesemia can be detrimental to cellular membranes and affect heart and neuromuscular functions. Insulin has anti-natriuretic effect on the kidneys leading to sodium and fluid retention and expansion of the extracellular fluid volume.

During rehabilitative phase, think of **refeeding syndrome** in case of deterioration of clinical condition after initial improvement. It needs early identification and nutritional support should be immediately stopped. The electrolyte abnormalities should be addressed along with supportive care.

## 7. Therapeutic Diets in the Outpatient Setting

Children with SAM who do not have any medical complication and well preserved appetite are managed as outpatients.[13] They are provided with Ready to Use Therapeutic Food (RUTF) as per their body weight until recovery.[14] Children started on RUTF should have access to safe drinking water as it does not contain water. Breastfeeding should be continued on demand. RUTF can be given in the presence of acute or persistent diarrhea but they need to be followed, to detect failure of response or complication which will warrant transfer to in-patient care. Active feeding should be encouraged but at the same time forced feeding avoided. In case of poor or suboptimal intake, they should be screened for sepsis or looked for other clinical complications. The cost of current standard ready-to-use therapeutic food (RUTF) is the major challenge to large scale implementation of community-based management of acute malnutrition. The evidence on the efficacy of RUTF comes from the observational studies, cross over studies, and comparative trials done in Africa.[39-41]

Presently there is no indigenously available RUTF in India.[42] An Indian study to compare the acceptability and energy intake of imported RUTF with cereal-legume based khichri among malnourished children 6–36 months demonstrated comparable acceptance for both the diets.[43] However the energy intake from RUTF was higher due to its better energy density. Literature review has suggested the potential benefits of adding whey or skimmed milk powder to fortified blended foods as it enhances the protein quality, allows a reduction in amount of soy/cereal that decreases the anti-nutrients, and provides micronutrients and bioactive factors that strengthens the immune system.[44,45] It also adds to the flavor of the meal that improves the acceptability. The decision regarding the type of diet used in the management can be made based on food accessibility and affordability.

### Modified Therapeutic Diets

The Cochrane review on the use of alternative diets (homemade RUTF-flour porridge) compared to standard RUTF in improving the clinical outcome of children with SAM in the outpatient setting is inconclusive.[46,47] A recent non-blinded, parallel-group, simple randomized controlled trial from Africa comparing the efficacy of soya-maize-sorghum RUTF (SMS-RUTF) with that of standard peanut paste-based RUTF (P-RUTF) revealed comparable recovery rate, weight gain, and length of stay using SMS-RUTF in children ≥ 24 months.[48] Another important observation from a recent systematic review is high prevalence of carbohydrate malabsorption (particularly lactose) in infants and children with SAM, which complicates their clinical course and outcome.[49] This generates the need to conduct multi-centric (from different geographical areas) clinical trials to study the outcome of children with SAM using modified therapeutic diets with reduced lactose content.

## 8. Delay Treatment with Iron

In SAM, iron is not utilized for hemoglobin synthesis due to reductive adaptation, rather it is stored. Hence the child continues to remain anemic even with extra iron stores. It is important to understand that the iron supplementation in the initial stabilization phase can be detrimental as it generates free iron radicals in the body. This free iron radical can damage the cell membranes and worsen the infections by promoting microbial proliferation. In addition, the body tries to convert free radicals to ferritin which diverts the substrates and energy from various vital activities. Therefore iron supplementation is not recommended in the initial stabilization phase and in presence of active sepsis.[15] However during rehabilitative phase as the process of repair and synthesis of new tissues begins, the stored iron is utilized for hemoglobin synthesis. This generates the need to replenish the stores and will thereby require iron supplementation. Both F-100 and RUTF have iron and there is no need to supplement additional iron.

## 9. Vitamin A Supplementation in Children with SAM

Vitamin A is an integral component of mucosal linings where it maintains the mucus barrier and prevents microbial adherence and invasion across the mucosal surface. This protective effect is seen at mucosal surfaces of respiratory, gastrointestinal, urinary, and the reproductive tract. It plays a crucial role in generation of appropriate immunological response *i.e.* both humoral and cell mediated immunity. In addition, Vitamin A is essential for visual function and regulation of cell growth and differentiation at the molecular level. The association of SAM and vitamin A deficiency has been demonstrated by various epidemiological studies. Vitamin A deficiency predisposes children 6–59 months to increased risk of blindness, infection[50], and mortality,[51] especially in children with history of measles and diarrhea.

Subclinical vitamin A deficiency (retinol <0.7 µmol/L) is highly prevalent in under-5 children in our country. The recommendation to supplement high dose vitamin A at admission in children with SAM or measles even in the absence of eye signs exists since 1999.[15] Literature review has demonstrated a high incidence of diarrhea[52] and mortality[53] associated with high dose vitamin A supplementation in children with edematous SAM. With the advent of therapeutic diets (F-75 and F-100) and RUTF fortified with vitamin A, concerns were raised regarding the efficacy and safety of giving high dose vitamin A (age appropriate) at admission except in presence of measles, severe diarrhea, and signs of vitamin A deficiency (eye signs).[54] The WHO 2013 guideline recommends daily vitamin A (@ 5000 IU/day) supplementation of children with SAM as a component of therapeutic diets or multivitamin supplements until treatment completion.[14] The use of high dose vitamin A at admission in children with SAM is indicated only in case the therapeutic diet does contain vitamin A.

## 10. Zinc Supplementation in SAM

Zinc is an essential trace mineral required for varied biological functions like growth, development, cognition, and immune modulation.[55] It is a limiting type II nutrient in various diets and plays a pivotal role in growth. Its role is indispensable in decreasing the severity and duration of the diarrheal episode and in preventing the recurrence of new episodes in the next 2–3 months.[56] Poor appetite is a cardinal sign of zinc deficiency which contributes to the weight loss in SAM. Zinc (10–20 mg per day) should be given to all children with SAM. WHO-recommended therapeutic diets (F-100/RUTF) already contain adequate zinc, and children with severe acute malnutrition receiving them do not require additional zinc. This amount permits repletion of deficit and promotes weight gain over 10 g/kg/d.[57]

## 11. Micronutrient Supplements

Children with malnutrition have significantly higher requirements for micronutrients because of increased metabolism associated with illness and the body being unable to extract the micronutrients from food consumed. Growth failure in malnutrition occurs primarily due to deficiency in Type II nutrients.[58] WHO recommended F-75 and F-100 diets are fortified with electrolyte, minerals, and vitamins required for optimum growth. In areas where the combined mineral and electrolyte enriched diets are not available, they have to be supplemented separately. All malnourished children should receive 5 mg of folic acid orally on day 1 and then 1 mg orally per day, thereafter. The rationale of vitamin A, zinc, potassium, and magnesium supplementation has been discussed above. Iron is added only in rehabilitative phase once the weight gain starts. The vitamin B complex (riboflavin, thiamine and pyridoxine) and other vitamins (ascorbic acid, and the fat-soluble vitamins D, E, and K) need to be added in twice the recommended daily allowance.

## 12. Sensory Stimulation

Children with SAM suffer from neurological sequelae of poor brain growth due to malnutrition. This is further compounded by poor interaction by the mother/ caregivers due to lack of time and attention. Such children often exhibit delayed motor skills, poor cognitive and social development, and continue to have low intelligence, behavior problems, and poor school achievement in later childhood.[59] Neonates and infants are most susceptible to effects of malnutrition due to rapid brain growth in infancy.

Psychosocial stimulation integrated with nutritional rehabilitation improved the growth and development of children with SAM in a time-lagged controlled study done in Bangladesh.[60] A randomized trial on Bangladeshi children 6–24 months with SAM revealed the favorable effects of psychosocial stimulation on mental development index scores and weight gain in a community based program.[61]

Sensory stimulation in the form of tender loving care and emotional support should begin in the stabilization phase. Structured play therapy (15–30 min/day) according to the level of child's development should be introduced in the rehabilitation phase using indigenous, simple, and inexpensive toys to help develop motor and language skills.[15] It should take place in a relaxed and stimulating environment. Mothers should be encouraged to play with their child using simple, homemade toys.

## 13. Discharge and Follow-up

The current WHO 2013 recommendation is to discharge children with SAM only when either weight-for height or length is more than or equal to −2 Z-score or mid-upper arm circumference is more than or equal to 125 mm, (depending upon admission criteria) and they have had no edema for at least 2 weeks.[14] They may not be kept in facility to achieve the above targets (anthropometric parameters) and may be shifted to the community based program wherever available when the following criteria are fulfilled:

   i. Appetite returned to normal (eats at least 75% of therapeutic food)
   ii. Medical complications resolved
   iii. No edema
   iv. Satisfactory weight gain (at least 5 g/kg/day) for 3 consecutive days.

Before discharge from facility, all children should receive age appropriate catch up immunization and treatment for helminthic infections. The mother/caregiver is well counseled about feed preparation and mode/frequency/amount of feeding, understands the need to play with the child, able to treat common illnesses like fever, diarrhea, and to identify the danger signs to seek immediate medical attention. The follow up plan should be explained to the mother and family.

## 6.8 MANAGEMENT OF INFANTS LESS THAN 6 MONTHS OF AGE WITH SEVERE ACUTE MALNUTRITION

### 1. Burden of SAM in Under-6 Months

The first 6 months of life are extremely important in an infant's life as it involves rapid physiological and physical changes that influence their age specific nutritional needs. Young infants with SAM carry a high risk of morbidity and mortality. Globally it is estimated that 4.7 million infants under 6 months of age are moderately wasted and 3.8 million are severely wasted.[62] An Indian research to determine the burden of under-nutrition in children < 6 months based on the secondary data analysis of NFHS-3, revealed prevalence of wasting, stunting, and under-weight as 31%, 20%, and 30% respectively.[63] They reported a significantly higher proportion of infants (< 6 months) with severe wasting (13%) as compared to those in the age group 6–59 months.

## 2. Etiology

Suboptimal feeding practices like delay in initiation of breastfeeding, lack of exclusive breastfeeding for 6 months, early introduction of complementary feeds; and inadequate feeding due to repeated episodes of diarrhea, pneumonia, and other illnesses are responsible for developing undernutri-tion. Besides, low birth weight, IUGR, prematurity, and perinatal insults also predispose the young infants to the above state. Severe malnutrition in the initial 6 months of life needs early identification and utmost attention to prevent the long term adverse consequences on health and neurodevelopmental outcome. Maternal factors influence the health of the infant in this phase, so it is essential to treat mother infant pair rather than infant alone. Currently there are no evidence based guidelines on the management of infants < 6 months with SAM. There is a need to conduct good quality research to fill the gap in this domain.

## 3. Clinical Course and Management Principles

The clinical course of infants < 6 months with SAM can be divided as uncomplicated and complicated as for the older age group. The WHO 2013 guidelines recommends managing infants in this age group as outpatients and inpatients, respectively.[14] Infants with uncomplicated SAM receive treatments as out patients that primarily includes feeding support and regular follow up. **Table 6.3** defines the criteria for admission and management in a health facility. The principles of management essentially remain the same as for children > 6 months with SAM and medical complications.

### Role of Breastmilk

All possible efforts should be directed towards establishment/re-establishment of effective exclusive breastfeeding by the mother. Breastmilk is the best source of nutrition in this age group. Breastmilk caters to the age specific nutritional needs of the young infant. It provides antibodies, hormones, enzymes, growth factors, and live cells which cannot be made available in the replacement feeds. In addition, the amino acid composition of the breastmilk cannot be replicated in formulas, even though the whey to casein ratio is adjustable.

Regular home visits by the health workers in the post-partum period helps to strengthen exclusive breastfeeding and address other social and family factors which have led to malnutrition.

**Supplementary Suckling Technique (SST)** can be utilized to support/re-establish lactation in small/weak infants. A substantial fraction of young infants with SAM suffer from consequences of low birth weight and merely supporting optimal feeding will help them to achieve catch up growth. An Indian study from Allahabad observed that SST was successful in re-establishing lactation in 55.7% infants <6 months with SAM.[64] In case of failure to re-establish lactation, donor human milk, if available, should be given. The biggest challenge is in infants where breastfeeding is not possible and in case of non-availability of a wet nurse or safe donor milk banks.

## If Breastfeeding is NOT Possible

In facility based management of infants with SAM where breastfeeding is insufficient/not possible and there is no edema, commercial generic infant formula or therapeutic diets F-75 or diluted F-100 (diluted by adding 30% water) may be given either alone or as a supplement to the breastfeed.[14] In case the young infant has edema, only F-75 is recommended to supplement the breast milk.[14] *The F-100 diets alone are never used in young infants due to high renal solute load and the risk of hypernatremic dehydration.*

All possible efforts should be directed towards safe preparation and use of replacement feeds. The rationale behind the use of infant formula/milk based therapeutic diets in the absence of breastfeeds is to provide optimal calories, proteins, and micronutrients that can be easily digested by the young infant for initial stabilization and later for catch up growth. The concerns regarding the use of cow's milk is its high solute load (increased protein load along with sodium, potassium and phosphorous), potential for developing iron deficiency, and allergic predisposition.

For successful management and to sustain the benefits of care to this vulnerable group, the evaluation and promotion of the physical and mental wellbeing of the mother/care giver is equally important. Transfer to the outpatient program is done when medical complications, including edema have resolved, the infant is clinically well, has good appetite and experiences weight gain on either exclusive breastfeeding or replacement feeds $\geq 5$ g/kg/day for at least 3 successive days. Before discharge from the health facility, ensure that the child is immunized for age and mother/caregiver is linked with community based follow up and support. Infants can be discharged from nutritional rehabilitation program only if they achieve weight-for-length $\geq -2$ Z-score on effective breastfeeding or with replacement feeds.

## 6.9 FUTURE RESEARCH

Children with SAM and edema are at increased risk of morbidity and mortality as compared to non-edematous SAM. The mechanism by which edema develops in SAM is still an enigma and several hypothesis have been proposed to explain its pathophysiology. One of the recent research has suggested the association of Gut Microbiota (GM) dysbiosis to edematous malnutrition.[65] Scientists have observed a greater diversity in the gut microbiota in children with SAM and edema than in those without edema but a causal relationship still needs to be established. In addition, this proposed mechanism encourages us to explore the efficacy of probiotics and prebiotics in the management of SAM by conducting good quality clinical research.

### References

1. World Health Organization. 10 facts on child health. Children: reducing mortality. Fact sheet No. 178. Updated September 2013. From: http://www.who.int/mediacenter/factsheets/fs178/en/. Accessed June 5, 2016.
2. International Institute for Population Sciences. National Family Health Survey 3, 2005-2006. Mumbai:IIPS;2006.
3. Black RE, Allen LH, Bhutta ZA, Caulfield LE, de Onis M, Ezzati M, *et al*. Maternal and Child Undernutrition Study Group. Maternal and child undernutrition: global and regional exposures and health consequences. Lancet. 2008;371:243–60.
4. Patrick J, Golden M. Leukocyte electrolytes and sodium transport in protein energy malnutrition. Am J Clin Nutr. 1977;30:1478–81.
5. Ashworth A. Khanum S, Jackson A, Shofield C. Guidelines for Inpatient Treatment of Severely Malnourished Children. Geneva: World Health Organization; 2003.
6. Ashworth A, Jackson A, Uauy R. Focusing on malnutrition management to improve child survival in India. Indian Pediatr. 2007;44:413–6.
7. Golden MH. The role of individual nutrient deficiencies in growth retardation of children as exemplified by zinc and protein. In: Waterlow JC, ed. Linear growth Retardation in Less Developed

Pediatric Countries. New York: Raven Press; 1988:143–63.

8. Golden MH. The nature of nutritional deficiency in relation to growth failure and poverty. Acta Paediatr Scand. 1991;374:95–110.

9. Golden MH. Evolution of nutritional management of acute malnutrition. Indian Pediatr. 2010;47:667–8.

10. Popkin BM, Richards MK, Montiero CA. Stunting is associated with overweight in children of four nations that are undergoing the nutrition transition. J Nutr. 1996;126:3009–16.

11. WHO Child Growth Standards and the Identification of Severe Acute Malnutrition in Infants and Children. A Joint Statement by the World Health Organization and the United Nations Children's Fund. Geneva: World Health Organization; 2009.

12. Community-based management of severe acute malnutrition. A joint statement by the World Health Organization, World Food Programme, United Nations Standing Committee on Nutrition, United Nations Children's Fund. Geneva: World Health Organization/World Food Programme/United Nations Standing Committee on Nutrition/United Nations Children's Fund; 2007.

13. UNICEF. Position Paper: Ready-to-Use Therapeutic Food for Children with Severe Acute Malnutrition. 2013. From: http://www.unicef.org/ media/files/Position_ Paper_Ready-to-use_ therapeutic_food_for_children_with_severe_acute_ malnutrition__June_2013. Accessed May 12, 2016.

14. WHO. Guideline: Updates on the management of severe acute malnutrition in infants and children. Geneva, World Health Organization; 2013. From: http://www.who.int/nutrition/ publications/guidelines/updates_management_ SAM_infantandchildren/en/. Accessed 25 November 2016.

15. Management of Severe Malnutrition: A Manual for Physicians and other Senior Health Workers. Geneva: World Health Organization; 1999.

16. Hossain MI, Dodd NS, Ahmed T, Miah GM, Jamil KM, Nahar B, Mahmood CB. Experience in managing severe malnutrition in a government tertiary treatment facility in Bangladesh. J Health Popul Nutr. 2009;27:72–80.

17. Ashworth A, Chopra M, McCoy D, Sanders D, Jackson D, Karaolis N, et al. WHO guidelines for management of severe malnutrition in rural South African Hospitals: effect on case fatality and the influence of operational factors. Lancet. 2004;363:1110–5.

18. Bhatnagar S, Lodha R, Choudhury P, Sachdev HPS, Shah N, Narayan S, et al. IAP Guidelines 2006 on hospital based management of severely malnourished children. Indian Pediatr. 2007;44:443–61.

19. Dalwai S, Choudhury P, Bavdekar SB, Dalal R, Kapil U, Dubey AP, et al. Indian Academy of Pediatrics. Consensus Statement of the Indian Academy of Pediatrics on integrated management of severe acute malnutrition. Indian Pediatr. 2013;50:399–404.

20. Singh K, Badgaiyan N, Ranjan A, Dixit HO, Kaushik A, Kushwaha KP, Aguayo VM. Management of children with severe acute malnutrition: experience of nutrition rehabilitation centers in Uttar Pradesh, India. Indian Pediatr. 2014;51:21–5.

21. Singh P, Kumar P, Rohatgi S, Basu S, Aneja S. Experience and outcome of children with severe acute malnutrition using locally prepared therapeutic diet. Indian J Pediatr. 2016;83:3–8.

22. WHO Training Course on the Management Of Severe Malnutrition. Geneva: World Health Organization; 2002 (updated 2009).

23. Isanaka S, Langendorf C, Berthé F, Gnegne S, Li N, Ousmane N, et al. Routine amoxicillin for uncomplicated severe acute malnutrition in children. N Engl J Med. 2016;374:444–53.

24. Alcoba G, Kerac M, Breysse S, Salpeteur C, Galetto Lacour A, Briend A, et al. Do children with uncomplicated severe acute malnutrition need antibiotics? A systematic review and meta-analysis. PLoS One. 2013;8:e53184.

25. The Treatment of Diarrhea: A Manual for Physicians and other Senior Health Workers. Geneva: World Health Organization; 2005.

26. Kumar R, Kumar P, Aneja S, Kumar V, Rehan HS. Safety and efficacy of low-osmolarity ors vs. modified rehydration solution for malnourished children for treatment of children with severe acute malnutrition and diarrhea: A randomized controlled trial. J Trop Pediatr. 2015;61:435–41.

27. Maitland K, Kiguli S, Opoka RO, Engoru C, Olupot-Olupot P, Akech SO, et al. Mortality after fluid bolus in African children with severe infection. N Engl J Med. 2011 30;364:2483–95.

28. Akech S, Karisa J, Nakamya P, Boga M, Maitland K. Phase II trial of isotonic fluid resuscitation in Kenyan children with severe malnutrition and hypovolaemia. BMC Pediatr. 2010;10:71.

29. Alleyne GAO. Studies on total body potassium in malnourished infants. Factors affecting potassium repletion. Br J Nutr. 1970;24:205–12.

30. Dørup I, Clausen T. Correlation between magnesium and potassium contents in muscle: role of Na(+)-K+ pump. Am J Physiol. 1993;264(2 Pt 1):C457-63.

31. Mehanna HM, Moledina J, Travis J. Refeeding syndrome: what it is, and how to prevent and treat it. Br Med J. 2008;336:1495–8.

32. Stanga Z, Brunner A, Leuenberger M, Grimble RF, Shenkin A, Allison SP, et al. Nutrition in clinical practice-the refeeding syndrome: illustrative cases and guidelines for prevention and treatment. Eur J Clin Nutr. 2008;62:687–94.

33. Waterlow JC, Golden MH. Serum inorganic-phosphate in protein-energy malnutrition. Eur J Clin Nutr. 1994;48:503–6.

34. Namusoke H, Hother AL, Rytter MJ, Kæstel P, Babirekere-Iriso E, Fabiansen C, et al. Changes in plasma phosphate during in-patient treatment of children with severe acute malnutrition: an observational study in Uganda. Am J Clin Nutr. 2016;103:551–8.

35. Smith IF, Taiwo O, Golden MH. Plant protein rehabilitation diets and iron supplementation of the protein-energy malnourished child. Eur J Clin Nutr. 1989;43:763–8.

36. Thakur N, Chandra J, Pemde H, Singh V. Anemia in severe acute malnutrition. Nutrition. 2014; 30:440–2.

37. Boateng A, Sriram K, Meguid MM, Crook M. Refeeding syndrome: treatment considerations based on collective analysis of literature case reports. Nutrition. 2010;26:156–67.

38. Gooda S, Wolfendale C, O Reilly J. The influence of feed rate on the risk of refeeding syndrome: a pilot study. J Hum Nutr Diet. 2009;22:592–3.

39. Briend A, Lacsala R, Prudhon C, Mounier B, Grellety Y, Golden MH. Ready-to-use therapeutic food for treatment of marasmus. Lancet. 1999;353:1767–8.

40. Briend A. Highly nutrient-dense spreads: a new approach to delivering multiple micronutrients to high-risk groups. Br J Nutr. 2001;85 Suppl 2:S175–9.

41. Diop EHI, Dossou NI, Ndour MM, Briend A, Wade S. Comparison of the efficacy of a solid ready-to-use food and a liquid, milk-based diet for the rehabilitation of severely malnourished children: a randomized trial. Am J Clin Nutr. 2003;78:302–7.

42. Gera T. Efficacy and safety of therapeutic nutrition products for home based therapeutic nutrition for severe acute malnutrition a systematic review. Indian Pediatr. 2010;47:709–18.

43. Dube B, Rongsen T, Mazumder S, Taneja S, Rafiqui F, Bhandari N, Bhan MK. Comparison of ready-to-use therapeutic food with cereal legume based Khichri among malnourished children. Indian Pediatr. 2009;46:383–8.

44. Hoppe C, Andersen GS, Jacobsen S, Mølgaard C, Friis H, Sangild PT, Michaelsen KF. The use of whey or skimmed milk powder in fortified blended foods for vulnerable groups. J Nutr. 2008;138:145S–161S.

45. Dror DK, Allen LH. The importance of milk and other animal-source foods for children in low-income countries. Food Nutr Bull. 2011;32:227–43.

46. Schoonees A, Lombard M, Musekiwa A, Nel E, Volmink J. Ready-to-use therapeutic food for home-based treatment of severe acute malnutrition in children from six months to five years of age. Cochrane Database System Rev 2013; 6:CD009000.

47. Lenters LM, Wazny K, Webb P, Ahmed T, Bhutta ZA. Treatment of severe and moderate acute malnutrition in low- and middle-income settings: a systematic review, meta-analysis and Delphi process. BMC Public Health. 2013;13(Suppl 3):S23.

48. Bahwere P, Balaluka B, Wells JC, Mbiribindi CN, Sadler K, Akomo P, Dramaix-Wilmet M, Collins S. Cereals and pulse-based ready-to-use therapeutic food as an alternative to the standard milk- and peanut paste-based formulation for treating severe acute malnutrition: a non-inferiority, individually randomized controlled efficacy clinical trial. Am J Clin Nutr. 2016;103: 1145–61.

49. Kvissberg MA, Dalvi PS, Kerac M, Voskuijl W, Berkley JA, Priebe MG, et al. Carbohydrate malabsorption in acutely malnourished children and infants: a systematic review. Nutr Rev. 2016;74:48–58.

50. Blomhoff R, Blomhoff HK. Overview of retinoid metabolism and function. J Neurobiol. 2006; 66:606–30.

51. Imdad A, Yakoob MY, Sudfeld C, Haider BA, Black RE, Bhutta ZA. Impact of vitamin A supplementation on infant and childhood mortality. BMC Public Health. 2011; 11(Suppl 3):S20.

52. Donnen P, Dramaix M, Brasseur D, Bitwe R, Vertongen F, Hennart P. Randomized placebo controlled clinical trial of the effect of a single high dose or daily low doses of vitamin A on the morbidity of hospitalized, malnourished children. Am J Clin Nutr. 1998;68:1254–60.

53. Donnen P, Sylla A, Dramaix M, Sall G, Kuakuvi N, Hennart P. Effect of daily low dose of vitamin A compared with single high dose on morbidity and mortality of hospitalized mainly malnourished children in Senegal: a randomized controlled clinical trial. Eur J Clin Nutr. 2007;61:1393–9.

54. Iannotti LL, Trehan I, Manary MJ. Review of the safety and efficacy of vitamin A supplementation in the treatment of children with severe acute malnutrition. Nutr J. 2013;12:125.

55. Prasad AS. Zinc: role in immunity, oxidative stress and chronic inflammation. Current Opin Clin Nutr Metabol Care. 2009;12:646–52.

56. Aggarwal R, Sentz J, Miller MA. Role of zinc administration in prevention of childhood diarrhea and respiratory illnesses: A meta-analysis. Pediatrics. 2007;119;1120.

57. Golden MH. Proposed recommended nutrient densities for moderately malnourished children. Food Nutr Bull. 2009;30:S267–343.

58. Golden MH. Specific deficiencies versus growth failure: type I and type II nutrients. J of Nutr Environmental Med. 1996;6:301–8.

59. Grantham-McGregor S1, Powell C, Walker S, Chang S, Fletcher P. The long-term follow-up of severely malnourished children who participated in an intervention program. Child Dev. 1994;65(2 Spec No):428–39.

60. Nahar B, Hamadani JD, Ahmed T, Tofail F, Rahman A, Huda SN, Grantham-McGregor SM. Effects of psychosocial stimulation on growth and development of severely malnourished children in a nutrition unit in Bangladesh. Eur J Clin Nutr. 2009;63:725–31.

61. Nahar B1, Hossain MI, Hamadani JD, Ahmed T, Huda SN, Grantham-McGregor SM, Persson LA. Effects of a community-based approach of food and psychosocial stimulation on growth and development of severely malnourished children in Bangladesh: a randomised trial. Eur J Clin Nutr. 2012;66:701–9.

62. Kerac M, Blencowe H, Grijalva-Eternod, C, McGrath M, Shoham J, Cole TJ, Seal A. Prevalence of wasting among under 6-month-old infants in developing countries and implications of new case definitions using WHO growth standards: a secondary data analysis. Arch Dis Child. 2011;96:1008–13.

63. Patwari AK, Kumar S, Beard J. Undernutrition among infants less than 6 months of age: an underestimated public health problem in India. Matern Child Nutr. 2015;11:119–26.

64. Singh DK, Rai R, Dubey S. Supplementary suckling technique for relactation in infants with severe acute malnutrition. Indian Pediatr. 2014;51:671.

65. Kristensen KH, Wiese M, Rytter MJ, Özçam M, Hansen LH, Namusoke H, et al. Gut microbiota in children hospitalized with oedematous and non-oedematous severe acute malnutrition in Uganda. PLoS Negl Trop Dis. 2016;10: e0004369.

# Community Based Management of Severe Acute Malnutrition

Praveen Kumar, Kirtisudha Mishra

Community based management of SAM (CSAM) or community-based rehabilitation refers to treatment that is implemented at home with external input, for example, from a health worker, or treatment that is given at a primary health clinic, a community day-care center, or a residential center in order to achieve catch-up growth.[1-4] It is one of the most effective interventions recommended by WHO and other international agencies.

## 7.1 EVOLUTION TO COMMUNITY MANAGEMENT OF SAM

### 1. Failure of In-Patient Management of SAM as the Sole Treatment Strategy

SAM is a life-threatening condition with median under-five case-fatality rate ranging from 30% to 50%. Despite elaborate in-patient management protocols laid down for children with SAM since 1970s, no appreciable decline has occurred in mortality among these children. The high cost and poor success rates of inpatient treatment have prompted debate over whether hospitals/ inpatient care alone are best places to treat SAM.[5,6]

The hospital-based approach was found to have several weaknesses **(Box 7.1)**.

- There is limited inpatient capacity and lack of enough skilled staff in hospitals to cater to the large number of children with SAM.[6,7]

**Box 7.1 Problems of Hospital-based Management of SAM as a Sole Strategy**

- Limited inpatient capacity
- Lack of enough skilled staff
- Late presentation of children with SAM to the hospitals
- Prolonged stay increases the hospital costs
- Increased chance of cross infection
- Other family members neglected and earnings affected
- Early discharge lead to high morbidity and mortality post discharge

- Children often present late to hospital due to lack of awareness and motivation in the community, often after they develop medical complications. Treatment outcomes are better if they are rehabilitated before development of medical complications.
- Prolonged admission in hospitals increases the hospital costs and also promotes cross infection among the immunosuppressed children with SAM resulting in high morbidity and mortality rates before and after discharge.[8-11]
- Moreover, families may request for early discharge of their children due to concern for the care of other family members and loss of earnings. Such children sent home before recovery remain malnourished because their home diet is inadequate for catch-up growth. Their immune function

remains impaired and thus prone to repeated infections leading to relapse and death.

## 2. The Community-based Therapeutic Care Model

Since the beginning of this century, there were moves to shift the focus of treatment of children with SAM away from hospitals to communities. Until 2001, emergency response to high levels of acute malnutrition was predominantly through Therapeutic Feeding Centers (TFCs). TFCs are large, in-patient centers where patients are admitted for 21 days or longer. To address some of the challenges of traditional TFCs, Valid International developed the concept of Community based Therapeutic care (CTC) model. Subsequently, more evidence emerged on the effectiveness of CTC in emergencies from Ethiopia, Malawi, Sudan, and Niger. WHO, UNICEF, WFP, and SCN published a joint statement describing community based approach to be effective in managing large number of SAM children in these communities.[12]

The core operating principles of the community based therapeutic model (CTC) are listed below:

a. *Maximum coverage and access:* Programs are designed to make services accessible for the highest possible proportion of a population in need.

b. *Timeliness:* Programs are aimed to identify the majority of cases of acute malnutrition before additional medical complications occur.

c. *Appropriate care:* Simple, effective outpatient care is conceived for those who can be treated at home and inpatient care for those who have complications.

d. *Care for as long as needed:* The children with SAM can stay in the program until they have recovered.

The major determinant for success of this model was to find and treat the cases of SAM,

overcoming the social and cultural barriers to access. The four main community based delivery systems tried were: (a) day-care nutrition centers; (b) residential nutrition centers; (c) primary health clinics; and (d) domiciliary rehabilitation. An extensive review was conducted by Ashworth, *et al.* assessing the effectiveness of rehabilitating severely malnourished children in the community settings. All four delivery systems were reported to be effective in this review of 34 studies. Effectiveness was defined as mortality of less than 5% or weight gain of more than 5 g/kg/day.[4, 13-16]

Following the successful implementation of the community based therapy model, a growing number of countries are adopting this model for children with SAM, reserving in-patient care for only the sickest children with complications. World Health Organization (WHO) has strongly recommended countries to adopt national policies for management of SAM having a strong community-based component that complements facility-based activities. It suggests making RUTF available to families of these children and encourages the local food industry to produce RUTF. It also calls for an integrated approach jointly working with other relevant sectors. Activities related with development and implementation of community management of SAM (CSAM) will be supported by WHO, UNICEF, WFP, and SCN.[12]

## 3. CSAM vs CMAM

It is important to note that CSAM refers to community based management of children with severe acute malnutrition (SAM); and it should not be confused with CMAM (community based management of acute malnutrition). Many times these two terms CSAM and CMAM have been used inter-changeably but there are fundamental differences between the two approaches:

a. CSAM programs aim to identify children with SAM and deliver services through

OTPs situated near the community. This was recommended by WHO and other agencies in their joint statement. This strategy has been piloted in different states of India.[12]

b. CMAM programs identify children with both SAM and MAM (moderate acute malnutrition). In these programs, the management of SAM children is similar to that described in this chapter. In addition, MAM children are enroled in a supplementary feeding program (SFP).[6] This strategy has been used by few organizations like Valid International during emergencies where SAM-MAM prevalence is >10%. CMAM strategy also has been used by few countries which have taken care of their SMA population.

In India, CMAM program may not be feasible and advisable at present, given the huge load it is likely to bring into the program. MAM children are attached to ICDS for feeding and growth monitoring.

## 7.2 EARLY IDENTIFICATION OF CHILDREN WITH SAM

Community based management will be effective only when it is able to provide services to the largest possible proportions of acute malnourished children before they develop medical complications. For achieving this, program needs to break the barriers to access and gain the faith of the community in the program. Two methods have been proposed for early identification of children with SAM: (a) community mobilization; and (b) screening.

### 1. Community Mobilization

The success of CSAM depends a lot on community participation (Box 7.2). To achieve this, the most important need is to minimize the barriers to access. Service providers need to understand the socio-cultural milieu of the community in which they operate. So it is preferable to employ local staff who can

---

**Box 7.2 Community Mobilization**

Community mobilization is a grass-root level process by which the community:
- Becomes aware of the problem and becomes more responsible
- Organizes and plans solutions together
- Develops healthy options
- Develops ownership of the program and helps in monitoring

---

effectively sensitize the population to ensure that people understand the services.

People who can play a critical part in community mobilization:
- Panchayat members including 'Sarpanch'
- Religious and local leaders
- Traditional healers, teachers
- *Mahila mandal*
- Local youth groups
- Mother's groups
- Other self-help groups of the community.

### Stages of Community Mobilization

i. *Assessing community capacity* Assessing community perceptions prior to community mobilization is necessary to identify the potential barriers to service access.

ii. *Community sensitization* Efforts should be made to create awareness among families in the community about malnutrition and its consequences. A sensitization campaign should introduce briefly the overall program, inform them what malnutrition means, what the dangers are to a malnourished child, and describe the physical characteristics of children with SAM based on local understanding and terminologies. The health workers should convince families about the need for growth monitoring, practicing good child care, cooperation, and bringing their children for examination. The families should be explained the importance of identifying children with SAM early (Box 7.3). Regular meetings should be planned and organized at places where it is convenient for community members to attend. Activities like group meetings, rallies, wall paintings, and posters can help create awareness and build a relationship with the community. This will ensure their participation in the program.

iii. *Case finding* There are two methods by which cases of SAM can be identified in the community: Screening and self-referral. Children with SAM can be identified in the community during regular home visits and campaigns, monthly CSAM clinics or weekly CSAM sessions, regular growth promotion and monitoring activities and OPDs of health facilities. Home visits and CSAM clinics can be run by ASHA or Anganwadi workers.

## 2. Screening Methods for Identification of Malnutrition in the Community

For maximum coverage, both active and passive screening should be established.

- *Active screening* at village level should be carried by AWW/ASHA/volunteers through house to house visit for all children (6–59 months).
- *Passive screening* is carried during growth monitoring/village health and nutrition days (VHND) for all children (6–59 months).

A number of anthropometric indicators have been used for identifying children with SAM like weight for age, height for age, weight for height, MUAC, MUAC-for-age, MUAC-for-height etc. The primary aim of most community based SAM management

programs is to prevent mortality. To achieve this, the most useful case definition will be the one which can identify children/individuals who are at high risk of death if they remain untreated but are likely to survive if they receive treatment in appropriate nutritional program.[17]

### Mid-upper Arm Circumference: Best Identification Tool in Community

Much research has been done to identify the best tool for screening malnourished children. Clinical assessment has generally been found to be subjective, difficult to standardize and difficult to express quantitatively. On the other hand, anthropometric indicators are both objective and quantitative. Multicomponent indicators (i.e., W/A, H/A, W/H, MUAC/A, and MUAC/H) usually require looking them up in multidimensional tables or plotting the values on a growth chart for location with regard to a reference curve.[18]

Velzeboer, *et al.*[19] reported that four of the five health volunteers in rural Guatemala could not perform W/H test unsupervised.[19] In contrast, Alam, *et al.*[20] reported that MUAC required only simple and inexpensive equipment and was faster and easier for minimally trained workers to perform in door-to-door screening, compared to any of the other anthropometric indicators. Further, Shakir recommended that a color-banded plastic strip simplified MUAC measurements and provided immediate classifications.[21] It was also reported by authors that MUAC measurement was far more acceptable and less unpleasant to children compared to weight and height measurements. Also, age independence for children aged 6 months–5 years makes MUAC an easy tool to use. MUAC alone performed better in terms of both sensitivity and specificity than all other anthropometric indicators in community setting.[22,23]

Mid-upper-arm circumference has been endorsed by WHO as the sole anthropometric indicator for screening and admission into therapeutic feeding programs.[23] It is a simple technique, requires no special equipment, and can be easily taught to community-based workers, making it practical for use in resource-poor settings. However in edematous malnutrition, MUAC alone may be unreliable. Hence most of the countries implementing CSAM program identify malnourished children between 6 months and 59 months in the community level by two methods:

i. By measuring mid upper arm circumference (MUAC); and

ii. By checking for bilateral pitting edema.

By combined use of MUAC and bilateral pitting edema, children are classified into following three categories:

- MUAC<11.5 cm and/or bilateral pitting edema—*Severe acute malnutrition*
- MUAC between 11.5–12.4 cm and no bilateral pitting edema—*Moderate acute malnutrition*
- MUAC ≥12.5 cm and no bilateral pitting edema—*Normal nutrition*

### 3. Self-referrals for Identification of Children with SAM

This can take place only when the community has been sensitized about undernutrition and its consequences. Once the people have obtained knowledge regarding undernutrition, they may be able to detect signs of undernutrition and seek the services of the health workers like ASHA, AWW, or ANM.

### 7.3 COMMUNITY-BASED MANAGEMENT OF SAM

There are 10 steps of enrolment and management of children with SAM in the CSAM program **(Box 7.4)**.

### 1. Anthropometric Assessment

All cases identified by community mobilizers, should be reassessed by health workers by MUAC at CSAM clinic to confirm that the referred child is having SAM.

---

**Box 7.4 The 10 Steps for Enrolment and Management of SAM Children in CSAM Program**

1. Anthropometric assessment
2. Medical assessment
3. Appetite assessment
4. Enrolment into C-SAM
5. Nutritional treatment
6. Medicines
7. Health education
8. Follow-up while in C-SAM program
9. Discharge criteria for C-SAM
10. Follow-up after discharge from C-SAM

### 2. Medical Assessment

All children referred to CSAM clinic need to be examined for any danger/emergency signs and common medical complications. If the child has any danger/emergency signs,he should be urgently referred to nutrition rehabilitation centers (NRC) or hospital.The mother/caregiver should be asked about complaints like cough, fever, diarrhea, lethargy, convulsions, skin infections, eye complaints etc. They should be examined for any signs suggesting medical complications or secondary causes.

### 3. Appetite Assessment

Appetite test **(Box 7.5)** is done to identify SAM children with medical complications. Many a times these children even with infections do not show clinical signs. Complications and infections lead to loss of appetite. Appetite test is carried out at each CSAM session/visit. Failure of an appetite test at any point of time is an indication for full assessment and referral to NRC.

### 4. Enrolment into CSAM

Whether the identified SAM child will require inpatient care or can be enroled in CSAM program should be decided by the age of the child, examination for medical complications, and appetite test **(Fig. 7.1)**.

Experiences from other countries have shown that in the presence of both facility and

## Box 7.5 Appetite Test

The appetite test has been standardized using Ready to use Therapeutic Food (RUTF). In absence of RUTF, few states have used Special feed to conduct appetite test.

### How to do appetite test?

- Do the test in a separate quiet area.
- Explain to the mother/caregiver how the test will be done.
- Child should not have received feed during last 2 hours
- The mother/caregiver should wash her hands.
- The mother sits comfortably with the child on her lap and offers therapeutic food.
- Child should be offered water freely during the test
- The test usually takes a short time but may take up to one hour.
- The child must not be forced to take the food offered.
- The child should be given a packet or a pot of RUTF to eat.

When the child has finished, the amount taken is judged or measure. If the child takes at least one third of a packet or three teaspoons from a pot of RUTF, he is labelled as **APPETITE TEST PASSED**

## Box 7.6 Measures to be Taken when Referral is Needed

- Mothers should be informed and counseled on the need for referral
- First dose of amoxicillin should be given
- Feed should be offered if the child has not received it in last 2 hours to prevent hypoglycemia
- Mother should be explained about keeping the child warm during transport.
- If diarrhea, tell mothers to give ORS on the way.

need referral to NRC for inpatient care. Measures to be taken when referral is needed are listed in **Box 7.6**.

## 5. Nutritional Treatment

Nutritional treatment is a critical component of SAM management. Community based rehabilitation have used three options:

a. Short-stay day-care residential nutrition centers with intensive rehabilitation

b. At home, with home or clinic visits without therapeutic foods

c. At home management with RUTF

There are strengths and weaknesses in all three options and a single system will not suit all situations. Some options may be better suited for urban families, rural population, or working mothers.[12]

Children with severe acute malnutrition need safe, palatable foods with a high energy content and adequate amount of vitamins and minerals. Children with SAM need more energy and proteins in addition to their normal energy and protein requirements, to rebuild the lost body mass. For successful rehabilitation, food provided should achieve intakes that will promote catch-up growth and improve immune function. Of the above three options, third option was found more suitable for the population where there is food insecurity, mothers are working, and other siblings are dependent on mothers.

RUTF have a nutrient composition similar to F-100, which is the therapeutic diet used in inpatient settings. However, RUTF are not

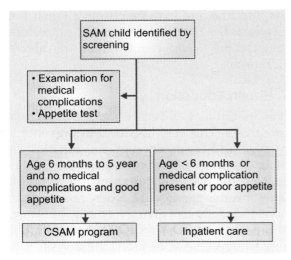

**Fig. 7.1** Decision tree for level of care

community management, approximately 85–90% of SAM children can be managed in the community. Only, 10–15% of children

water-based, meaning that bacteria cannot grow in them. These foods due to this advantage can be used safely at home without facility of refrigeration and even in areas where the hygiene is sub-optimal.[4]

## RUTF vs Home-based Recipes

Some studies on home-based treatment of SAM compared the effectiveness of RUTF with home-made traditional recipes. Manary, et al.[24] studied 282 children in Malawi and found that children receiving RUTF were more likely to reach weight for height Z-score of normal children than those receiving home-made blended maize/soy flour, with an average weight gain of 5.2 g/kg/day in the RUTF group compared to 3.1 g/kg/day in the maize/soy flour group. A recent Cochrane review on RUTF versus other forms of therapeutic food, however, could not find high quality evidence for definitive conclusions. The authors concluded that either RUTF or flour porridge could be used to treat children at home depending on availability, affordability, and practicality.[25]

## RUTF at Home

RUTF packets should be given to mothers every week and they should be advised that it is a medicinal food and not to be shared with other children in the house. The amount of food given to the child should be sufficient to take care of the caloric requirement of 200 kcal per kilogram of body weight per day. Mothers/caretakers should be told the exact amount to be given in each feed, as per child's weight, with a total of around 6–8 feeds/day. Child should be given water freely when they are eating RUTF. In addition, breastfeeding and homemade food should continue as per the child's appetite. In case of diarrhea, RUTF feeding should continue. Mothers should be asked to bring back the empty packets of RUTF during the next follow up visit.[12]

## 6. Medicines

Some essential medicines should be provided along with RUTF, like antibiotics and anti-helminthic drugs. The caretakers should be taught how to give each of the medicines.

### A. Antibiotics

Children with SAM are usually immuno-suppressed. The usual signs of infection such as fever are often absent and infections remain hidden. Majority of community based programs have used oral co-trimoxazole for all enrolled children. There is concern regarding emergence of resistance to this drug and most counties are now using oral amoxicillin for 5–7 days. Oral amoxicillin is also effective in reducing overgrowth of bacteria in the GI tract.

However these recommendations are based on assumptions. There are contradictory reports of its effect on weight gain and recovery rate.[26,27] A recent randomized controlled trial from Niger could not find any benefit of routine amoxicillin in children with uncomplicated SAM.[28]

### B. Antihelminthics

Children with SAM are often infested with worms. Albendazole is actively absorbed from the intestine and is more effective when the GI tract is free of other infections. It is therefore given on the second visit to all children above 12 months.

## 7. Health Education

It is essential to educate the mothers and caregivers. This step is critical in preventing relapse and occurrence of malnutrition in other children of the family.When the child is first enrolled in the program, information about need of therapeutic foods, how to give, need and method of giving medicines at home, and basic hygiene is required. At the end of subsequent CSAM session/clinic visit, it is vital to check whether caretakers have understood the advice.

Education during subsequent sessions should include the following:
• Appropriate feeding practices;

- Advantages of continued breastfeeding;
- Feeding during illness;
- Management of common illnesses like diarrhea;
- Characteristics of good complementary foods;
- How to improve quality and energy density of locally available food items;
- Importance of timely immunizations; and
- Recognize danger signs.

## 8. Follow-up while in the CSAM Program

Children are called for follow-up every week in CSAM sessions.During every follow-up visit, the following need to be done:
- Measure MUAC and weight, and perform appetite test.
- If weight gain is satisfactory and appetite is good, mother should be praised for their good care.
- If weight is static or there is weight loss:
  - Take medical history, assess for danger signs or medical complication.
  - Assess compliance to medicines and RUTF intakes

Routine home visits for follow-up between the CSAM sessions are not required in all cases. It may be required if mother/caregiver misses follow-up visits or child has poor weight gain.

## 9. Discharge Criteria

The child should be discharged from the CSAM program when he achieves an MUAC > 12.5 cm. Exit outcomes are classified in following categories:
- *Discharged cured:* MUAC ≥12.5 cm
- *Discharged Not recovered:* Children with SAM who do not meet discharge criteria even after 4 months of CSAM program with compliance to diet and medicines or medical referrals who do not return back in the program.
- *Defaulted:* Children who left the program before achieving the discharge criteria or

those who were absent for three consecutive weeks.
- *Transferred to NRC:* Children who required inpatient care due to medical complications or not gaining weight under CSAM program.

## 10. Follow-up after Discharge from CSAM Program

It is advisable to follow-up every child discharged from the CSAM program at least four times during the first 12 months after discharge. The first visit should be 1 month after discharge; the second visit at 3 months after discharge; third visit at 6 months after discharge and the fourth visit at 12 months after discharge. The children must be enroled in Supplementary Nutrition Programs of the ICDS. Children, who could not recover (not met the discharge criteria) even after four months in the program, should be referred to the nutrition rehabilitation center for medical examination. Every follow-up visit should involve weighing the child, measuring MUAC, medical examination, and recording medical history regarding any illness between the intervening periods from the last visit.

## 7.4 CURRENT STATUS OF CSAM PROGRAMS

This CSAM model has been deemed a success worldwide, performing consistently well, achieving high cure rates (>90%), low death rates (<2%), and low default (<10%) rates.It is now widely implemented as part of routine government services and in humanitarian emergencies across Africa, Asia, and South America.[29]

### A. Global Experience

A recent paper has been published reviewing the coverage data from CSAM programs in 21 countries in Africa, Afghanistan, Haiti, Nepal, Pakistan, and the Philippines, collected between July 2012 and June 2013. The standard coverage assessment methods used were the semi-quantitative evaluation of access and coverage (SQUEAC) in 43 assessments and Simplified Lot Quality Assurance Sampling Evaluation of Access and Coverage (SLEAC) method used in one case.[30] This analysis shows that the mean level of estimated coverage achieved by the programs was 38.3%. For rural programs, it was 34.6%, for urban 40.9%, and for camp settings, 74.2%. Such a pattern is much lower than that achieved by the early version of the CTC models which reported coverage levels ranging between 56% and 82% with an average of 72.5%. Roger, et al.[31] elicited that the most commonly reported barriers for access were lack of awareness of malnutrition, lack of awareness of the program, high opportunity costs, inter-program interface problems, and previous rejection.

## B. Bihar Experience

India too has been brewing to begin the CSAM program for quite some time. The first conventional CSAM program in India was carried out in Biraul block of Darbhanga district in Bihar. The caregivers of the children with uncomplicated SAM were given a 1-week supply of WHO-standard, pre-packaged F100-equivalent, lipid-based, ready-to-use, therapeutic paste. An observational, retro-spective study of 8274 children admitted in this program was done by Burza, et al., which showed that 4595 (55%) children were discharged as cured while 77 (0.9%) died.[32]

However, the use of RUTF got entangled in many controversies in India, following an unsanctioned use of imported ready to use therapeutic food by several international organizations in 2008. Concern was raised regarding its misuse and commercial exploitation.

## C. The Odisha Experience

In recent years, CSAM program was launched in few states as pilot project. In Odisha, in the tribal-dominated Kandhamal district, CSAM program was launched through the existing system of anganwadi centers under the guidance of women and child development and health and family welfare departments. The pilot project is funded by DFID India and supported by Valid International. Over 2,000 community-level workers have been trained to diagnose SAM, provide basic medical screening, and prescribe the correct dose of ready to use therapeutic food to any children found to be suffering from SAM. A small RUTF production facility run by a local women's self-help group has been established which has the capacity to supply energy dense nutrient rich food to the entire district.[33]

## D. CSAM in Rajasthan

Similar community based programs have also begun in Rajasthan under the name of Poshan. A cluster of villages from 41 blocks in 10 high priority districts and 3 tribal Districts were identified for enrolment into the project. A total of 23,000 children from these villages were screened by medical staffs. Those with severe health issues or cases of malnutrition were referred to local malnutrition treatment centers where they were given an Energy Dense Nutrition Supplement (EDNS), locally known as Poshan Amrit, for 8 to 10 weeks. On completion of Phase 1 of this project in June 2016, it was found that more than 95% of the 9640 children enroled for this treatment had recovered and discharged. There were less than 0.3% deaths and around 2.5% children could not recover, which is below the global acceptable limits for similar programs. Boosted by the success of this first phase, the Government of Rajasthan plans to scale up the CSAM project to more districts aiming to reach 25,000 children.[34]

## 7.4 CONCLUSIONS

Considering that vast numbers of children with SAM reside in the Indian subcontinent and the grossly appalling hospital bed: patient ratios, in-patient management of all cases of SAM is not operationally feasible. Home-based treatment of children with SAM is the need of the hour. Several workshops and meetings by Government and non-governmental groups have been conducted in the country and there is a growing consensus within India that the adoption of community-based management of acute malnutrition is crucial to achieve widespread, effective coverage, and treatment of children with SAM.

Malnutrition remains a disturbing reality of India. With its mammoth magnitude in this country, no program is expected to succeed without incorporating a component of community based care. The operational steps described above provide a feasible means of establishing CSAM program in India, in order to tackle the menace of malnutrition.

## References

1. WHO. Community based management of severe acute malnutrition. From: http://www.who.int/nutrition/topics/Statement_community_based_man_sev_acute_mal_eng.pdf. Accessed 5 Aug 2016.

2. International Food Policy Research Institute. 2016. Global Nutrition Report 2016: From Promise to Impact: Ending Malnutrition by 2030. Washington, DC From: http://dx.doi.org/10.2499/9780896295841.Accessed 20 Nov 2016.

3. Raykar M,Majumder M, Laxminarayan R, Menon P. India Health Report: Nutrition 2015, New Delhi, India: Public Health Foundation of India; 2015.

4. Ashworth A. Efficacy and effectiveness of community-based treatment of severe malnutrition. Food Nutr Bull. 2006;27(suppl):S24–48.

5. Lawless J, Lawless MM. Admission and mortality in a children's ward in an urban tropical hospital. Lancet. 1966;2:1175–6.

6. Gueri M, Andrews N, Fox K, Jutsum P, St Hill D. A supplementary feeding program for the management of severe and moderate malnutrition outside hospital. J Trop Pediatr. 1985;31:101–8.

7. Brewster D. Improving quality of care for severe malnutrition. Lancet. 2004;363:2088–9.

8. Cook R. Is hospital the place for the treatment of malnourished children? J Trop Pediatr. Environ Child Health.1971;17:15–25.

9. Roosmalen-Wiebenga MW, Kusin JA, de With C. Nutrition rehabilitation in hospital-a waste of time and money? Evaluation of nutrition rehabilitation in a rural district hospital in southwest Tanzania:I, short-term results. J Trop Pediatr.1986;32:240–3.

10. Roosmalen-Wiebenga MW, Kusin JA, de-With C. Nutrition rehabilitation in hospital-a waste of time and money? Evaluation of nutrition rehabilitation in a rural district hospital in South-west Tanzania: II, long-term results. J Trop Pediatr. 1987; 33:24–28.

11. Reneman L, Derwig J. Long-term prospects of malnourished children after rehabilitation at the Nutrition Rehabilitation Center of St Mary's Hospital, Mumias, Kenya. J Trop Pediatr. 1997;43:293–96.

12. Prudhon C1, Prinzo ZW, Briend A, Daelmans BM, Mason JB. Proceedings of the WHO, UNICEF, and SCN Informal Consultation on Community-Based Management of Severe Malnutrition in Children. Food Nutr Bull. 2006;27(3 Suppl):S99–104.

13. Diop EI, Dossou NI, Briend A, Yaya MA, Ndour MM, Wade S. Home-based rehabilitation for severely malnourished children using locally made ready-to-use therapeutic food (RTUF). Report from the 2nd World Congress of Pediatric Gastroenterology, Hepatology and Nutrition. Paris, July 3-7, 2004 Medimond, Monduzzi Editore (International Proceedings) pp.101–5.

14. Sandige H, Ndekha MJ, Briend A, Ashorn P, Manary MJ. Home-based treatment of malnourished Malawian children with locally produced or imported ready-to-use food. J Pediatr Gastroenterol Nutr. 2004;39:141–6.

15. Manary MJ, Ndekha MJ, Ashorn P, Maleta K, Briend A. Home based therapy for severe malnutrition with ready-to-use food. Arch Dis Child. 2004;89:557–61.

16. Navarro-Colorado C, McKenney P. Home based rehabilitation in severe malnutrition vs inpatient care in a post-emergency setting. A randomised clinical trial in Sierra Leone.Report 2003. Presented at an Inter-Agency Workshop, Emergency Nutrition Network, Dublin, 8-10 October 2003.

17. Collins S, Sadler K, Dent N, Khara T, Guerrero S, Myatt M, Saboya M, Walsh A. Key issues in the success of community-based management of severe malnutrition. Food Nutr Bull. 2006 Sep;27(3 Suppl):S49–82.

18. Myatt MI, Khara T, Collins S. A review of methods methods to detect cases of severely malnourished children in the community for their

admission into community-based therapeutic care programs. Food Nutr Bull. 2006;27(3 Suppl):S7–23.

19. Velzeboer MI, Selwyn BJ, Sargent F, Pollitt E, Delgado H. The use of arm circumference in simplified screening for acute malnutrition by minimally trained health workers. J Trop Pediatr. 1983;29:159–66.

20. Alam N, Wojtyniak B, Rahaman MM. Anthropometric indicators and risk of death. Am J Clin Nutr. 1989;49:884–8.

21. Shakir A. Arm circumference in the surveillance of protein-calorie malnutrition in Baghdad.Am J Clin Nutr. 1975;28:661–5.

22. Briend A, Zimicki S. Validation of arm circumference as an indicator of risk of death in one to four year old children. Nutr Res. 1986;6:249–61.

23. Trowbridge FL, Sommer A. Nutritional anthropometry and mortality risk. Am J Clin Nutr. 1981; 34:2591–2.

24. Manary MJ. Local production and provision of ready-to-use therapeutic food (RUTF) spread for the treatment of severe childhood malnutrition. Food Nutr Bull. 2006;27(3 Suppl):S83–9.

25. Schoonees A, Lombard M, Musekiwa A, Nel E, Volmink J. Ready-to-use therapeutic food for home-based treatment of severe acute malnutrition in children from six months to five years of age. Cochrane Database Syst Rev. 2013;6:CD009000.

26. Lazzerini M, Tickell D. Antibiotics in severely malnourished children: Systematic review of efficacy, safety and pharmacokinetics. Bull World Health Organ. 2011; 89:594–607.

27. Trehan I, Amthor RE, Maleta K, Manary MJ. Evaluation of the routine use of amoxicillin as part of the home-based treatment of severe acute

malnutrition. Trop Med Int Health. 2010;15:1022–8.

28. Isanaka S, Langendorf C, Berthe F, Gnegne S, Li N, Ousmane N, et al. Routine amoxicillin for uncomplicated severe acute malnutrition in children. N Engl J Med. 2016;374:444–53.

29. Guerrero S, Rogers E. Access for All, Volume 1: Is community-based treatment of severe acute malnutrition (SAM) at scale capable of meeting global needs? 2013. Coverage Monitoring Network, London.Available from:http://www.coverage-monitoring.org/wp-content/uploads/2013/07/AAH-Policy-Paper-Comp.pdf.Accessed 20 Nov, 2016.

30. UNICEF. Global SAM management update: Summary of findings. UNICEF, New York: 2013. Available from: http://reliefweb.int/sites/reliefweb.int/files/resources/Global%20SAM%20Management%20Update.pdf.Accessed 20 Nov 2016.

31. Rogers E, Myatt M, Woodhead S, Guerrero S, Alvarez JL. Coverage of community-based management of severe acute malnutrition programs in twenty-one countries, 2012-2013. PLoS One. 2015;10:e0128666.

32. Burza S, Mahajan R, Marino E, Sunyoto T, Shandilya C, Tabrez M, et al. Community-based management of severe acute malnutrition in India: new evidence from Bihar. Am J Clin Nutr. 2015;101:847–59.

33. Valid.Indian CMAM Pilot.From: http://www.validinternational.org/indian-cmam-pilot/. Accessed 8August 2016.

34. National Health Mission Department of Medical, Health and Family Welfare Government of Rajasthan.Poshan: CMAM status. From: http://poshanraj.org/cmamstatus.aspx.Accessed 8 August 2016.

# 8

# Ready to Use Therapeutic Food

Umesh Kapil, Neha Sareen

WHO and UNICEF recommend the following two approaches for the treatment of children with severe acute malnutrition (SAM) (*i*) Inpatient care/facility-based approach for management of complicated SAM; and (*ii*) community/home based approach for children without medical complications, with the use of ready-to-use therapeutic food (RUTF).[1,2] In India, several hospitals and non-government organizations are engaged in community-based management of severe acute malnutrition using locally available foods along with nutrition education.[3] These institutions treat undernourished children with foods that are available at low cost. In this chapter, we will discuss the concept of ready to use therapeutic food (RUTF) and its application for integrated management of severe acute malnutrition in the current scenario.

## 8.1 CONCEPT OF READY TO USE THERAPEUTIC FOOD (RUTF)

*RUTF is a generic name given to all the products which are available in a ready-to-eat form, off the shelf, and designed to treat children with severe malnutrition, by meeting their nutritional deficits and also the current nutritional requirements.* WHO recommended nutritional components for RUTF are listed in **Table 8.1**.

RUTF is recommended to be used for management of SAM children who are not suffering from complication and have adequate appetite as proven by the Appetite Test. There are many characteristics (discussed in Section 8.2) which should be present in an RUTF to make it efficacious and acceptable by the community. RUTF is safe to use at the family level. It also ensures rapid weight gain in SAM children. These characteristics also make RUTF operationally feasible in management of SAM children with high percentage of success. The development and use of RUTF has modified the management of SAM children.

## A. WHO Recommendations on RUTF

A consensus statement has been developed for community based management of SAM by WHO/UNICEF/SCN.[4,5] According to this, children with SAM and without complication should be managed at the family level; and RUTF can be used for management of these children in communities which have limited access to local diets for nutritional rehabilitation. When families have access to nutrient dense foods, these SAM children should be managed with carefully designed diets using low cost family foods. In these diets, vitamins and minerals are to be added. Also, when we are treating SAM children with RUTF, we must ensure that breastfeeding and infant and young child feeding should be promoted. Children below 6 months of age

**Table 8.1** WHO Recommended Nutritional Composition of RUTF

| Nutritional component | Quantity |
|---|---|
| Moisture content | 2.5% maximum |
| Energy | 520–550 kcal/100 g |
| Proteins | 10%–12% total energy |
| Lipids | 45%–60% total energy |
| Sodium | 290 mg/100 g maximum |
| Potassium | 1,110–1,400 mg/100 g |
| Calcium | 300–600 mg/100 g |
| Phosphorous (excluding phytate) | 300–600 mg/100 g |
| Magnesium | 80–140 mg/100 g |
| Iron | 10–14 mg/100 g |
| Zinc | 11–14 mg/100 g |
| Copper | 1.4–1.8 mg/100 g |
| Selenium | 20–40 µg |
| Iodine | 70–140 µg/100 g |
| Vitamin A | 0.8–1.1 mg/100 g |
| Vitamin D | 15–20 µg/100 g |
| Vitamin E | 20 mg/100 g minimum |
| Vitamin K | 15–30 µg/100 g |
| Vitamin $B_1$ | 0.5 mg/100 g minimum |
| Vitamin $B_2$ | 1.6 mg/100 g minimum |
| Vitamin C | 50 mg/100 g minimum |
| Vitamin $B_6$ | 0.6 mg/100 g minimum |
| Vitamin $B_{12}$ | 1.6 µg/100 g minimum |
| Folic acid | 200 µg/100 g minimum |
| Niacin | 5 mg/100 g minimum |
| Pantothenic acid | 3 mg/100 g minimum |
| Biotin | 60 µg/100 g minimum |
| n-6 fatty acid | 3%–10% of total energy |
| n-3 fatty acid | 0.3%–2.5% of total energy |

*Note:* Although RUTF contains iron, F-100 does not. The composition of F-100 can be found in "Management of Severe Malnutrition: A manual for physicians and other senior health workers, World Health Organization, Geneva, 1999."

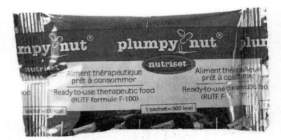

Fig. 8.1: Plumpy'Nut: The first commercial RUTF

vegetable fat, peanut butter, skimmed milk powder, lactoserum, maltodextrin, sugar, mineral and vitamin complex. Plumpy'Nut® **(Fig. 8.1)** was the first RUTF developed in 1996. It has been extensively used in Africa. It is an energy dense homogenous paste of lipids and micronutrients; the composition is similar to therapeutic food recommended by the World Health Organization. The nutrient and energy composition of Plumpy'Nut® is depicted in **Table 8.2**.[6] RUTF has also been produced locally in several countries like Malawi and Niger.[4]

## 8.2 ADVANTAGES AND DISADVANTAGES OF RUTF[4]

### A. Advantages of RUTF

i. RUTF provides all the nutrients required for recovery;

ii. RUTF leads to faster recovery rate and higher acceptability than F-100;

iii. It can be stored at room temperature for long periods of time;

iv. It has a long shelf life, even without refrigeration (24 months) and does not spoil easily even after opening;

v. The quantity distributed to each child is easy to calculate and is based on the weight;

vi. Sachet is opened by cutting one corner and child can eat the paste directly;

vii. No preparation or cooking is required;

viii. RUTF does not need to be diluted with water (this eliminates risk of contamination);

should not be given RUTF or any solid food. They should be on exclusive breastfeeding.

### B. Commercial RUTF

Commercial RUTF is being used in many developing countries, and many brands of RUTF are available. These are usually packaged in individual sachets. The sachet contains a paste of groundnut composed of

**Table 8.2** Nutrients and Energy Composition of Plumpy Nut®: A Commercial RUTF

| Nutrient | Quantity sachet of 92 g | Nutrient | Quantity sachet of 92 g |
|---|---|---|---|
| Energy | 500 kcal | Vitamin A | 840 mcg |
| Proteins | 12.5 g | Vitamin D | 15 mcg |
| Lipids | 32.86 g | Vitamin E | 18.4 mg |
| Calcium | 276 mg | Vitamin C | 49 mg |
| Phosphorus | 276 mg | Vitamin $B_1$ | 0.55 mg |
| Potassium | 1002 mg | Vitamin $B_2$ | 1.66 mg |
| Magnesium | 84.6 mg | Vitamin $B_6$ | 0.55 mg |
| Zinc | 12.9 mg | Vitamin $B_{12}$ | 1.7 mcg |
| Copper | 1.6 mg | Vitamin K | 19.3 mcg |
| Iron | 10.6 mg | Biotin | 60 mcg |
| Iodine | 92 mcg | Folic acid | 193 mcg |
| Selenium | 27.6 mcg | Pantothenic acid | 2.85 mg |
| Sodium | < 267 mg | Niacin | 4.88 mg |

ix. The risk of bacterial growth is very limited, and consequently it is safe to use without refrigeration at household level;

x. It can be used at home with supervision from the local health center staff;

xi. It reduces length of stay in hospital or therapeutic feeding center;

xii. It reduces number of staff necessary for preparation and distribution of therapeutic food to SAM children;

xiii. It is liked by children; and is safe and easy to use without close medical supervision; and

xiv. It can be used in combination with breastfeeding and other best practices for infant and young child feeding.

## B. Disadvantages of RUTF

i. RUTF costs several times more than per capita costs for preventing malnutrition through community-based approaches compared to utilizing local foods. A full course of treatment costs around $80-100 per child. In India and other developing countries, the use of RUTF is currently supported by external development agencies;

ii. RUTF use erodes the traditional best practices for infant and child feeding, particularly, it may adversely impact the breastfeeding practices which are prevalent in the community;

iii. RUTF leads to dependence on imported products of developed countries by the poor population of developing countries. RUTF has a potential for commercial exploitation of poor communities beyond the treatment of severe acute malnutrition;

iv. The high cost of management of SAM children can lead to diversion of resources for routine health care of children;

v. Foods made with peanut commonly get contaminated with aflatoxin if adequate quality control measures are not taken during manufacturing;

vi. RUTF has a high renal solute load and therefore, there is a need of more water by the child;

vii. The high sugar content of RUTF may encourage the child to consume or develop liking for sweet foods;

viii. RUTF treats the child, however, the determinants which caused SAM continue to remain in the family and there is high probability that children who have been cured of SAM may revert back to SAM status due to adverse influence of determinants present in the family;

ix. RUTF is a vertical treatment approach by which the family skills are not improved for preventing the child to develop SAM; and

x. RUTF has a specified expiry-time and the data is not available regarding what happens to the product after the expiry of the RUTF packets.[7]

## 8.3 LOCAL RUTF (L-RUTF) AND TRADITIONAL THERAPEUTIC FOODS

Traditionally, management of severe acute malnutrition has been done in India with the therapeutic food (local RUTF). Many locally produced/recipes foods that are culturally acceptable and relatively low cost are being used for management of SAM for many decades by academic and medical institutions as well as by nongovernmental groups.[8] **Table 8.3** provides details of some of this L-RUTF.[8]

These local RUTF are modified family foods utilized for treatment of severe acute malnutrition. A mix of energy dense *khichri*, milk, dal, sugar, fruit, fruit juice, and egg has been used successfully to treat SAM children both in hospital and home settings. In Tamil Nadu, a mix of 80 g rice, 10 g dal, 2 g oil, 50 g of vegetables and condiments has been administered to SAM children to each child between 2 and 4 years of age successfully.[9] This provides 358.2 calories and 8.2 g protein per child.[10] Other experiments by NGOs such as mobile crèches have used local RUTF including eggs, soya products, and milk for management of SAM children at a cost of Rs 8 per child per day.[8]

Shelf life is not required for these local RUTF as they are prepared in required quantities only needed by local women's groups under the supervision of the respective hospital or Non-Government Organization.

### Advantages of Local RUTF (Traditional Therapeutic Foods)

Production of local RUTF from the foods available in the community helps to promote local agricultural practices and locally available foods. Local production of RUTF may also promote livelihoods amongst the families which may be harboring SAM children. Production of local RUTF may use the existing women's groups and self help groups (SHGs) as well as small scale industry available in the community. It allows greater community participation.

## 8.4 CURRENT EVIDENCE ON EFFICACY AND EFFECTIVENESS OF RUTF

### 1. Schoonees, *et al.* Cochrane Review 2013

A Cochrane review on RUTF for home-based treatment for severely malnourished children between six months to five years concluded that the "Current scientific evidence is limited and, therefore it cannot be concluded that there is a difference between RUTF and flour porridge as home treatment for severely malnourished children, or between RUTF given in different daily amounts or with different ingredients. Either RUTF or standard diet such as flour porridge can be used to treat severely malnourished children at home. Decisions should be based on availability, cost, and practicality." In order to determine the effects of RUTF, more high-quality studies are needed. According to this Cochrane review, the impact of RUTF and flour porridge was almost similar.[10]

### 2. Mamidi, *et al.* Indian Pediatrics 2010

Another study conducted by National Institute of Nutrition, Hyderabad[11] reported that the diet based on local energy dense foods was suitable for the nutrition rehabilitation of severely malnourished children though the rate of weight gain was moderate.

### 3. Dube, *et al.* Indian Pediatrics 2009

An acceptability trial was conducted in urban low to middle socioeconomic neighbourhoods in Delhi to compare the acceptability and energy intake of ready-to-use therapeutic food (RUTF) with cereal legume based *khichri*

**Table 8.3** Traditional Therapeutic Foods used for Management of Severe Acute Malnutrition in India

| Name of mix | Composition and calorific value | State |
|---|---|---|
| Davangere mix | Laddoos made of equal quantities of groundnuts, roasted Bengal gram, jaggery and ragi. Each 100 g gives 400 calories and 15 g protein. | Medical College, Davangere, Karnataka |
| Shakti nutrimix | Rice, wheat, whole gram (chana), groundnut, sugar, salt, cardamom, black pepper, vitamins and minerals. Each 100 g. of mix provides 10.4 g protein, 5.3 g fat, and 402 calories | Shibipur People's Care Organisation, Howrah, West Bengal |
| Nutrimix | Wheat (400 g), rice (400 g), grams (75 g), moong (75 g), groundnut (50 g); sprouted, dried, roasted and powdered 2 heaped spoons in glass of water or milk with sugar twice a day | Development Research Communication and Service Center, Kolkata, West Bengal |
| Nutrimix | Wheat/rice and Bengal gram/ moong in ratio 4:1. Used for treating SAM, for preparing F-75, F-100, as starter and catch up foods. Each 100 g cooked provides 120–150 kcal and protein 2–3 grams. Can be made more energy dense by adding seasonal fruits, and micronutrient rich by adding electolyte mineral solution | CINI (Child In Need Institute), Kolkata, West Bengal |
| LAPSI | Green millet, peanut, jaggery. Successfully used for quick recovery from SAM | Bharat Agro Industries Foundation and CAPART, Maharashtra |
| SAT Mix | Roasted and ground rice, wheat, black gram and sugar in ratio 1:1:1:2. Provides 380 calories per 100 g. | Sree Avittom Thirunal Hospital, Kerala |
| HCCM (high calorie cereal milk) | 15 g flour of mother's choice or availability in home. 5 mL cooking oil of mother's choice, 2 teaspoons of sugar. Cooked like payasam. 100 mL HCCM =187 calories. Provision of at least 300 extra calories per day in addition to the food from the family pot (= HCCM made with < 200 mL of milk) | Christian Medical College, Vellore, Tamil Nadu |
| Sattu Maavu | Wheat flour 42%, maize flour 10%, malted Ragi flour 5% Bengal gram flour 12%, jaggery 30% vitamin premix 1%. Each 100 g provides protein 9 to 10% and calories 360 kcal. | Nutrition monitoring program, Tamil Nadu |

among malnourished children.[12] Thirty one children between 6-36 months with moderate wasting, with no clinical signs of infection or edema were included. Children were offered weighed amounts of RUTF and *khichri* in unlimited amounts for 2 days, one meal of each on both days. Water was fed on demand. It was found that the proportion of children who accepted RUTF eagerly was 58% as against 77% for khichri. The energy intake from RUTF was higher due to its extra energy density.

## 4. Burza, et al. *American Journal of Clinical Nutrition 2015*

In Bihar, uncomplicated SAM cases were treated as outpatients in the community by using a WHO-standard, ready-to-use, therapeutic lipid-based paste produced in India; complicated cases were treated as inpatients by using F75/F100 WHO-standard milk until they could complete treatment in the community. A total of 8274 children were admitted including 6613 (79.9%) children aged 6–23 months. Of 3873 children admitted under the old criteria, 41 children (1.1%) died, 2069 children (53.4%) were discharged as cured, and 1485 children (38.3%) defaulted. Of 4401 children admitted under the new criteria, 36 children (0.8%) died, 2526 children (57.4%) were discharged as cured, and 1591 children (36.2%) defaulted.[13]

## 5. Thakur, et al. *Indian Pediatrics 2013*

This trial was conducted in Pediatric ward of tertiary care public hospital in Central India to compare the efficacy of locally-prepared ready-to-use therapeutic food (L-RUTF) and locally-prepared F-100 diet in promoting weight-gain in children aged 6 to 60 months, with severe acute malnutrition. The control cohort received F-100 while the intervention cohort enrolled received L-RUTF. There were 49 subjects in each group. Rate of weight-gain was found to be 9.59 ± 3.39 g/kg/d in L-RUTF group and 5.41 ± 1.05 g/kg/d in locally prepared F-100 group. The rate of weight gain was significantly better in L-RUTF group (P<0.0001; 95% CI 3.17–5.19). No serious adverse effect was observed with use of L-RUTF. L-RUTF promoted more rapid weight-gain when compared with F-100 in patients with SAM.[14]

## 6. Singh, et al. *Indian Pediatrics 2010*

A trial was conducted in pre-schools run by the Department of Community Health in Kaniyambadi administrative block, Vellore, India to evaluate the effectiveness of a locally made ready-to-use therapeutic food (RUTF) in decreasing mild to moderate malnutrition. Children aged 18–60 months with weight-for-age less than –2 Z-score were included. A locally produced energy-dense supplement (RUTF), and the current standard of care, teaching caregivers how to make a fortified cereal-milk supplement called High Calorie Cereal Milk (HCCM) was given to children. Increase in weight-for-age status was the main outcome for the study. The mean (SD) weight gain at 3 months was higher in the RUTF group: RUTF (n = 51): 0.54 kg; (95% CI = 0.44–0.65) vs HCCM (n = 45): 0.38 kg (95% CI = 0.25–0.51), P = 0.047. The weight gain per kilogram of body weight was directly proportional to the severity of malnutrition. Community-based treatment showed weight gain in both groups, the weight gain being higher with L-RUTF.[15]

## 8.5 RUTF IN INDIA: A CRITICAL APPRAISAL

In India, at present, Government of India policy is not to use RUTF for management of children with SAM. However, as Health and Nutrition are State's Subject as per the Constitution of the country, Rajasthan State has initiated the use of RUTF in management of SAM children.

### The Rajasthan Experience

Use of RUTF in the Rajasthan state is being sponsored by GAIN, an international voluntary organization. This initiative is actively supported by UNICEF, an organization which is known for its philanthropic activities. It is not clear from the publication available that for how many years GAIN would continue to provide support of supply of RUTF for the management of SAM children. It can be documented that the treatment of SAM children with RUTF is like mopping the floor in a room without plugging the leaking tap. There is a little effort on educating the mothers of SAM children, improving their skills and enabling them to treat the causes of undernutrition prevalent in the family. The aim of this program is to distribute as many packets as possible to the children. The distribution of RUTF for management of SAM has not been based on any scientific evidence available from the country. The efficacy of RUTF which has been documented as evidence on SAM children is essentially from the African countries which are affected by wars or famines. In these countries the children had nothing to eat and when they were provided RUTF, children consumed it in entire quantity as they were starving. The situation in India is different, almost all the families have availability of foods, although, it may not be nutrient dense and micronutrient rich.

Funding of the Rajasthan program is being done by International organization and their aim is to prove that RUTF is efficacious in treatment of SAM children so that they are able to motivate other state governments to adopt use of RUTF in management of SAM. There are many unanswered questions which needs to be looked into:

i. Anganwadi Workers (AWWs) will have to take care of the storage and distribution of the RUTF but the knowledge and skills of the AWW are low to ensure the safe and secure storage and distribution of the RUTF;

ii. The climatic condition varies greatly from North to South and East to West, and hence the storage of the RUTF can be a great challenge. In the desert area, there is a high temperature of 48°C while in Himachal Pradesh and Jammu and Kashmir, the temperature goes 30°C below 0°C. We do not have any scientific data on impact of extremes of temperatures on quality of RUTF;

iii. The Food Safety Standard Authority of India (FSSAI) has till date not given permission for large scale manufacturing and its use in India; and

iv. Also, it is not clear if RUTF is to be used with a health claim for treatment of

**Box 8.1 Concerns of Indian Scientist on RUTF use in India**

1. Due cognizance should be given to the demonstrated efficacy and safety of RUTF for its use in treatment of children with severe acute malnutrition.

2. RUTF is likely to be substantially expensive, over the energy dense home available foods i.e local RUTF.

3. Safety of unregulated use of RUTF, especially in relation to following needs to be monitored:
   • RUTF has high fat content which may lead to an increased adiposity, which is likely to increase the epidemic of non-communicable diseases in future adulthood.
   • RUTF has more solute content; the possible impact on renal function has not been studied in detail.
   • There is lack of evidence on acceptability by SAM children;
   • Use of RUTF may lead to displacement of traditional optimal Infant and Young Child Feeding practices;
   • The evidence on the fate of the children who have recovered with use of RUTF is not known when they go the families without access to food security
   • An undue emphasis is being given to a medicalised and therapeutic model instead of promoting the available sustainable preventive model for treatment of SAM children using L-RUTF.

children suffering from SAM, then it would be equated with a drug and then RUTF should be required to undergo the same stringent regulatory clearances as for other drugs utilized in the country.

Concerns of Indian scientists over the use of RUTF in SAM are summarized in **Box 8.1**.

## The Way Forward

Presently in India, we have about 8 million SAM children. We do have policy and guidelines for management of SAM children who are hospitalized. These guidelines are based on WHO/UNICEF guidelines. It would be extremely difficult to admit all the SAM children to the hospital due to shortage of beds/unwilling parents. When a child is admitted to a hospital, the entire family has to move to the hospital as child needs mother to take care and there are siblings of the SAM child who also have to be looked after by the mother.

There is evidence that SAM children are being treated successfully using the traditional foods in the country. However, there has been no clinical trial conducted to assess the impact of these traditional foods on treatment of SAM. There is a need to undertake carefully designed trial with traditional foods so that we are able to establish their effectiveness. The traditional foods are locally available, they are cost effective, do not require shelf-life, can be prepared locally, acceptable by the community, and avoids dependence on external agencies to provide them.

In the wisdom, it is important that we should use our local resources. We should take advantages of scientific evidence available globally, however, we should act locally for the benefit of our community.

## References

1. WHO Child Growth Standards and the Identification of Severe Acute Malnutrition In Infants and Children. A Joint Statement by the World Health Organization and the United Nations Children's Fund. 2009. Available from: http://www.who.int/nutrition/publications/severemalnutrition/9789241598163/en/index.html. Accessed 3 September 2016.

2. Management of Children with Severe Acute Malnutrition (SAM) is a National Priority to Achieve Reduction in Under Five Mortality: SAM Expert Group India. Available from: http://cyberlectures.indmedica.com/show/246/1/Management_of_Children_with_Severe_Acute_Malnutrition_%28SAM%29__is__a_National_Priority_to_Achieve_Reduction_in_Under_Five_Mortality. Accessed on 28 September 2016.

3. Prasad V, Holla R, Gupta A. Should India use commercially produced ready to use therapeutic foods (RUTF) for severe acute malnutrition (SAM). Soc Med. 2009;4:52–5.

4. UNICEF. Position paper. Ready to use therapeutic food for children with severe acute malnutrition. 2013. Available from: (http://www.unicef.org/media/files/Position_Paper_Ready-to-use_therapeutic_food_for_children_with_severe_acute_malnutrition__June_2013.pdf). Accessed on 20th September 2016.

5. UNICEF. Community based management of severe acute malnutrition. A Joint Statement by the World Health Organization, the World Food Programme, the United Nations System Standing Committee on Nutrition and the United Nations Children's Fund. Available from: http://www.unicef.org/publications/files/Community_Based_Management_of_Sever_Acute_Malnutrition.pdf. Accessed on 20th August 2016.

6. Management of Malnutrition in Children Under Five Years. Available from: http://motherchild-nutrition.org/malnutrition-management/info/rutf-plumpy-nut.html. Accessed on 21th September 2016.

7. Results from the Initial Demonstration of RUTF for the Treatment of Acute Malnutrition in Cambodian Children. National Nutrition Program, Cambodia Clinton Foundation HIV/AIDS Initiative, 2009. Available from: http://www.cmamforum.org/pool/resources/use-of-rutf-for-treating-acute-malnutrition-in-cambodia-2009.pdf. Accessed 12th September 2016.

8. Working Group for Children under Six. How should India approach the management of severe acute malnutrition? A Position Paper. Social Medicine. 2009;4:40–4.

9. Rajivan AK. History of Direct Nutrition Programmes in Tamil Nadu. Available from: http://www.righttofoodindia.org/data/anuradha.pdf. Accessed on 25 November, 2016.

10. Schoonees A, Lombard M, Musekiwa A, Nel E, Volmink J. Ready-to-use therapeutic food for home-based treatment of severe acute malnutrition in children from six months to five years of age. Cochrane Database System Rev. 2013;6:CD009000.

11. Mamidi RS, Kulkarni B, Radhakrishna KV, Shatrugna V. Hospital based nutrition rehabilitation of severely undernourished children using energy dense local foods. Indian Pediatr. 2010;47:687–93.

12. Dube B, Rongsen T, Mazumder S, Taneja S, Rafiqui F, Bhandari N, et al. Comparison of ready-to-use therapeutic food with cereal legume-based khichri among malnourished children. Indian Pediatr. 2009;46:383–8.

13. Burza S, Mahajan R, Marino E, Sunyoto T, Shandilya C, Tabrez M, Kumari K, et al. Community-based management of severe acute malnutrition in India: new evidence from Bihar. Am J Clin Nutr. 2015;101:847–59.

14. Thakur GS, Patel C. Locally-prepared ready-to-use therapeutic food for children with severe acute malnutrition: A controlled trial. Indian Pediatr. 2013;50:295–9.

15. Singh AS, Kang G, Ramachandran A, Sarkar R, Peter P, Bose A. Locally made ready to use therapeutic food for treatment of malnutrition: a randomized controlled trial. Indian Pediatr. 2010;47:679–86.

# 9 Facility Based Management of Children with Severe Acute Malnutrition

Praveen Kumar, Shivani Rohatgi

Malnutrition is a preventable cause in approximately 35–45% of under-five mortality occurring worldwide.[1,2] Children who have severe acute malnutrition (SAM) have approximately 8–9 times higher risk of mortality with common illnesses like pneumonia, diarrhea, and malaria. Besides increasing the risk of mortality, malnutrition also causes growth retardation and impaired psychosocial and mental development. There is strong scientific evidence to suggest that if children having SAM with medical complications receive protocol based management, their survival improves significantly. This is one of the key cost-effective interventions to improve child survival.

This chapter describes facility based management of children with severe acute malnutrition who are between 6–59 months. Management of infants with SAM who are under 6 months is described in another chapter.

## 9.1 INDICATIONS FOR FACILITY BASED MANAGEMENT

As described in Chapters 4 and 5, several physiological and metabolic changes occur in children with severe acute malnutrition which is also known as reductive adaptation.[3,4] These changes make many treatments inappropriate which may be otherwise appropriate for children with normal nutritional status **(Box 9.1)**. In 1990s, reported mortality rates in children with severe acute malnutrition varied between 5–50% which was largely due to differences in the management practices. Mortality was reported lower in centers which managed clinical problems in a considered order. In 1999, World Health Organization issued guidelines for better identification of SAM and improving its treatment outcome.[3] Until 2001, even emergency response to high levels of acute malnutrition was predominantly through Therapeutic Feeding Centers (TFCs) which are large, in-patient centers where SAM patients were admitted for 21 days or longer.[5] Subsequently, more evidence emerged on effectiveness of community therapeutic

> **Box 9.1 Reasons for High Mortality in Severe Acute Malnutrition**
> 1. Inability to distinguish between acute and rehabilitation phases
> 2. Excessive use of intravenous fluids
> 3. Fluid overload due to lack of monitoring during rehydration
> 4. Use of diuretics for edema
> 5. Use of albumin for edema
> 6. Not keeping the child warm and euglycemic
> 7. Low index of suspicion for infection
> 8. Early use of diets high in protein and sodium
> 9. Failure to monitor food intake
> 10. Early treatment of anemia with oral iron.

centers implemented in several countries like Ethiopia, Malawi, Sudan, and Niger. WHO, UNICEF, WFP and SCN published a joint statement in 2006 describing community based approach to be effective in managing large number of SAM children in their communities.[6]

In the presence of good community-based management, the vast majority (85–90%) of children with SAM may be managed in the community while only a minority, those with poor appetite and/ or medical complications (10–15%), will need hospitalization or facility-based care **(Table 9.1)**.[7,8] **Figure 9.1** depicts management algorithm from screening to discharge and follow-up in presence of CSAM program in place.

Under the National Health Mission (NHM), different states have opened special centers which are known as **nutrition rehabilitation centers** (NRC) or **malnutrition treatment centers** (MTC). At these centers, children with SAM are admitted with well-defined admission criteria and receive standard protocol based management.

## 9.2 PRINCIPLES OF FACILITY BASED MANAGEMENT

### A. Objectives of Facility-based Care

1. To provide protocol based treatment and improve survival of children with severe acute malnutrition, particularly those with medical complications;

2. To recuperate undernourished children through supplemental feeding;
3. To promote physical and psychosocial growth of children with severe acute malnutrition (SAM); and
4. To empower mothers to improve their feeding and child caring practices.

### B. Steps of Management

A good history, physical examination **(Table 9.2)**, and appetite test help to decide the level of care for an individual child. As per WHO 2013 update, children with medical complications (presence of general danger signs, or pink classification of IMNCI), or poor appetite should be treated in a facility.[9] Children who are initially managed in facility (NRC/MTC), can also be transferred to community based care when their medical complications are resolved, have a good appetite, and are clinically well and alert. However, if community based management is not available, all children with severe acute malnutrition should be admitted in a health facility/ Nutrition Rehabilitation Center. Only basic investigations are required in majority of children. These are enlisted in **Box 9.2**.

### C. Essential Components of Care

World Health Organization has recommended 10 essential steps for SAM management **(Table 9.3)** to take care of physiological and metabolic changes of these children. These guidelines have been adapted by Indian

| Table 9.1 Modalities of SAM Treatment | | |
|---|---|---|
| *Criteria* | *Poor appetite OR medical complication* | *Good appetite and no medical complication* |
| | ↓ | ↓ |
| Type of therapeutic feeding | **Facility based** F-75 → F-100/ EDNS and 24 hour medical care | **Community based** EDNS and basic medical care |
| Discharge criteria (transition criteria from facility to community based care) | Reduced edema Good appetite (with acceptable intake of EDNS) | W/H >-2 Z-score Or MUAC >12.5 cm No edema for last 2 weeks |

EDNS: Energy dense nutritional supplement

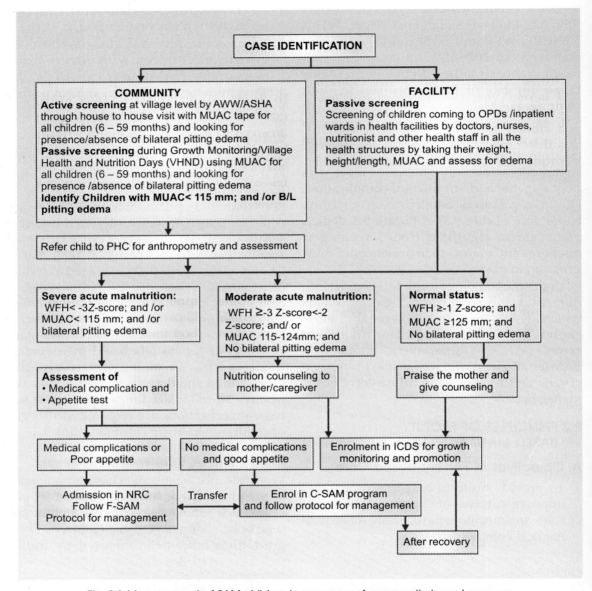

**Fig. 9.1** Management of SAM children in presence of community based program

Academy of Pediatrics in their consensus statement.[10,11] and Ministry of Health and Family Welfare, GOI.[8]

There are three phases of treatment:

- First phase is *stabilization phase* in which focus is on stabilizing the patient by careful initiation of feeding, identifying and treating life threatening complications like hypothermia, hypoglycemia, dehydration etc (Steps 1 to 7 in **Table 9.3**). The stabilization phase usually takes 2–7 days.
- Second phase also known as *rehabilitation phase* involves increasing the energy and nutrient content of feeds.
- Third phase is *follow-up after discharge* which aims to prevent relapses.

**Table 9.2** History and Examination in Severe Acute Malnutrition

*Take a history concerning*

- Duration of sickness
- Recent intake of food and fluids
- Usual diet (before the current illness)
- Breastfeeding
- Complementary feeds- introduction time, quality, quantity
- Duration and frequency of complaints if any: diarrhea (watery/bloody), vomiting (number), fever, cough
- Loss of appetite
- Contact with open case of tuberculosis
- History of measles in last 3 months
- Known or suspected HIV infection
- Immunization status
- Health of parents and family circumstances

*On examination, look for*

- Look for emergency signs
- Anthropometry- weight, height or length, mid upper arm circumference
- Baseline pulse, heart rate, respiratory rate
- Sensorium
- Signs of dehydration if history of diarrhea (general condition, sunken eyes, skin pinch and thirst)
- Edema, lymphadenopathy
- Signs of shock (cold hands, slow capillary refill, weak and fast pulse)
- Palmar pallor
- Eye signs of vitamin A deficiency
- Localizing signs of infection, including ear and (to understand the child's social background) throat infections, skin infection or pneumonia
- Fever (temperature >37.5°C or 99.5°F)
- Hypothermia (axillary temperature <35°C or 95 °F)
- Mouth ulcers/ Oral thrush
- Skin changes: Hypo or hyperpigmentation, desquamation, ulceration
- Systemic examination: hepatosplenomegaly, any murmur or deformities, hypertonia (cerebral palsy)
- Signs of meningeal irritation
- Exudative lesions (resembling severe burns) often with secondary infection (*Candida*).

## 9.3 HYPOGLYCEMIA: TREAT AND/OR PREVENT

In children with SAM, hypoglycemia is defined as blood glucose less than 54 mg/dL.

**Box 9.2 Laboratory Tests Required for Facility Based Care**

1. Blood glucose
   - At admission
   - During stabilization; if child is hypothermic or lethargic
2. Hemoglobin or packed cell volume in all children
   - Peripheral smear, if child has anemia
3. Serum electrolytes (sodium, potassium, and calcium whenever possible)
4. Screening for infections:
   - Total and differential leukocyte count, blood culture
   - Urine microscopy and culture
   - Chest X-ray
   - Mantoux test
   - Blood smear for malaria; if febrile
5. Additional investigations depending on clinical situation and availability
   - Screening for HIV (in presence of recurrent infections, presence of oral thrush, lymphadenopathy, unexplained death of parents, persistent diarrhea, parotid enlargement)
   - Any other specific test e.g. anti-tissue transglutaminase antibody test for celiac disease

All severely malnourished children are at risk of developing hypoglycemia. Hypoglycemia has been reported as an important cause of mortality in SAM children with medical complications.[12,13] It has been recommended to measure blood sugar on admission and subsequently in children who become lethargic. If the blood glucose measurement facility is not available immediately then hypoglycemia should be assumed to be present and treatment should be initiated. Hypoglycemia and hypothermia are also signs that indicate possibility of underlying infections.[14]

### A. Hypoglycemia with Lethargy, Unconsciousness, or Convulsion

- Give IV 10% glucose 5 mL/kg followed by 50 mL of 10% glucose or sucrose by nasogastric (NG) tube.
- If IV dose cannot be given immediately, NG glucose or dextrose 50 mL should be given immediately.

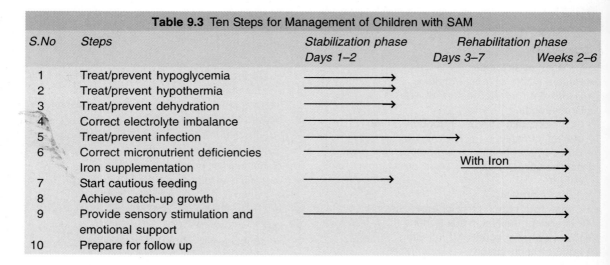

**Table 9.3** Ten Steps for Management of Children with SAM

| S.No | Steps | Stabilization phase Days 1–2 | Rehabilitation phase Days 3–7 | Weeks 2–6 |
|---|---|---|---|---|
| 1 | Treat/prevent hypoglycemia | ⟶ | | |
| 2 | Treat/prevent hypothermia | ⟶ | | |
| 3 | Treat/prevent dehydration | ⟶ | | |
| 4 | Correct electrolyte imbalance | ⟶ | | |
| 5 | Treat/prevent infection | ⟶ | | |
| 6 | Correct micronutrient deficiencies | ⟶ | | |
| | Iron supplementation | | With Iron ⟶ | |
| 7 | Start cautious feeding | ⟶ | | |
| 8 | Achieve catch-up growth | | ⟶ | |
| 9 | Provide sensory stimulation and emotional support | ⟶ | | |
| 10 | Prepare for follow up | | ⟶ | |

- Give appropriate antibiotics and start feeding with starter diet.
- Check blood sugar again after 30 minutes and repeat 10% glucose or sugar solution, if hypoglycemia persists.

## B. Asymptomatic Hypoglycemia (Not Lethargic, Conscious)

- Give the first feed of starter diet or 50 mL of 10% glucose or sugar solution (4 rounded teaspoon of sugar in 200 mL of water) orally or by nasogastric tube, followed by the starter feed as soon as possible.
- Give 2-hourly feeds, day and night, at least for the first day.
- Give appropriate antibiotics.
- Check temperature and prevent hypothermia.

## 9.4 HYPOTHERMIA: TREAT AND/OR PREVENT

Hypothermia in SAM child is defined as axillary temperature < 35°C or rectal temperature < 35.5°C. Following measures have been recommended to treat and prevent hypothermia:

- Make sure the child is clothed properly (including the head). Cover with a warmed blanket and place a heater (not pointing directly at the child) or lamp nearby, or put the child on the mother's bare chest or abdomen (skin-to-skin) and cover them with a warmed blanket and/or warm clothing.
- Feed the child immediately.
- Give appropriate antibiotics.

*If there is severe hypothermia (<32°C), more aggressive approach is required.*

- Give warm humidified oxygen.
- Give 5 mL/kg of 10% dextrose IV immediately or 50 mL of 10% dextrose by nasogastric route (If intravenous access is difficult).
- Give intravenous antibiotics dose immediately.
- Rewarm with radiant warmer till child's temperature rises to 35°C.
- Give warm feeds immediately orally or by NG tube.
- If there is feed intolerance or contra-indication for nasogastric feeding, start maintenance IV fluids.
- If there is history of diarrhea or evidence of dehydration, rehydrate using warm fluids immediately.
- Take the child's temperature 2-hrly until it rises to more than 36.5°C. Take it half-hourly if a heater is being used.
- Check for hypoglycemia whenever hypothermia is found.

## Prevent Hypothermia

- Place the bed in a warm, draught-free part of the ward and keep the child covered.
- Change wet nappies, clothes, and bedding to keep the child and the bed dry.
- Avoid exposing the child to cold (e.g. after bathing, or during medical examinations).
- Let the child sleep with the mother.
- Feed the child 2-hourly, starting immediately.
- Give 2 hourly feed both day and night till the time temperature is stable.

## 9.5 DEHYDRATION: TREAT AND/OR PREVENT

Diarrhea is a common morbidity in children with SAM. Many of the signs that are normally used to assess dehydration are unreliable in a child with severe malnutrition, making it difficult or impossible to detect dehydration reliably or determining its severity. A severely malnourished child is usually apathetic when left alone and irritable when handled. In severely malnourished child, the loss of supporting tissue and absence of sub-cutaneous fat make the skin thin and loose. It flattens very slowly when pinched, or may not flatten at all. As a result, dehydration tends to be overdiagnosed and its severity over-estimated.

Ask the mother if the child has watery diarrhea or vomiting. If the child has watery diarrhea or vomiting, assume dehydration and give ORS. Since signs of dehydration are not very reliable, rehydration orally or through a nasogastric tube is recommended. IV rehydration is indicated only if the child has signs of shock and is lethargic or unconscious.

### A. Rehydration of Children without Shock

Keeping physiological changes in mind, most of guidelines recommend following regimen for rehydration.[3,8,9]

Case fatality decreased from 17% to 9% when a standardized protocol, based on the WHO guidelines was introduced in

| How often to give ORS | Amount to be given |
|---|---|
| Every 30 minutes for first 2 hours | 5 mL/kg weight |
| Alternate hours for up to 10 hours* | 5–10 mL/kg** |

*Starter (F-75) diet and ORS given in alternate hours
**The amount offered in this range should be based on child's willingness to drink and amount of ongoing losses

Bangladesh.[15] The main changes were slower rehydration, avoidance of intravenous fluids whenever possible, giving antibiotics in all cases, immediate feeding, and giving potassium, magnesium, and micronutrients as recommended by WHO guidelines.

### Which ORS to be used?

WHO has recommended a special ORS known as **ReSoMal** (Rehydrating Solution for severely malnourished children) for rehydrating children with SAM which contains less sodium (45 meq/L), has added potassium (40 meq/L), and minerals as compared to low osmolarity ORS. As per WHO 2013 update, *ReSoMal continues to be recommended for children with severe acute malnutrition*. There are two indications for rehydration with low osmolarity ORS—cholera and profuse watery diarrhea.[9]

However, these recommendations are not based on strong scientific evidence. A systematic review which examined the effectiveness of different interventions like H-ORS, a modified WHO-ORS (ReSoMal), an ORS containing glucose, glucose plus ARS or rice powder and supplementation with zinc concluded that ReSoMal did not perform better over standard WHO-ORS in rehydrating these children.[16-18] Rice-ORS appeared to be more favorable than glucose - ORS in treating children with cholera.[19] Supplementation with 40 mg elemental zinc in addition to standard ORS resulted in a significantly shorter duration of diarrhea and better recovery rate.[18] A recent study compared the safety and efficacy of low-osmolarity ORS *vs.* modified ReSoMal for treatment of children with SAM and diarrhea. This study reported comparable success rate of rehydration in both the groups. Though the children in modified ReSoMal group achieved early rehydration but a higher proportion (15.4%) developed hyponatremia as compared to 1.9% on low osmolarity ORS.[20]

*If ReSoMal is not available*

Where ReSoMal is not available, It has been recommended by WHO to prepare ReSoMal by dissolving 1 low-osmolarity ORS sachet in 2000 mL water in place of 1000 ml and adding 50 g of sugar and 40 mL of mineral mix solution. To avoid rapid changes in homeostasis in children with SAM, the dehydration correction is done orally (or through nasogastric tube) and slowly alternating with feeds (F-75 therapeutic diet) over 10–12 hours with intensive monitoring of vitals. The fluid requirements can change during the course of rehydration depending upon the ongoing losses, ability to drink, vomiting, and appearance of signs of overhydration.[9]

*Monitoring is Important for the Child who is Taking ORS*

Baseline respiratory rate, pulse rate, urine output, and frequency of stools and vomiting should be monitored every 30 minutes. Increasing respiratory rate by 5/min and pulse rate by 15/min indicates overhydration. ORS should be stopped immediately in this case and child should be reassessed after 1 hour **(Fig. 9.2)**.

ORS should be stopped when the child has 3 or more of the signs of improved hydration status *i.e.* child no longer thirsty, less lethargic, slowing of respiratory and pulse rates from previous high rate, improvement in skin turgor, and reappearance of tears. If an admitted child develops diarrhea, ORS should be stopped once he/she reaches the recorded weight before the onset of diarrhea. After rehydration, offer 50 mL ORS after each loose stool to children less than 2 years and 100 mL to children who are 2 years or older.

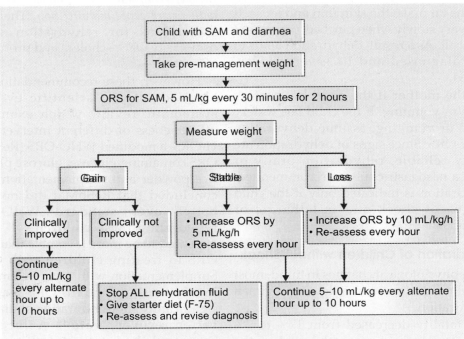

**Fig. 9.2** Fluid management in SAM children with diarrhea

## B. How to Manage SAM Children with Shock?

The severely acute malnourished child is considered to have shock if he/she has cold hands AND slow capillary refill (longer than 3 seconds), AND weak and fast pulse.

The management of shock in children with severe malnutrition remains very controversial due to lack of strong scientific evidence. Shock can evolve due to fluid losses in case of diarrhea or as part of septic shock or may have both the components. The differentiation is difficult due to unreliability of clinical signs of dehydration.At the same time, these children are susceptible to risk of over-hydration, heart failure, pulmonary edema, and clinical deterioration if rapid and large volumes of fluid are used for management of shock as done in well-nourished children. A randomized controlled trial conducted in Kenya that compared the efficacy of Ringer's lactate isotonic fluid (RL), half-strength Darrow's in 5% dextrose (HSD/5D), and 4.5% human albumin solution (HAS) in SAM children with shock was prematurely terminated due to high mortality and inadequate correction of shock in all study arms.[21] There are no well conducted randomized controlled trials to guide us on the best possible fluid to resuscitate, rate of infusion, and outcome in terms of mortality or recovery in children with malnutrition.In presence of shock or lethargy/unconscious-ness, WHO recommends rehydration with either half-strength Darrow's solution with 5% dextrose, or Ringer's lactate solution with 5% dextrose, or 0.45% saline with 5% dextrose. Initially 15 mL/kg is given over one hour with meticulous monitoring of vital parameters. Once the shock improves, rest of the fluid rehydration is carried out orally or via nasogastric tube as in case of *Some dehydration* over next 10–12 hours. Feeds are initiated at earliest alternating with oral fluids as the child recovers from shock **(Fig. 9.3)**. Although previous guidelines recommended second bolus of 15/mL/kg over 1 hour to children who respond to first bolus, recently published ETAT module advise to shift to oral rehydration after one bolus.[22]

## 9.6 CORRECT ELECTROLYTE IMBALANCE

Children with SAM have deficiency of potassium and magnesium while they have excess sodium in their cells. So they need higher potassium, magnesium to make up for what is lost and restricted sodium intake.[23-25] Magnesium is essential for potassium to enter the cells and be retained. In a descriptive study, authors concluded that electrolyte changes were common in grade II and III malnourished patients, particularly who presented with diarrheal episode of variable duration.[23]

### A. Role of Magnesium

Magnesium plays an essential role in numerous cellular reactions including oxidative phosphorylation, enzymatic reactions, nucleic acid metabolism, and protein synthesis. Magnesium depletion in malnourished children may be asymptomatic or may produce symptoms like anorexia, nausea, muscular weakness, lethargy, tremors, athetoid movement, seizures, and psychomotor changes. WHO and IAP consensus guidelines recommend potassium supplementation for at least 2 weeks at 3–4 mmol/kg/day. On day 1, 50% magnesium sulfate should be given IM once (0.3 mL/kg up to a maximum of 2 mL). Thereafter, extra magnesium (0.4–0.6 mmol/kg daily) may be supplemented orally. Injection magnesium sulfate may be given *orally* mixed with feeds.

### B. Role of Potassium

A randomized, double blind, placebo controlled, clinical trial by Manary, *et al.*[26] has proven efficacy of high potassium supplementation in improving the outcome of edematous children. This study reported lesser case fatality in children who received higher potassium supplementation (7.7 mmol/kg/

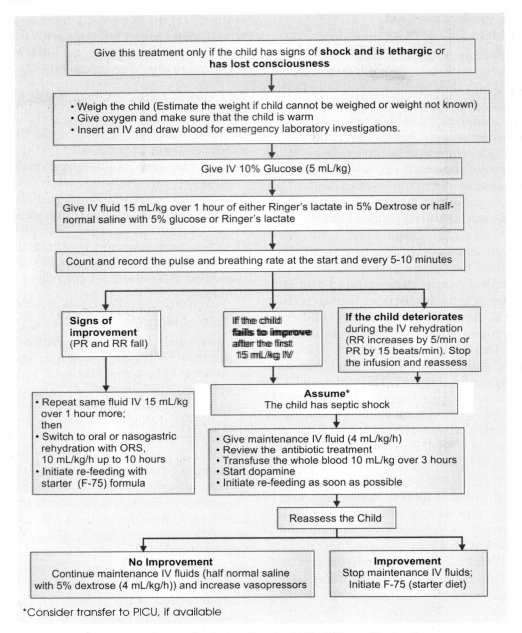

Give this treatment only if the child has signs of **shock and is lethargic** or **has lost consciousness**

- Weigh the child (Estimate the weight if child cannot be weighed or weight not known)
- Give oxygen and make sure that the child is warm
- Insert an IV and draw blood for emergency laboratory investigations.

Give IV 10% Glucose (5 mL/kg)

Give IV fluid 15 mL/kg over 1 hour of either Ringer's lactate in 5% Dextrose or half-normal saline with 5% glucose or Ringer's lactate

Count and record the pulse and breathing rate at the start and every 5-10 minutes

**Signs of improvement** (PR and RR fall)

If the child fails to improve after the first 15 mL/kg IV

**If the child deteriorates** during the IV rehydration (RR increases by 5/min or PR by 15 beats/min). Stop the infusion and reassess

- Repeat same fluid IV 15 mL/kg over 1 hour more; then
- Switch to oral or nasogastric rehydration with ORS, 10 mL/kg/h up to 10 hours
- Initiate re-feeding with starter (F-75) formula

**Assume\***
The child has septic shock

- Give maintenance IV fluid (4 mL/kg/h)
- Review the antibiotic treatment
- Transfuse the whole blood 10 mL/kg over 3 hours
- Start dopamine
- Initiate re-feeding as soon as possible

Reassess the Child

**No Improvement**
Continue maintenance IV fluids (half normal saline with 5% dextrose (4 mL/kg/h)) and increase vasopressors

**Improvement**
Stop maintenance IV fluids; Initiate F-75 (starter diet)

\*Consider transfer to PICU, if available

**Fig. 9.3** Management algorithm for SAM children with shock

day) as compared to controls who received a standard potassium intake (4.7 mmol/kg/day).[26] The study recommended that the standard potassium supplement for the initial phase of treatment of kwashiorkor be increased from 4 to 8 mmol/kg/day. In a study conducted by Khalil, *et al.*[27] it was found that magnesium level was lower than normal in severely malnourished children. Magnesium supplemented group of patients show better improvement of appetite, reduction of vomiting, and improving of hypotonia.[27,28]

## 9.7 GIVE ANTIBIOTICS

Infection and malnutrition have always been intricately linked. Studies have documented high prevalence of pneumonia, bacteremia, and urinary tract infections in children with severe acute malnutrition, which often may not be symptomatic. Small bowel bacterial overgrowth is common in children with severe acute malnutrition.[29] Bagga, et al.[30] reported significant bacteriuria in SAM children (15.2% vs. 1.8% in controls). The incidence of bacteriuria in malnourished and normally nourished subjects with fever was 28.6% and 5.7%, respectively. Authors concluded that malnourished children, particularly those with fever, are at risk for UTI.

Children admitted with severe acute malnutrition and complications such as septic shock, hypoglycemia, hypothermia, skin infections, or respiratory or urinary tract infections, or who appear lethargic, should be given parenteral (IM orIV) antibiotics. Children admitted with severe acute malnutrition and with no apparent signs of infection and no complications should be given an oral antibiotic like amoxicillin. IAP and GOI guidelines recommended antibiotics are summarized in **Table 9.4**.

### Duration of Antibiotic Therapy

It depends on the diagnosis i.e.: 7 days in suspected sepsis, 10–14 days in culture proven sepsis, at least 14–21 days in meningitis, and 4 weeks for deep seated infections. Antimalarials should be given if blood smear or RDT is positive for malaria parasites. Antitubercular therapy should be added if tuberculosis is diagnosed as per RNTCP recommended criteria.

### Response to Treatment for Infection

If there is good response to antibiotics, child becomes alert, active, gains weight >5 g/kg/day and there is no further episodes of complications like hypoglycemia or hypothermia.

### 9.8 CORRECT MICRONUTRIENT DEFICIENCIES

All SAM children have vitamin and mineral deficiencies. They need higher vitamin A, multivitamins, folic acid, zinc, and copper for their optimal recovery. They also need additional iron during *rehabilitation phase*.

**Table 9.4** Recommended Antibiotics for Children with SAM

| Status | Antibiotics |
|---|---|
| All admitted case without medical complication and good appetite | • Give Oral amoxicillin 15 mg/kg /dose three times per day for 5 days |
| All admitted cases with any complications other than shock, meningitis and dysentery | • Inj. Ampicillin 50 mg/kg/dose 6 hourly and Inj. Gentamicin 7.5 mg/kg once a day for 7 days<br>• Add inj. Cloxacillin 100 mg/kg day 6 hourly if staphylococcal infection is suspected.<br>• Revise therapy based on sensitivity report |
| For septic shock or worsening/ no improvement in initial hours | • Give third generation cephalosporins like Inj. Cefatoxime 150 mg/kg/day in 3 divided doses or Ceftriaxone100 mg/kg/day in 2 divided doses along with Inj. Gentamicin 7.5 mg in single dose.<br>Do not give second dose of Gentamicin until child is passing urine |
| Meningitis | • IV Cefatoxime 50 mg/kg/dose 6 hourly or Inj. Ceftriaxone 50 mg/kg 12 hourly plus Inj. Amikacin 15 mg kg/day divided in 8 hourly doses |
| Dysentery | • Give cefixime 8–10 mg/kg in 2 divided doses/day for 5 days. If the child is sick, give Inj. Ceftriaxone 100 mg/kg once a day or divided in 2 doses for 5 days |
| On discharge | • 200 mg albendazole for children aged 12–23 months, 400 mg albendazole for children aged 24 months or more. |

## A. Vitamin A Supplementation

Vitamin A plays an important role in maintaining epithelial lining. In addition to impairing immune responses, vitamin A deficient children have less capacity to produce mucus, which enables bacterial adherence and invasion of pathogenic microbes. Untreated vitamin A deficiency in children, more so in severely malnourished children may cause blindness and increased susceptibility to infection and mortality. Several observational studies have reported vitamin A deficiency in severe acute malnutrition.[31-34] Lower serum retinol concentrations in children with severe acute malnutrition have been shown to increase diarrheal morbidities.[34]

Earlier guidelines recommended one dose of oral vitamin A to all children with SAM unless they have received vitamin A dose in last 1 month or has edema. For all children with edema, one dose of vitamin A was recommended to be given after disappearance of edema **(Table 9.5)**. Oral supplementation or treatment with vitamin A is preferred over injections. For oral administration, an oil based formulation is preferred. For IM treatment, only water-based formulation and half of oral dose should be used.

### Revised Recommendations

WHO 2013 update based on studies from sub-Saharan Africa and Bangladesh has revised recommendations regarding vitamin A supplementation:[35,36]

- Low-dose vitamin A supplementation (5000 IU) given daily to children with severe

**Table 9.5** Recommended Oral dose of Vitamin A according to Child's Age

| Age | Vitamin A dose |
|---|---|
| <6 months | 50 000 IU |
| 6–12 months or if weight <8 kg in children >12 months | 100 000 IU |
| >12 months and weight >8 kg | 200 000 IU |

3 doses in case of Signs of Vitamin A deficiency on Day-1, Day-2 and Day-15 to all children with SAM

acute malnutrition is more effective than single high dose vitamin A supplementation in reducing the mortality of children with edema by reducing the incidence and severity of severe diarrhea and respiratory infection.

- High-dose vitamin A supplementation appears to confer some benefit in children with severe acute malnutrition who present with severe diarrhea or shigellosis or with signs of vitamin A deficiency. High-dose vitamin A supplementation also reduces mortality in children with severe acute malnutrition and post measles pneumonia.

## B. Other Micronutrients

Copper and zinc play an important role in preventing lipid peroxidation and cell membrane damage. Malnourished children are also deficient in riboflavin, ascorbic acid, pyridoxine, thiamine, and the fat-soluble vitamins D, E and K. Hence, SAM children should be given *multivitamin supplement* which contains vitamin A, C, D, E and vitamin $B_{12}$ and not just vitamin B-complex. Recommended dose is twice of recommended daily allowance. They also should be given Folic acid 5 mg on day 1, then 1 mg/day; Elemental Zinc-2 mg/kg/day; and Copper-0.3 mg/kg/day. Iron should be started after two days of the child being on Catch up formula (F-100). Give whole blood or packed cell transfusion only if Hb is < 4 g/dL or if Hb is 4–6 g/dL and child has respiratory distress. Blood transfusion should not be repeated within 4 days unless there is ongoing bleeding.

## 9.9 INITIAL FEEDING

Feeding is a critical part for the management of children with SAM. During stabilization phase SAM children with medical complications and or poor appetite are given a special diet known as F-75 diet.

Basic principles of initial feeding are as follows:

- Feeding should be initiated as early as possible which is given every 2 hourly.

- Feed should have low osmolarity, low lactose, and low proteins.
- Feeds should be given during rehydration.
- Use nasogastric feed if oral acceptance is poor.
- Encourage mothers to continue breast-feeding wherever possible.
- Ensure night feeds.

## A. F-75: The Starter Diet

F-75 is a therapeutic formula to be used during initial management. F-75 formula is specially made to meet the child's needs without overloading the body's systems in the initial stage of treatment. F-75 diet provides 75 calories/100 mL and 0.9 g of protein/100 mL. It contains dried skim milk, oil, complex of minerals vitamins mix (CMV), and dextromaltose. Composition of WHO recommended F-75 diet is given in **Table 9.6**.

*When commercial F-75 is used there is no need to give electrolytes (potassium, magnesium), micronutrients, or vitamins separately as F-75 also contains all essential electrolytes, micronutrients, and vitamins.*

If commercial F-75 is not available, it is recommended to prepare starter diet with milk, sugar, rice powder, and vegetable oil

**Table 9.6** Composition of WHO Recommended Therapeutic Diets

| Constituents | F-75 Diet | F-100 Diet |
|---|---|---|
| Energy | 75 Calories | 100 Calories |
| Protein | 0.9 g | 2.9 g |
| Lactose | 1.3 g | 3 g |
| Potassium | 3.6 mmol | 5.9 mmol |
| Sodium | 0.6 mmol | 1.9 mmol |
| Magnesium | 0.43 mmol | 0.73 mmol |
| Zinc | 2.0 mg | 2.3 mg |
| Copper | 0.25 mg | 0.25 mg |
| *Percentage of energy* | | |
| Protein | 5.0% | 12% |
| Fat | 32.0% | 53% |
| Osmolarity | 333 mOsmol/L | 419 mOsmolL |

**(Table 9.7)**. However, this preparation will not be able to meet electrolytes, micronutrients, and vitamins requirements. These will need to be supplemented separately.

Starter diet (F-75) is always calculated using admission weight *i.e.* by 130 mL/kg/day. And for children with severe edema; the volume is calculated by 100 mL/kg/ day. Feed the child F-75/starter diet orally, or by nasogastric tube; if necessary.

It is recommended to feed the child with a cup and spoon encouraging the child to finish

**Table 9.7** Local Preparation of Therapeutic Diets[8]

| Contents (Per 100 ml) | Starter (F-75) diet Amount for 100 mL | Starter (F-75) diet (Cereal Based) Amount for 100 mL | Catch-up (F-100) diet Amount for 100 mL | Catch-up (F-100) diet (Cereal Based) Amount for 100 mL |
|---|---|---|---|---|
| Milk (mL) (cow milk) | 30 | 30 | 90 | 75 |
| Sugar (g) | 10 | 7 | 7.5 | 2.5 |
| Vegetable oil (g) | 2 | 2 | 2 | 2 |
| Puffed Rice (*Murmura*) (g) | -- | 3.5 | _ | 7 |
| Water to make (mL) | 100 | 100 | 100 | 100 |
| Energy (kcal/100 mL) | 75 | 75 | 100 | 100 |
| Protein (g/100 mL) | 0.9 | 1.1 | 2.9 | 2.9 |
| Lactose (g/100 mL) | 1.2 | 1.2 | 4.2 | 3 |

*Adapted from IAP Guidelines 2006

**Powdered puffed rice may be replaced by commercial pre-cooked rice preparations (in same amounts)

***Important note about adding water: Add just the amount of water needed to make 100 mL of formula. Do not simply add 100 mL of water, as this will make the formula too dilute. A mark for 100 mL should be made on the mixing container for the formula, so that water can be added to the other ingredients up to this mark.

the feed. Mothers should be encouraged to breastfeed on demand between F-75 feeds. Despite coaxing and patience, many children will not take sufficient diet by mouth during the first few days of treatment. Common reasons include a very poor appetite (does not take 80% of the offered than feed in 2 consecutive feeds), weakness, oral ulcers, and painful stomatitis. Such children should be fed using a nasogastric (NG) tube until child takes 2–3 complete feeds orally.

*Criteria for increasing volume/decreasing frequency of feeds*
Feeding should be continued 2 hrly atleast for 24 hours and frequency may be changed based on the criteria described below.
1. Feed interval should be changed from 2 hourly to 3 hourly if child finishes most feeds, there is no vomiting and modest diarrhea (i.e., <5 watery stools per day).
2. If there is vomiting or diarrhea, or poor appetite, continue 2-hourly feeds.
3. If there is no vomiting, no diarrhea, and most feeds are consumed, change to 4 hourly after keeping on 3 hourly feed for at least 24 hours.

## B. Recording and Monitoring

It is important to record amount offered, consumed, any vomiting or diarrhea because shifting from 2 hourly to 3 hourly and then 4 hourly is guided by amount consumed, vomiting, and diarrhea. It has been recommended to use the admission weight to determine volume of feed during stabilization even if the child's weight changes. For edematous child with SAM, the child's starting weight (admission weight) should be used to determine the amount of Starter (F-75) diet, even if edema disappears.

## 9.10 ACHIEVE CATCH-UP GROWTH

Once general condition stabilizes, child needs more energy and protein to rebuild wasted tissue. This phase of treatment is known as rehabilitation phase. However this change goes through a phase called transition phase. WHO recommends changing from F-75 to F-100, once general condition stabilizes, usually indicated by a return of appetite.F-100 diet contains 100 kcal/100 mL and 2.9 g of protein per 100 mL. In absence of commercial preparation, catch up diet (F-100) may be prepared locally **(Table 9.7)**.

## A. Recognize Readiness for Transition

The child is ready to enter in this phase when he is accepting orally well, shows clinical improvement (more alert, smile etc.), has no signs of hypoglycemia and hypothermia, and no shock. In edematous children, edema starts disappearing. This phase shall continue for at least 48 hours and till the child shows signs of recovery. If transition is too rapid, heart failure may occur.

## B. How to Feed during Transition Phase

- The F-100 should be given every 4 hours in the same amount as given in F 75 for next 2 days (48 hours).
- On day 3 after entering transition phase feed should be increased by 10 mL in each feed up to a upper limit of 30 mL/kg or some feed is left in cup. If the child does not finish a feed, offer the same amount at the next feed; then increase by 10 mL.

*During this phase, monitor for following signs of heart failure:*
- Increase in respiratory rate by 5 breaths per minute or more AND
- Increase in pulse rate by 15 beats per minute or more.

*Criteria to move back from transition phase to phase 1 when:*
- If child looks sick, lethargic; or
- Child develops complications like hypoglycemia, hypothermia; or
- If there is increase in edema; or
- A child with no edema initially and who develops it now; or
- Rapid increase in the size of liver; or

- Any other signs of fluid overload; or
- Develops abdominal distension; or
- If the child has significant re-feeding diarrhea (>5 loose stools in last 24 hours); or
- The child takes less than 75% of the feed in two or more feeds in transition phase.

## C. Rehabilitation Phase

After three days on transition, If child accepts and finishes feed offered during transition phase (F-100 feed), has modest diarrhea (4 or less and not watery), and no vomiting, then child shall be given F-100 diets freely (upper limit of 220 mL/kg/day). If the child is still hungry after taking all the feed, more shall be given.

During this phase, the feed volume is determined as per the current weight of the child. During rehabilitation phase, the child should be fed amount which provides energy ranging from 150 to 220 kcal/kg/day and 4–6 g of proteins/kg/day.If the child is breastfed, continue to breastfeed between feeds. When child has satisfactory weight gain for three consecutive days (>5 g/kg/day) then he may be shifted on to mixed diet. He can be given a semisolid food item (energy density of 1 kcal/g) like *khichari*, premixes, *halwa* so that child receives three feeds of catch up diet and three feeds of semisolid. Also when the child is growing well and there is no risk of hypoglycemia or hypothermia, then 1 night feed can be omitted to ensure undisturbed sleep during night.

## D. RUTF Diet during Transition and Rehabilitation

The WHO 2013 update has given option of using RUTF (ready to use therapeutic food)/ EDNS (energy dense nutritional supplement) in children above 6 months during transition and rehabilitation phase. Child should be allowed to drink as much water he/she wants to drink. Many states in India use locally prepared special feeds (SF) in place of RUTF which contain adequate calories and proteins. However SF lacks electrolytes and micronutrients which should be given additionally to meets the child's requirement.

## 9.11 PROVIDE SENSORY STIMULATION AND EMOTIONAL SUPPORT

Children with SAM have delayed motor, behavioral, mental, and emotional development. They do not play, cry, smile, complain, or show normal emotions—they become lethargic and feeble. Stimulation and physical activity may help in developing skills. Recovery is faster in children who receive sensory stimulation and are involved in play daily. Daily play session should include language and motor activities, and activities with toys. In addition to informal group play, the aim should be to play with each child individually, for 30 minutes, two sessions each day. Also emphasize the importance of regular play sessions at home after discharge. In addition to informal group play; the aim should be to play with each child individually, for 30 minutes, two sessions each day. Each play session should include language and motor activities, and activities with toys. Mothers should be counseled to continue play therapy at home after discharge.

## 9.12 PREPARE FOR DISCHARGE AND FOLLOW-UP

It is important to encourage mother of these children to feed, comfort, hold and play with the child. She must be involved in these daily care activities during her stay at the facility. She must be given full discharge instruction and explained the importance of follow-up after discharge.

## Monitoring Progress during Treatment

Progress is monitored by calculating daily weight gain. If child on F-100 diet gains weight > 10 g/kg/day it is said to be good weight gain while 5–10 g/kg/day is moderate and <5 g/kg/day is poor. In case of moderate weight gain there is a need to check intake, supplements, and antibiotics. If there is poor weight gain, full reassessment is required including underlying infections like tuberculosis, HIV etc.

SAM children with medical complications usually need 10 to 15 days, to achieve this phase depending on each child's medical condition. All discharged children require follow up for another 2–3 months for ensuring full recovery. Criteria for labelling primary failure are given in **Table 9.8**. Criteria for discharge in presence and absence of community based management are summarized in **Boxes 9.3** and **9.4**.

*The child is discharged from program when:*

- Clinically well; and
- Weight for height is ≥ –2 Z-score / MUAC ≥125 mm and
- No edema for two consecutive follow up visits (if child had edema on admission).

Anthropometric criteria used for admission should be followed for discharge criteria. If the child had edema on admission then either W/H or MUAC can be used.

## 9.13 HOW EFFECTIVE IS CURRENT MANAGEMENT PROTOCOL

Several studies have reported decline of mortality when WHO recommended protocol was followed.[37-39] In a critical appraisal of inpatient care by Brewster,[40] following eight possible measures have been suggested to improve treatment outcome.

1. Use of low lactose, low osmolality milk feeds during the early stage of treatment

**Box 9.3 Discharge from Nutrition Rehabilitation Center when Community based Program is not available**

*Child*
- Edema has resolved
- Child has satisfactory weight gain for 3 consecutive days (>5 g/kg/day)
- All infections and other medical complications have been treated
- Child has received micronutrients supplementation for 10–14 days
- Immunization is updated
- Child is eating an adequate amount of food

*Mother/caregiver*
- Knows how to prepare energy dense foods and how to feed the child
- Knows how to give prescribed medications, vitamins, folic acid and iron at home
- Knows how to make appropriate toys and play with the child
- Knows how to give home treatment for diarrhea, fever and acute respiratory infections, and how to recognize danger signs for which medical assistance must be sought
- Follow-up plan is discussed and understood

*Failure to Respond (in NRC)*

| Criteria | Approximate time after admission |
|---|---|
| • Failure to regain appetite | Day 4 |
| • Failure to start losing edema | Day 4 |
| • Edema still present | Day 10 |
| • Failure to gain atleast 5 g/kg/day for 3 successive days after feeding freely on catch up diet. | |

*After discharge from NRC each child must come for follow up visit every fortnightly (15 days) for 2 months in the NRC.*

especially in HIV-exposed infants and diarrheal cases;

2. More cautious use of high carbohydrate loads (ORS, ReSOMal, 10% dextrose);

3. More careful grading up and down of feed volumes according to the child's responses during the early rehabilitation phase;

4. Rapid rehydration of children in shock with Ringer's lactate with closer monitoring for heart failure;

**Table 9.8 Failure to Respond to Treatment**

| | Time |
|---|---|
| *Primary failure* | |
| Failure to regain appetite | Day 4 |
| Failure to start to loose edema | Day 4 |
| Edema still present | Day 10 |
| *Secondary failure* | |
| Failure to gain at least 5 gm/kg of body weight per day during rehabilitation for 3 successive days. | |

**Box 9.4 Discharge from Nutrition Rehabilitation Center when Community Based Program is Functioning**

Where Community Based Care Program is well functional, child should be transferred from the facility care to community based care if following criteria is fulfilled:

- Child has completed antibiotic treatment
- Medical condition resolved/stabilized
- Has good appetite (eating at least 120-130 cal/kg/day)
- Has good weight gain ( at least 5 g/kg/day for three consecutive days) on exclusive oral feeding
- No edema
- Caretakers sensitized to home care and education through counseling sessions has been completed
- Immunization is up-to-date

After discharge from CSAM, each child must be followed up in the community for four times—after 15 days; 1 month; 3 months; and 6 months of discharge.

5. Greater use of third generation cephalosporin and fluoroquinolones antibiotics to treat sepsis owing to resistant organisms;

6. Consider adding glutamine-arginine as gut protective agents in addition to zinc and vitamin A;

7. The addition of phosphate to existing potassium and magnesium supplements for those at risk of refeeding syndrome;

8. Introduce better tools for diagnosis and improving management of HIV-tuberculosis co-infected children.

## CONCLUSIONS

Facility based care has a definite place in management of children with severe acute malnutrition. In presence of community based management also; 10–15% with medical complications or poor appetite will require inpatient care. Adherence to WHO recommended 10 steps decreases mortality significantly in these children.

## References

1. UNICEF, WHO, World Bank. UNICEF-WHO-World Bank Joint child malnutrition estimates. New York, Geneva and Washington DC:UNICEF, WHO & World Bank;2012.

2. Raykar M, Majumder M, Laxminarayan R, Menon P. India Health Report: Nutrition 2015, New Delhi, India: Public Health Foundation of India; 2015.

3. Management of Severe Acute Malnutrition: A manual for physicians and other senior health workers. Geneva; World Health Organization; 1999.

4. Guidelines for Inpatient Treatment of Severely Malnourished Children. Geneva:World Health Organization; 2003.

5. Ashworth A. Efficacy and effectiveness of community-based treatment of severe malnutrition. Food Nutr Bull. 2006;27(suppl):S24–48.

6. Prudhon C1, Prinzo ZW, Briend A, Daelmans BM, Mason JB. Proceedings of the WHO, UNICEF, and SCN Informal Consultation on Community-Based Management of Severe Malnutrition in Children. Food Nutr Bull. 2006;27(3 Suppl):S99–104.

7. Sandige H, Ndekha MJ, Briend A, Ashourn P, Manary MJ. Home-based treatment of malnourished Malawian children with locally produced or imported ready-to-use food. J Pediatr Gastroenterol Nutr. 2004;39:141–6.

8. Ministry of Health and Family Welfare, Government of India. Operational guidelines on facility-based management of children with severe acute malnutrition. New Delhi:National Rural Health Mission, Ministry of Health and Family Welfare; 2011.

9. WHO. Guideline: Updates on the Management of Severe Acute Malnutrition in Infants and Children. Geneva: World Health Organization; 2013.

10. Bhatnagar S, Lodha R, Choudhury P, Sachdev HPS, Shah N, et al. IAP Guidelines 2006 on hospital based management of severely malnourished children. Indian Pediatr. 2007;44:443–61.

11. Dalwai S, Choudhury P, Bavdekar SB, Dalal R, Kapil U, et al. Indian Academy of Pediatrics. Consensus Statement of the Indian Academy of Pediatrics on integrated management of severe acute malnutrition. Indian Pediatr. 2013;50:399–404.

12. Ashworth A, Chopra M, McCoy D, Sanders D, Jackson D, Karaolis N, *et al*. WHO guidelines for management of severe malnutrition in rural South African hospitals: effect on case fatality and the influence of operational factors. The Lancet. 2004;363:1110–15.

13. Schofield C, Ashworth A. Why mortality rates for severe malnutrition remained so high? Bull WHO. 1996;74:223–9.

14. Government of Madhya Pradesh. Facility-based Management of Children with Severe Acute Malnutrition.Madhya Pradesh:National Rural Health Mission, Integrated Child Development Scheme and UNICEF;2014.

15. Ahmed T, Ali M, Ulla MM. Mortality in severely malnourished children with diarrhea and use of a standardized management protocol. Lancet. 1999;353:1919–22.

16. Alam S, Afzal K, Maheshwari M, Shukla I. Controlled trial of hypo-osmolar versus World Health Organization oral rehydration solution. Indian Pediatr.2000;37:952–60.

17. Alam NH, Islam S, Sattar S, Monira S, Desjeux JF. Safety of rapid intravenous rehydration and comparative efficacy of 3 oral rehydration solutions in the treatment of severely malnourished children with dehydrating cholera. J Pediatr Gastroenterol Nutr. 2009;48:318–27.

18. Dutta P, Mitra U, Datta A, Niyogi SK, Dutta S, *et al*. Impact of zinc supplementation in malnourished children with acute watery diarrhoea. J Trop Pediatr. 2000;46:259–63.

19. Alam NH, Hamadani JD, Dewan N, Fuchs GJ. Efficacy and safety of a modified oral rehydration solution (ReSoMaL) in the treatment of severely malnourished children with watery diarrhea. J Pediatr. 2003;143:614–19.

20. Kumar R, Kumar P, Aneja S, Kumar V, Rehan HS. Safety and efficacy of low-osmolarity ORS vs. modified rehydration solution for malnourished children for treatment of children with severe acute malnutrition and diarrhea: A randomized controlled trial. J Trop Pediatr. 2015;61:435–41.

21. Maitland K, Kiguli S, Opoka RO, Engoru C, Olupot-Olupot P, *et al*. Mortality after fluid bolus in African children with severe infection. N Engl J Med. 2011;364:2483–95.

22. WHO ETAT Guidelines. Emergency Triage and Treatment. Geneva: World Health Organization; 2016.

23. Memon Y, Majeed R, Ghani MH, Shaikh S. Serum electrolytes changes in malnourished children with diarrhoea. Pak J Med Sci. 2007;23:760–64.

24. Williams AF. Pediatric Nutrition. *In:* The Nutrition Society Textbook Series, Clinical Nutrition. United Kingdom: Blackwell Publishing; 2005. p.378–411.

25. Alleyne GAO. Studies on total body potassium in malnourished infants. Factors affecting potassium repletion. Br J Nutr. 1970;24:205–12.

26. Manary MJ, Brewster DR. Potassium supplementation in kwashiorkor. J Pediatr Gastroenterology Nutr. 1997;24:194–201.

27. Khallil MI, Baki AA, Akhter N, Azad M, Zafreen F, *et al*. Magnesium Supplementation of children with severe protein energy malnutrition. JAFMC Bangladesh. 2008;4:10–13.

28. Zieve L. Role of cofactors in the treatment of malnutrition as exemplified by magnesium. Yale J Bio Med. 1975;48:229–37.

29. Heinkens GT, Bunn J, Amadi B, Manary M, Chhagan M, *et al*. Case management of HIV infected severely malnourished children: challenges in the area of highest prevalence. The Lancet. 2008;371:1305–7.

30. Bagga A, Tripathi P, Jatan V, Hari P, Kapil A, *et al*. Bacteriuria and urinary tract infections in malnourished children. Pediatr Nephrol. 2003; 18:366–70.

31. Imdad A, Yakoob MY, Sudfeld C, Haider BA, Black RE, *et al*. Impact of vitamin A supplementation on infant and childhood mortality. BMC Public Health. 2011; 11(Suppl. 3):S20.

32. Stephensen C, Franchi LM, Hernandez H, Campos M, Gilman RH, *et al*. Adverse effects of high-dose vitamin A supplements in children hospitalized with pneumonia. Pediatrics, 1998;101:E3.

33. De Fátima Costa, Caminha M da Silva, Diniz A, Falbo AR, de Arruda IK, Serva VB, de Albuquerque LL, de Freitas Lola MM, Ebrahim GJ *et al*. Serum retinol concentrations in hospitalized severe protein energy malnourished children. J Trop Pediatr. 2008;54:248–52.

34. Ashour M, Salem SI, El- Gadban HM, Elwan NM, Basu TK. Antioxidant status in children with protein-energy malnutrition (PEM) living in Cairo, Egypt. Eur J Clin Nutr. 1999;53:669–73.

35. Donnen P, Sylla A, Dramaix M, Sall G, Kuakuvi N, *et al*. Effect of daily low dose of vitamin A compared with single high dose on morbidity and mortality of hospitalized mainly malnourished children in Senegal: a randomized controlled clinical trial. Eur J Clin Nutr. 2007;61:1393–9.

36. Donnen P, Dramaix M, Brasseur D, Bitwe R, Vertongen F, *et al*. Randomized placebo controlled clinical trial of the effect of a single high dose or daily low doses of vitamin A on the morbidity of hospitalized, malnourished children. Am J Clin Nutr. 1998; 68:1254–60.

37. Bemal C, Velasquez C, Alcaraz G, Botero J. Treatment of severe malnutrition in children: Experience in implementing the World Health Organization guideline in Turbo, Colambia. J Pediatr Gastroenterol Nutr. 2008;46:322–8.

38. Prudhon C, Golden MH, Briend A, Mary JY. A model to standardise mortality of severely malnourished children using nutritional status on admission to therapeutic feeding centres. Eur J Clin Nutr. 1997;51:771–7.

39. United Nations Interagency Group for Child Mortality Estimation. Levels and trends in child mortality. Report 2012. New York:United Nations Children's Fund;2012.

40. Brewster DR. Inpatient management of severe malnutrition: time for a change in protocol and practice. Ann Trop Paediatr. 2011;31:97–107.

# Discharge and Follow-up of Children with Severe Acute Malnutrition

Ajay Gaur

Discharge of children with severe acute malnutrition (SAM) requires a strict vigilance and regular monitoring so that each child could be discharged at the most appropriate time. Both the early and late discharge might be dangerous. As categorization to SAM is based on weight/height less than –3 Z-score, visible severe wasting, mid upper arm circumference less than 11.5 cm, and bilateral pitting edema, discharge criteria should be such that it incorporates all of the above mentioned four criteria. However, discharge also depends upon local and individual circumstances. In a consensus statement of Indian Academy of Pediatrics (IAP) on Severe Acute Malnutrition, it was recommended that management of SAM should not be a stand-alone program; it should be integrated with community management therapeutic programs along with judicious use of therapeutic foods.[1]

## 10.1 CRITERIA FOR DISCHARGE FROM NUTRITION REHABILITATION CENTER

### A. Criteria, when Community based Program for Management of Severe Acute Malnutrition (CSAM) is Available for Ongoing Care

If a community based program (CSAM) is available for management of children with severe acute malnutrition, then children discharged from the nutrition rehabilitation center (NRC) may be shifted to such unit after fulfilling the following criteria:[2-4]

1. Appetite returned to normal (eating at least 75% of therapeutic food);
2. Medical complications resolved;
3. No edema; and
4. Satisfactory weight gain (at least 5 g/kg/day) for at least 3 consecutive days.

All children thus transferred to the CSAM program should be given locally produced therapeutic foods and followed.

### B. Criteria, if CSAM is Not Available

Anthropometric indicators like target weight-for-height or MUAC should not be used as deciding factors for the transfer of child from inpatient to outpatient care, rather this decision should be based on the clinical condition of the child. Before discharging from the facility based care, it should be ensured that the child is clinically well, active and alert, free from medical complications, showing good appetite and weight gain, received immunization up to date, and treated for helminthic infections with albendazole, 200 mg for children aged 12–23 months and 400 mg for children more than 24 months.[2-4] Criteria for discharge from the program are listed in **Box 10.1**. The algorithm for discharge is shown in **Fig. 10.1**.

**Box 10.1 Criteria for Discharging a Child with SAM**

*Child*

1. Achieved weight gain of >15% (target weight) and has satisfactory weight gain for 3 consecutive days (>5 g/kg/day)
2. Edema has resolved
3. Child is eating adequate amount of nutritious food that the mother can prepare at home
4. All infections and other medical complications have been treated
5. Immunization is updated

*Mother/ Caregiver*

1. Knows how to prepare appropriate foods and feed the child
2. Knows how to make toys and play with the child
3. Knows how to give treatment at home for diarrhea, fever, and acute respiratory tract infections
4. Knows how to recognize signs for which they should seek medical assistance
5. Follow up plan has been explained to them

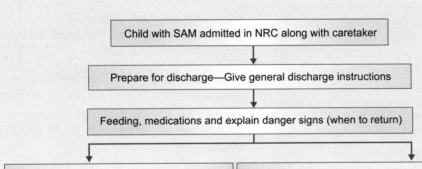

Child with SAM admitted in NRC along with caretaker

Prepare for discharge—Give general discharge instructions

Feeding, medications and explain danger signs (when to return)

**Discharge from NRC—CSAM Program is available:**
1. Appetite returned to normal (eats at least 75% of therapeutic food)
2. Medical complications resolved
3. No edema
4. Satisfactory weight gain (at least 5 g/kg/day) for 3 consecutive days
5. Follow up as per schedule and care at home

**Discharge from NRC – No CSAM Program:**
**For Child:**
1. Achieved weight gain of >15% (target weight) and has satisfactory weight gain for 3 consecutive days (5g/kg/day)
2. Edema has resolved
3. Child is eating adequate amount of nutritious food that the mother can prepare at home
4. All infections and other medical complications have been treated
5. Immunization is updated

**For Mother:**
1. Knows how to prepare appropriate foods and feed the child
2. Knows how to make toys and play with the child
3. Knows how to give treatment at home for diarrhea, fever and acute respiratory tract infections
4. Knows how to recognize signs for which they should seek medical assistance
5. Follow up plan has been explained to them

**Fig. 10.1** Algorithm for discharge and follow up of children with severe acute malnutrition

## C. Merits and Demerits of Using Target Weight Gain

In 2006, IAP proposed guidelines for the hospital based management of severely malnourished children which were adapted from WHO guidelines and recommended that child should be discharged when the weight for height is 90% of the NCHS median.[5] However, as per the WHO guidelines on severe acute malnutrition published in 2009,[6] discharge criteria based only on a minimum weight-for-height are not applicable to programs using mid-upper arm circumference (MUAC) as admission criteria because some children selected using MUAC already fulfil this weight-for height discharge criteria on admission into the program. This is particularly a problem in large scale community programs where MUAC is used rather than weight-for-height for categorizing a child into SAM. So it was recommended that the discharge criterion be based on percentage weight gain because it has the advantage of easy applicability both to children admitted based on MUAC as well as weight for height. It was recommended that for simplicity, 15% weight gain could be used as a discharge criterion. When weight for height is used as an admission criterion, it is advisable to continue to discharge children at weight-for-height −1 Z-score.

For edematous SAM, if after disappearance of edema, weight for height is above −3 Z-score or MUAC above 11.5 cm, discharge after 2 weeks of disappearance of edema is usually sufficient to prevent relapse. However the current evidence fails to support it as it results in the more severely malnourished children getting the shortest duration of treatment and being discharged when still malnourished.[3]

Thus, *WHO in 2013,[7] recommended the following:*

1. A children with severe acute malnutrition should be discharged from treatment when their:
   a. Weight-for-height/length is ≥ −2 Z-score and they have had no edema for at least 2 weeks, or
   b. Mid upper arm circumference is ≥125 mm and they have had no edema for at-least 2 weeks.
2. The same anthropometric indicator that is used to confirm severe acute malnutrition should also be used to assess whether a child has reached nutritional recovery, *i.e.* if mid-upper arm circumference is used to identify that a child has severe acute malnutrition, then mid-upper arm circumference should be used to assess and confirm nutritional recovery.
3. Children admitted with only bilateral pitting edema should be discharged from treatment based on whichever anthropometric indicator, mid upper arm circumference or weight-for-height is routinely used in programs.
4. Percentage weight gain should not be used as a discharge criterion.

## D. Precautions before Discharging a Child of SAM from Facility

1. *Immunization* Before discharge from facility, all children with SAM should be immunized up to the age.
2. *Treatment of helminthiasis* Treatment for helminthiasis should be given to all children with SAM before discharge:
   a. Albendazole 200 mg, single dose, orally for children 12–23 months of age
   b. Albendazole 400 mg, single dose, orally for children aged 24 months or more
3. *General instructions to mother/caregiver* In addition to feeding, following general instructions will need to be given to the mother:
   a. *For how long to continue any needed medication*
      • Folic acid for 2 weeks
      • Micronutrient supplements
      • Iron for 2–3 months at home
   b. *Signs to bring the child back for medical assistance*
      • Not able to drink or breastfeed
      • Stops feeding

- Develops fever
- Breathes fast or difficulty in breathing
- Convulsions
- Diarrhea for more than one day, or
- Blood in stool

## E. What to do if Early Discharge is Unavoidable

If the discharge of a SAM child is unavoidable before reaching −2 Z-score, then it is necessary to make special arrangements for the follow-up of the child. Special visits by health care workers like ASHA, AWW, ANM to the child's home or the visit of the child to a health facility or in the CSAM program must be ensured. Special training should be given to the mother to prepare feeds and regarding supplements like iron, folic acid, and multivitamins at home.

## 10.2 FOLLOW-UP AFTER DISCHARGE

Before discharge, condition of the child and need to follow-up should be discussed with the mother/caregiver. Following written plan should be given to them:

1. Follow-up every 15 days for up to 2 months (four follow-up visits), then
2. Monthly until weight-for-height Z-score reaches −1 or above
3. If any problem arises, visits should be more frequent until it is resolved.

*At each follow-up visit*

1. Child should be examined for medical complications
2. Child should be weighted, MUAC measured, and results should be recorded
3. Mother's should be asked about the child's recent health, feeding practices, and play activities
4. Training of mother should focus on areas that need to be strengthened, especially feeding practices and mental and physical stimulation of the child.

*Follow-up of children discharged before recovery*
A proper plan must be laid out for the child who has been discharged early from the in-patient treatment. Mark the worker that will be responsible for the supervision of the child. Health worker must be appointed to take care of the child at home. A discharge note must be given to the mother/caretaker containing information regarding in-patient treatment, any continuing treatments, child's weight on discharge, feeding recommendations, and measures expected from the health care worker. If there is failure to gain weight over a 2-week period or weight loss between any two measurements, the child should be referred back to hospital.

## 10.3 DISCHARGE CRITERIA FOR A COMMUNITY-BASED THERAPEUTIC CARE (CTC) PROGRAM

For emergencies, CTC approach and manual was designed by the CTC Research and Development Program, in collaboration between Valid International and Concern Worldwide to maximize coverage and access to the treatment of severe acute malnutrition.[8,9]

In practice, this means prioritizing providing care for the majority of the acutely malnourished over inpatient care for a few extreme cases. Three forms of treatment are provided according to the severity of the child's condition:

1. Those with moderate acute malnutrition and no medical complications are supported in a supplementary feeding program (SFP) which provides dry take-home rations (THR) and simple medicines.
2. Those with SAM with no medical complications are treated in an outpatient therapeutic program (OTP), which provides ready to use therapeutic food (RUTF) and routine medicines to treat simple medical conditions.
3. Those who are acutely malnourished and have medical complications are treated in an in-patient stabilization center (SC) until

they are well enough to continue with out-patient care.

## 1. Criteria for Admission to Supplementary Feeding Program (SFP)

Children are admitted to the SFP if they:
- have MUAC<125 mm;
- are less than 80% of median weight-for-height;
- have been discharged from the OTP.

## 2. Criteria for Discharge from the Supplementary Feeding Program

Children are discharged from the SFP when they:
- are more than 85% of median weight-for-height for two consecutive program distributions (for MUAC admissions, a fixed length of stay may be required, as for OTP);
- are non-responding, *i.e.* the child does not reach the target weight after four months of treatment;
- after being discharged from OTP, have received at least two months follow up in the SFP and have been more than 85% of

the median weight-for-height for two consecutive program distributions.

## 3. Outcome of Outpatient Therapeutic Program

A child, after gone through the OTP, can be labelled as discharged cured, defaulted, not cured, or transferred to inpatient care. These terms are defined in **Table 10.1**.

*Modifications to admission and discharge criteria in the absence of SFP.* In these situations, admission and/or discharge criteria of OTP may be increased. Admission criteria can be increased to MUAC 115 mm to ensure that children at risk are identified and to prevent further decline. Discharge criteria can also be increased to a longer minimum length of stay (or 85% of median weight-for-height where national guidelines require), in order to ensure recovery and avoid readmission.

## 4. Discharge Criteria from a Stabilization Center

The child is discharged from a stabilization center (SC) when the appetite has returned (eats at least 75% of RUTF); medical

**Table 10.1** Outcome Definitions of an Outpatient Therapeutic Program for SAM[8]

| | |
|---|---|
| Discharged cured | Minimum stay of two months* in the program, MUAC >115 mm, no edema for two consecutive weighing, sustained weight gain** and clinically well.*** |
| Defaulted | Absent for three consecutive weeks |
| Died | Died during time registered in OTP |
| Transferred to inpatient care | Condition has deteriorated and requires inpatient care |
| Non-cured | Has not reached discharge criteria within four months.**** |

\* All OTP discharges should be sent to the SFP where they stay for a minimum of two months (longer if they have not attained the SFP discharge criteria by that time).

\*\* Sustained weight gain is a gain in weight every week for two consecutive weeks.

\*\*\* Where national guidelines require the use of WHM for admission, discharge should be when the child reaches 80% weight for height and no edema for two consecutive weighing and is clinically well.

\*\*\*\* Before this time, children must have been followed-up at home and should be transferred to SC inpatient care for investigations where possible. Discharged non-cured children should be sent to the SFP; they can be readmitted to the OTP if they fulfil entry criteria again and are therefore once more at high risk of mortality. No child should be discharged as non-cured if their MUAC is still <110 mm.

complications are controlled; and the edema is resolving, eating 75% of the RUTF ration would provide the child with the minimum requirement of 150 kcal/kg/day. When a medical condition is chronic, the symptoms should be controlled by giving appropriate medical treatment in the outpatient setting.

## 5. Exit Indicators

Indicators for exiting the CTC program[9] provide information about the proportion of patients completing the treatment successfully or not successfully (recovered, defaulter, death). They are calculated as a percentage of the total number of exits (discharges) during the reporting month.

- *Recovery (or cured) rate:* Number of beneficiaries that have reached discharge criteria within the reporting period divided by the total exits.
- *Defaulter rate:* Number of beneficiaries that defaulted during the reporting period divided by the total exits. Defaulter will be a child with SAM admitted to the ward but absent (from the ward) for three consecutive days without been discharged.
- *Non-respondent:* This exit category includes those beneficiaries who fail to respond to the treatment *e.g.* the patient remains for a long period of time under the target weight.

## 6. Fixed Length of Stay Discharge Criteria

Adherence to stringent technical standards, service delivery, and the achievement of high coverage takes precedence over individual responses to the delivered intervention. From this perspective, it may be reasonable to adopt a fixed length of treatment for CTC programs. In such programs, patients admitted with edema but with a weight-for-height percentage of median above 80% are, typically, retained in the program for a fixed period after loss of edema. Preliminary analysis of data from CTC programs in Malawi and Ethiopia suggests that an episode length of 60 days would result in approxi-mately 50% of discharges achieving at least a 15% weight gain at discharge.[9]

## 7. Follow-up

Children's progress is monitored on a weekly basis at the program site. It can also be monitored for particular cases, where required, through visits by outreach workers or volunteers, so that issues can be discussed in the home environment. In some cases, follow-up is called for to check whether a child should be referred back to the clinic between visits and to discuss aspects of the home environmentthat may be affecting the child's progress in the OTP.

## 10.4 FOOD AND NUTRITION TECHNICAL ASSISTANCE (FANTA) PROJECT DISCHARGE CRITERIA

Food and Nutrition Technical Assistance Project (FANTA)[10] strengthens nutrition and food security policies, strategies, programs and systems in developing countries. FANTA collaborates with national governments, non-governmental organizations, and other partners on a wide range of food and nutrition related activities. The FANTA module provides an orientation to inpatient care for the management of severe acute malnutrition with medical complications. It also covers admission and discharge processes and criteria as well as the basic principles of medical treatment and nutrition rehabilitation. When a child having SAM is ready for discharge from in-patient to out-patient care in a FANTA project facility, following steps must be undertaken:

1. Clinical status, bilateral pitting edema, mid-upper arm circumference (MUAC), weight, and height must be assessed and appetite must be tested with ready-to-use therapeutic food (RUTF). RUTF has been introduced gradually in the past days and the child is expected to eat more than 75% of its daily diet with RUTF.
2. The out-patient referral slip must be completed, providing a summary of the

medical interventions and treatment given to the child.

3. Mother/caretaker must be informed about the follow-up day and date to the nearest out-patient care and must be given sufficient RUTF (at-least of 1 week duration).
4. Measures about basic hygiene and use of RUTF must be discussed with the mother/ caregiver. She should also be given instructions regarding the use of remaining medications.
5. Child must not be kept waiting for transition from in-patient to out-patient facility. It should be done as early as the condition of child permits.
6. She should be informed about the danger signs and what she should do if they occur before the next follow-up session.

Discharge criteria from in-patient to out-patient care are listed in **Table 10.2**.

## 10.5 IMNCI DISCHARGE CRITERIA FOR SEVERE ACUTE MALNUTRITION

Integrated Management of Childhood illness (IMCI) guidelines for management of the child with serious infection or severe malnutrition in 2000[11] proposed that a child who is having 90% of weight for length (equivalent to −1 Z-score) can be considered to have recovered. The child is likely to have low weight for age because of stunting.Children with SAM must be discharged only when full recovery is ensured, to prevent relapse and death after discharge. However sometimes early discharge is inevitable. Such children will need continuing care as an out-patient to complete rehabilitation and prevent relapse.

### 1. Criteria for Discharge before Completion of Recovery

Early discharge may be considered if some effective alternative supervision is available. Home treatment may be considered only on the fulfilling of the following criterion:

*For child*
  i. age 12 months or more;
  ii. has completed antibiotic treatment;
  iii. has good appetite;
  iv. has good weight gain;
  v. edema lost if previously present; and
  vi. completed 2 weeks of potassium, magnesium, vitamin and minerals supplements.

*For mother/caretaker*
  i. not employed outside the home;
  ii. received sufficient training on appropriate feeding regarding type, amount and frequency;
  iii. financially capable to feed the child; and

| Table 10.2 Discharge Criteria of SAM in FANTA Project[10] | |
|---|---|
| *Children 6–59 months* | *Criteria for discharge* |
| 1. Children referred to in-patient care because of medical complications | 1. Pass RUTF appetite test<br>2. Medical complications resolved<br>3. Bilateral pitting edema decreasing<br>4. Clinically well and alert |
| 2. Children referred to in-patient care because of Marasmic-Kwashiorkar | 1. Bilateral pitting edema resolved<br>2. Pass RUTF appetite test<br>3. No medical complications<br>4. Clinically well and alert |
| 3. Children whose mother/ caregiver choose in-patient care over out-patient care or whose medical condition requires prolonged hospitalization | 1. Child stays in the in-patient care till the mother-care giver is confident enough to take care of the child in out-patient care or until regains his full weight.<br>2. Discharge criteria are same as above |

iv. ready to follow the instructions or advice given.

*Local health workers:* Must be trained to provide domiciliary care.

## 2. Care of Children at Home After Discharge

Energy dense and protein rich meals must be given to children who are being treated at home. Following considerations must be ensured:

1. At-least 150 kcal/kg/day and protein intake of at least 4 g/kg/day must be aimed.
2. Feeding the child at least 5 times per day with food items containing at least 100 kcal and 2–3 grams of protein per 100 grams of food.
3. Home based food items should be used with simple modifications.
4. Appropriate quantity and quality of foods should be given at least 5 times daily.
5. High energy snacks like milk, banana, bread, biscuits should be given between meals.
6. Child should be encouraged and assisted in completion of each meal.
7. Child should be asked to eat separately so that his intake could be checked.
8. Required electrolytes and micronutrient supplements should be provided.
9. Breastfeeding should be continued as long as child wants.

## 10.6 THE INDIAN EVIDENCE

In India, a study was conducted in Bihar on the community based management of SAM children to report the characteristics and outcome of 8274 children of SAM, treated between February 2009 and September 2011.[12] Between February 2009 and June 2010, the program admitted children with a weight-for-height Z-score (WHZ) <–3 and/or mid-upper arm circumference (MUAC) <110 mm and discharged those who reached a WHZ >–2 and MUAC >110 mm. These variables changed in July 2010 to admission on the basis of an MUAC <115 mm and discharge at an MUAC ≥120 mm. In this study, uncomplicated SAM cases were treated as outpatients in the community by using a WHO-standard, ready-to-use, therapeutic lipid-based paste produced in India whereas complicated cases were treated as inpatients by using F-75/F-100 WHO-standard milk until they could complete treatment in the community.

It was observed that out of 3873 children admitted under the old criteria, 41 children (1.1%) died, 2069 children (53.4%) were discharged as cured, and 1485 children (38.3%) defaulted. Out of 4401 children admitted under the new criteria, 36 children (0.8%) died, 2526 children (57.4%) were discharged as cured, and 1591 children (36.2%) defaulted. For children discharged as cured, the mean (±SD) weight gain and length of stay were 4.7 ± 3.1 and 5.1 ± 3.7 g and 8.7 ± 6.1 and 7.3 ± 5.6 wk under the old and new criteria, respectively (P < 0.01).[12] This study showed that the introduction of MUAC<115 mm and/or edema as sole admission criteria resulted in higher number of admissions and it also lead to lower threshold severity, with the result that more children were included who are at lower risk of death and have a smaller WHZ deficit to correct than children identified with old criteria. This has lead to early recovery and discharge. Moreover increased emphasis on ASHA training and involvement could be an effective step towards decreasing defaulter rate and increasing follow up.

Another study was conducted in Uttar Pradesh, India,[13] to study the output indicators of a nutrition rehabilitation center to assess its performance on 182 children of SAM between 6 and 59 months of age. It found that the recovery rate, death rate, defaulter rate, mean (SD) weight gain and mean (SD) duration of stay in the nutritional rehabilitation center were 68%, 2.2%, 4.4%, 13.0 (9.0) g/kg/d, 12.7 (6.8) days, respectively.[13] This study came out with the fact that a high number of incomplete follow up could be because of discharge of patients on request or other social regions, which could be reduced with the involvement of ASHA (accredited social health activist) and ANM (auxilliary nurse midwife). Also NRCs should be attached with the community health schemes for proper management and follow-ups.

## 10.7 LINKING ICDS WITH THE COMMUNITY-BASED THERAPEUTIC CARE

The Government of India has initiated a linkage between the community based care Programs for undernourished children under 6 years of age and ICDS program via *Sneha Shivir* approach, which is a community based approach for the prevention and management of moderate and severe acute malnutrition.[14] Sneha Shivir has been introduced in 200 high burden districts of the country and is to be served through an additional Anganwadi Worker/Nutrition Counsellor at the anganwadi center. Key interventions of *Sneha Shivirs* organized during the 12 day session would largely include the following:

- Selection of moderate and severe undernourished children (preferably not more than 15 per AWC/cluster);
- Orientation of mothers and caregivers of selected children;
- Weight monitoring of the selected children;
- Deworming of these children;
- Ensure iron folic acid administration and complete immunization for these children;
- 12 day hands-on practice sessions for mothers and caregivers to promote improved feeding and child care practices;
- Recording of weight on first day, 12th day and after 18 days;
- Theme based education using IEC on feeding, health, hygiene, and psychosocial care on each of the 12 days, using mother child protection card package;

*Health check-up and referral services;*
- 18 days home based practices;
- Repeat of session for each child till child becomes normal; and

- Monitoring progress-child-wise, AWC-wise as well as at the block and district levels.

Such linkages between ICDS and community based care programs would result in better growth monitoring of SAM and SAM children and will keep a check over these children before they would land up in SAM again. A detailed description of SnehaShivir and other similar initiatives is provided in Chapter 16.

## REFERENCES

1. Dalwai S, Choudhury P, Bavdekar SB, *et al.* Consensus Statement of the Indian Academy of Pediatrics on integrated management of severe acute malnutrition. Indian Pediatr. 2013;50:399–404.
2. National Health Mission, Madhya Pradesh (India). Facitity-based Management of Children with Severe Acute Malnutrition. Training of Medical Officers/ Staff Nurses Participant Manual. National Health Mission, Madhya Pradesh (India); 2014.
3. Kumar P, Singh P. Severe Acute Malnutrition. *In*: Gupta P, Menon PSN, Ramji S, Lodha R. PG Textbook of Pediatrics. 1st ed. Vol 1; New Delhi: Jaypee; 2015.p. 841–48.
4. Ministry of Health and Family Welfare, Government of India. Operational guidelines on facility based management of children with severe acute malnutrition. National Rural Health Mission. New Delhi, India: Ministry of Health and Family Welfare; 2011.
5. Bhatnagar S, Lodha R, Choudhury P, *et al.* IAP guidelines 2006 on hospital based management of severely malnourished children. Indian Pediatr. 2007;44:443–61.
6. World Health Organization (WHO). WHO child growth standards and identification of severe acute malnutrition in infants and children. A joint statement by the World Health Organization and the United Nation Children's Fund. Geneva: World Health Organization; 2009.
7. World Health Organization (WHO). WHO Guidelines Approved by the Guidelines Review Committee. Guidelines Updates on the Management of Severe Acute Malnutrition in Infants and Children. Geneva: World Health Organization; 2013.
8. Community based Therapeutic Care (CTC) Research and Development Program. Community

based Therapeutic Care (CTC): A Field Manual. Oxford, UK: Valid International; 2006.

9. Collins S, Sadler K, Dent N, Khara T, Guerrero S, Myatt M *et al.* Key issues in the success of community-based management of severe malnutrition. Technical background paper. Geneva: World Health Organization; 2005;42–9.

10. Inpatient care for the management of SAM with Medical Complications in the context of CSAM. Module-5, Community Based Management of Acute malnutrition: FANTA Project; 2008. Available from:http://www.fantaproject.org/sites/default/files/resources/CSAM_Training_Mod5_ENGLISH_Nov2008.pdf. Accessed: on 15 August 2016.

11. World Health Organization (WHO). Management of the Child with a Serious Infection or Severe Malnutrition: Guidelines for care at the first referral level in developing countries. Department of Child and Adolescent Health and Development. Geneva: World Health Organization; 2002.

12. Burza S, Mahajan R, Marino E, Sunyoto T, Shandilya C, Tabrez M *et al.* Community-based management of severe acute malnutrition in India: new evidence from Bihar. Am J Clin Nutr. 2015;101:847–59.

13. Maurya M, Singh DK, Rai R, Mishra PC, Srivastava A. An experience of facility-based management of severe acute malnutrition in children aged between 6-59 months adopting the World Health Organization Recommendations. Indian Pediatr. 2014;51:481–3.

14. Ministry of Women and Child Development, Government of India. Integrated Child Development Services (ICDS) Scheme. Available from: http://icds-wcd.nic.in/icds/icds.aspx. Accessed on 29 September 2016.

# Severe Acute Malnutrition in Infants Less than 6 Months Age

AK Rawat

## 11.1 INTRODUCTION

Severe acute malnutrition (SAM) is increasingly being recognized in infants who are less than 6 months of age.[1] The velocity and intensity of growth, development, and maturation is maximum during first six months of life. Neurodevelopment in young infancy is especially sensitive to undernutrition. Severe acute malnutrition in infants less than 6 months will thus affect their future physical, social, and mental development. There are fundamental differences in criteria for identification, admission criteria, and management protocol due to physiological differences between young infants and older children. These differences justify separate management of severe acute malnutrition in infants less than 6 months of age.[2,3]

### Diagnosis

An infant less than 6 months is having SAM if his/her weight-for-length is <–3 Z-score or has bilateral pitting edema without any other cause. For infants whose length is less than 45 cm, presence of visible severe wasting is alone sufficient for the diagnosis of severe acute malnutrition.[4] *Mid-upper arm circumference, used as one of the criteria for diagnosis of SAM in children between 6 and 59 months, is not used as a diagnostic criterion for SAM in children younger than 6 months.*

## 11.2 BURDEN OF SEVERE ACUTE MALNUTRITION IN INFANTS LESS THAN 6 MONTHS

Infants less than six months of age have a target diet of exclusive breastfeeding and since exclusive breastfeeding provides adequate nutrition and protection against infection, there is a misconception that severe acute malnutrition is rare in children less than six months of age. As per estimates, approximately 4.7 million infants under 6 months of age worldwide are moderately wasted and 3.8 million are severely wasted.[2]

Patwari, *et al.*[3] in a recent study,reported the secondary analysis of National Health and Family Survey-3 to compare the prevalence of wasting, stunting, and underweight in infants less than 6 months and 6–59 months. The prevalence of wasting was higher (31%) in infants less than 6 months as compared with children between 6 and 59 months. Thirteen per cent of infants less than 6 months had severe wasting, 30% were underweight, and 20% were stunted. Most infants (69%) were exclusively breastfed for the first 2 months, but exclusive breastfeeding dropped to 50% at 2–3 months and to 27% at 4–5 months. There was no statistically significant difference in wasting and stunting in the exclusively breastfed infants and not exclusively breastfed groups.[3]

## 11.3 RISK FACTORS

Factors ranging from underlying infant disease to poor maternal physical or mental health, and social factors can contribute to malnutrition in infants younger than 6 months. Episodes of common childhood illnesses also influence the nutritional intake and increase the risk of undernutrition. Important factors operating at various levels for instigating nutritional deficit in infants younger than 6 months are described below:[4]

1. *Low birth weight and/or fetal malnutrition at birth.* Preterm newborns are too weak to suckle, unable to stimulate breastmilk production and get inadequate nutrition. Additionally, their requirement is high to meet catch-up growth.

2. *Non-availability of breastmilk due to illness or death of mother or any other reason.* Such newborns are prone to poor weight gain, diarrhea, pneumonia, and sepsis; and some of them may develop SAM, particularly if they were born premature or with low birth weight.

3. *Infections* increase susceptibility to SAM due to decreased intake and increased demand of nutrients.

4. *Inappropriate feeding practices* have significant role in malnutrition. These may consist of delay in initiation or infrequent breastfeeding. Early initiation of animal milk or other food items will predispose to infections and lead to decreased suckling efforts, resulting in decreased breastmilk production.

5. *Intrauterine infections*, congenital malformations, and systemic diseases may also predispose to SAM in young infants.

## 11.4 PRINCIPLES OF MANAGEMENT

Infants less than 6 months have problems in thermoregulation, and have immature renal and gastrointestinal functions as compared to those of older children. Clinical signs of infection and hydration status may also be more difficult to identify and interpret in the younger infant. As a result, criteria for admitting and discharging infants with severe acute malnutrition have not been adequately defined. There are also differences in management protocol.

## 1. Initial Evaluation

Temperature and vitals should be immediately recorded in each infant. After triaging and managing emergency signs, history and examination should be completed. As described earlier, risk factors and causes of severe acute malnutrition are predominantly related to maternal health, antenatal, natal, and postnatal events. Hence it is important to record age of mother, educational and socioeconomic status, living conditions, house environment, drinking water source, access to toilets, and occupations of parents. General health and any short or long-term illness (TB, HIV) in mother, number of antenatal checkup, iron and folic acid supplementation should also be recorded. Detailed feeding history including assessment of attachment and positioning (while breastfeeding) is required. The presenting complaints and relevant clinical examination of the infant should also be recorded. An Indian study has reported acute diarrhea (35.2%) as the most common presenting complaint in young infants presenting with SAM, followed by complaint of failure to gain weight (26.9%).[5]

## 2. Admission Criteria for Inpatient Care

Ministry of Health and Family Welfare, Government of India guidelines and earlier WHO guidelines recommended admission and inpatient care for all infants less than 6 months.[4,6] However, during last few years, arguments have been raised against these recommendations,[7] because infants with uncomplicated SAM may run an unnecessary risk of acquiring infection, if hospitalized. Moreover, mother and caregivers are often reluctant for inpatient care. Loss of family-wages during hospitalization is another factor

**Box 11.1 Revised Guidelines for Hospitalization in Infants <6 months with Severe Acute Malnutrition**

Infants who are less than 6 months of age with severe acute malnutrition and any of the following complicating factors should be admitted for inpatient care:

- Any serious clinical condition or medical complication
- Recent weight loss or failure to gain weight and who have not responded to nutrition counseling and support
- Ineffective feeding (attachment, positioning and suckling) directly observed for 15–20 min, ideally in a supervised separated area
- Any pitting edema
- Any medical or social issue needing more detailed assessment or intensive support (e.g. disability, depression of the caregiver, or other adverse social circumstances).

that may hinder and defer hospitalization by the family. Therefore WHO has suggested to change the admission criteria for these infants, as outlined in **Box 11.1**.

### 3. Community Based Management for Uncomplicated SAM

During last 10 years, management of children aged 6–59 months with SAM has seen major change in management with introduction of community-based management for children with severe acute malnutrition (CSAM) without medical complications and having good appetite. However key intervention of CSAM program i.e., ready to use therapeutic food (RUTF) is not applicable for infants less than 6 months.[7,8] World Health Organization in its 2013 update recommends that uncomplicated severe acute malnutrition in infants less than 6 months should be recognized and outpatient treatment should be offered as first line of treatment. Feeding needs to be supported by the community health workers. This outpatient approach is believed to be more practical, more acceptable to families, is likely to decrease risk of nosocomial infections, and decrease cost of treatment due to long hospital stay.[9]

## 11.5 INPATIENT MANAGEMENT OF SEVERE ACUTE MALNUTRITION FOR CHILDREN < 6 MONTHS AGE

Basic principles of management of infants <6 months with SAM, who have medical complications or poor feeding history, is similar to older children with medical complications or poor appetite. These children should receive same general medical care as older infants and children, i.e. treatment of hypoglycemia, hypothermia, dehydration, electrolyte imbalance, infection, micronutrient supplementation, initiation of feeding, catch-up feeding, sensory stimulation, and discharge. All admitted patients should be given parenteral antibiotics like ampicillin and gentamicin to treat sepsis, micronutrients, **(Box 11.2)** and appropriate treatment for other medical conditions like tuberculosis, HIV etc. However, dietary management of children in this age group is labor intensive and requires a different approach from that needed for older children.

Feeding management may be broadly divided into two categories: (a) For those, with prospects of breastfeeding; and (b) For those, without prospects of breastfeeding.

### 1. Feeding of Infants with Prospects of Breastfeeding

Maternal factors influence the health of the infant in this phase, so it is essential to treat

**Box 11.2 Antibiotics and Micronutrients for Infants <6 months age with SAM**

- Amoxicillin oral 30 mg/kg two times a days (total 60 mg/kg/day) for 5 days; to treat bacterial growth in intestines to infants without medical complications. Injection ampicillin along with an aminoglycoside (gentamicin) should be started in infants with medical complications
- Multivitamin supplements – fat and water soluble are given in amount double of RDA
- Vitamin A 50,000 IU once only (age group 1–6 months)
- Folic acid 5 mg once only
- Ferrous sulfate 1 mg/kg/day (elemental iron) once general condition is stable and weight gain starts

## Box 11.3 Method for Supplementary Suckling Technique (SST)

- The supplementation is given via a No-8 nasogastric tube.
- The tip is cut back beyond the side ports approximately 1 cm.
- Supplemented milk is put in a cup. The mother holds the cup with one hand initially 5–10 cm above the breast. The end of the tube is put in a cup.
- The tip of the tube is put on the breast at the nipple and the infant is offered the breast. Health staff can hold the cup/*katori* and support the mother. It may take one or two days for the infant to get used of the tube and it is important to continue this for few days.
- When the infant sucks on the breast with the tube in mouth, the milk from the cup is sucked up through the tube and taken by the infant.
- The cup/katori is placed **at least 10 cm below** the level of the breast so the milk does not flow too quickly and distress the infant.

technique (SST) which stimulates milk production by stimulating prolactin **(Box 11.3)**.

### Choice of Supplementary Food

For supplementary feed, WHO 2013 update has recommended expressed breastmilk (EBM) as the first choice. If EBM is not available, commercial infant formula, diluted F-100 (volume of 100 mL diluted to 135 mL by adding 35 mL of plain water), or F-75 can be used for infants without edema. The amount of diluted F-100 for different body weights is shown in **Table 11.1**. This recommendation is based on possible adverse effect of high solute load on infant kidney.[11] Once the child is on SST, child weight should be monitored **(Fig. 11.1)**. SST is stopped gradually after satisfactory weight gain is achieved.[12] Infants with SAM and edema should be given infant formula or F-75, if breastmilk is not available.

mother infant pair rather than the infant alone. All possible efforts should be directed towards establishment of exclusive breastfeeding by the mother. Mother and family members should be counseled about advantages of breastfeeding. Infants should be breastfed and mother should be supported during breastfeeding, also support should be given to mother to relactate. If not possible, wet nursing should be encouraged. Breastmilk is stimulated by supplementary suckling

### Tips for Supplementary Sucking Technique

- Before SST the infant is allowed to take breastfeed and then SST is done, this is practiced every 3 hourly for 8 feeds.
- Once weight gain (20 g/day) starts and sustained for 2–3 days, then the amount of F-100D is halved. If weight gain continues for 2–3 days the SST is stopped and is observed for 2–3 days whether weight gain

| Table 11.1 Amounts of EBM/F100 Diluted for Infants on SST | | |
|---|---|---|
| Weight (kg) | Total mL of EBM/F100 diluted | Quantity of EBM/F100 diluted per feed in mL (8 feeds/day) |
| >=1.2 kg | 200 | 25 |
| 1.3 to 1.5 kg | 240 | 30 |
| 1.6–1.7 | 280 | 35 |
| 1.8–2.1 | 320 | 40 |
| 2.2–2.4 | 360 | 45 |
| 2.5–2.7 | 400 | 50 |
| 2.8–2.9 | 440 | 55 |
| 3.0–3.4 | 480 | 60 |
| 3.5–3.9 | 520 | 65 |
| 4.0–4.4 | 560 | 70 |

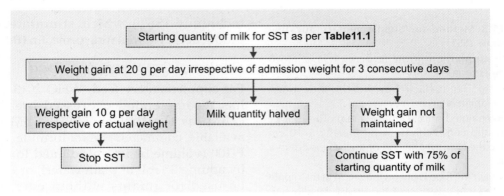

**Fig. 11.1** Decision flow for infants <6 months on supplementary sucking technique (SST)

is sustained or not. If weight gain is not sustained on reducing F-100D then its amount is increased.

- In majority, SST will be successful. If this is not successful in 10–14 days, then the process may be discontinued after counseling mother and families. SST may be continued if mother is willing.

## 2. Feeding of Infants without Prospects of Breastfeeding

One of the biggest challenges is how to support infants who cannot be breastfed because either the mother is dead or is not available for breastfeeding. If there are no realistic prospects of being breastfed, infant should be given appropriate and adequate replacement feeds. WHO recommends F-75

(75 kcal/100 mL) during initiation of treatment phase and therapeutic F-100 diluted (F-100D) during transition and rehabilitation phase by cup **(Table 11.2)**. Indications for nasogastric feeding, routine supplements, and treatment of complications are similar to older children.

*Feeding of Infants who do not Require Inpatient Care or Whose Caregivers Decline for Admission*

The mother or the other caregiver must be counseled and supported for optimal infant and young child feeding, based on general recommendations for feeding infants and young children, including for low-birth-weight infants.[13] It is important to monitor weight gain weekly to observe changes. In

| Weight (kg) | Stabilization phase F-75 (Non Cereal) (mL) | Transition phase F-100 D (mL) | Rehabilitation phase F-100 D (mL) |
|---|---|---|---|
| ≤1.5 | 30 | 30 | 40–50 |
| 1.6–1.8 | 35 | 35 | 45–60 |
| 1.9–2.1 | 40 | 40 | 50–70 |
| 2.2–2.4 | 45 | 45 | 60–80 |
| 2.5–2.7 | 50 | 50 | 70–90 |
| 2.8–2.9 | 55 | 55 | 80–100 |
| 3.0–3.4 | 60 | 60 | 90–110 |
| 3.5–3.9 | 65 | 65 | 100–120 |
| 4.0–4.4 | 70 | 70 | 110–130 |
| 4.5–4.9 | 80 | 80 | 120–140 |

**Table 11.2** Amount of Feed to be Offered to Infants Without Prospects of Breastfeeding

case of weight loss or static weight while the mother or caregiver is receiving support for breastfeeding, then he or she should be referred to inpatient care; it is recommended that assessment of the physical and mental health status of mothers or caregivers should be promoted and relevant treatment or support provided.

## 3. Sensory Stimulation

Due to lack of interaction and play, children with SAM have delayed mental and behavioral development. Play therapy is intended to develop language and motor skills aided by simple, inexpensive toys. It should take place in a loving, relaxed, and stimulating environment. Physical activity should be stimulated as soon as the child is well.

## 4. Health Education of Mothers

All mothers should be educated about feeding and child care practices before discharge. They should be motivated and supported so that they can sustain exclusive breastfeeding till six months of age. Mothers also should be counseled to start appropriate complementary foods when child completes 180 days, and explained the importance of timely immunization and care during common illnesses.

## 5. Discharge Criteria

*Discharge from inpatient Care*

WHO 2013 guidelines suggest that infants who have been admitted to inpatient care can be transferred to outpatient care when:

a. All clinical conditions or medical complications, including edema, are resolved[5]

b. The infant has good appetite, is clinically well and alert,

c. Weight gain on either exclusive breastfeeding or replacement feeding is satisfactory, > 5 g/kg/day for at least 3 successive days,

d. The infant has been checked for immunizations and other routine interventions and

e. Danger signs (when to return) is understood by mother. The danger signs include the following: unable to take feed, vomits everything, convulsions, lethargic or unconscious, high grade fever, and fast breathing

f. The mothers or caregivers are linked with needed community-based follow-up and support like anganwadi.

*Discharge Criteria from All Care*

a. Infant is breastfeeding effectively or feeding well with replacement feeds

b. Infant has adequate weight gain of 15–20% after edema disappears

c. Infant has achieved a weight-for-length ≥–1 Z-score.

## 11.6 PREVENTION

- All efforts should be made in the antenatal period to prevent low birth weight and preterm deliveries.

- Initiation of breastfeeding soon after delivery (not later than 60 minutes) in normal deliveries and as soon as possible in cesarean deliveries.

- Exclusive breastfeeding for 6 months, minimum 8–10 feeds in day and night on demand, alternating breasts in subsequent feeds, and feeding for approximately 20 minutes in each feed.

- Skilled help for mothers having difficulties in breastfeeding or who feel that her milk is not enough.

- Counsel mothers for their own well-being, for diet, and for fluid intake.

- Monitor growth by regular weighing weekly in first month, fortnightly in 2nd month and then monthly till 6 months of age. If at any time the weight is found to be static (beyond 10th postnatal day in full-term, 14 days in preterm infants) or actual weight loss beyond 7th day in full term or 10th day in preterm, assessment should be done to find out cause and it should be corrected.

# References

1. Caballero B. Early nutrition and risk of disease in the adult. Public Health Nutr.2001;4:1335–6.

2. WHO. Guideline: Updates on the Management of Severe Acute Malnutrition in Infants and Children. Geneva: World Health Organization; 2013.

3. Patwari AK, Kumar S, Beard J.Undernutrition among infants less than 6 months of age: an underestimated public health problem in India. Matern Child Nutr. 2015;11:119–26.

4. Kerac M, Blencowe H, Grijalva-EternodC, McGrath M, Shoham J, Cole TJ, Seal A. Prevalence of wasting among under 6-month-old infants in developing countries and implications of new case definitions using WHO growth standards: a secondary data analysis. Arch Dis Child. 2011;96:1008–13.

5. Singh DK, Rai R, Mishra PC, Maurya M, Srivastava A. Nutritional rehabilitation of children < 6 mo with severe acute malnutrition. Indian J Pediatr.2014;81:805.

6. Ministry of Health and Family Welfare, Government of India. Operational guidelines on facility-based management of children with severe acute malnutrition. National Rural Health Mission.New Delhi:Ministry of Health and Family Welfare;2011.

7. Bried A, Maire B, Fontaine O, Garenne M. Mid-upper arm circumference and weight for height to identify high- risk malnourished under-five children. Matern Child Nutr. 2012;8:130–3.

8. Collins S. Treating severe acute malnutrition seriously. Arch Dis Child. 2007;92:453–61.

9. World Health Organization. Relactation: review of experience and recommendations for practice. Geneva:WHO;1998.

10. Stewart RC. Maternal depression and infant growth: a review of recent evidence. Matern Child Nutr. 2007;3:94–107.

11. Hoetjes M, Rhymer W, Matasci-Phelippeau L, van der Kam S. Emerging cases of malnutrition amongst IDPs in Tal Abyad district, Syria. Field Exchange. 2014;48:133–7.

12. Wilkinson C, Isanaka S. Diluted F100 vs infant formula in treatment of severely malnourished infants <6 months. Field Exchange, 2009; 37:8. Available from: http://fex.ennonline.net/37/diluted.aspx.Accessed 5 October 2016.

13. WHO. Infant and Young Child Feeding Counselling: An Integrated Course. Geneva: World Health Organization; 2006.

14. WHO. Severe Malnutrition: Report of a Consultation to Review Current Literature, 6–7 September 2004. Geneva: World Health Organization; 2005.

# Management of Moderate Acute Malnutrition

AK Patwari

## 12.1 DEFINITION

Moderate acute malnutrition (MAM) is defined as "a weight-for-age between −3 and −2 Z-score below the median of the WHO child growth standards without edema" and/or mid-upper arm circumference (MUAC) between 11.5–< 12.5 cm without edema. It can be due to a low weight-for-height (wasting) or a low height-for-age (stunting) or to a combination of both.

In 2010, it was estimated that 55 million preschool-age children were wasted, of whom about 40 million had moderate acute malnutrition (MAM).[1,2] Five years later, the scenario has not improved significantly, with over 90 million children under age five who are underweight.[3]

MAM is a precursor of severe acute malnutrition (SAM) and is associated with a large proportion of nutrition-related deaths. Nutrition programs for the management of MAM in children have remained virtually unchanged for the past 30 years[4] resulting in persistence of morbidity and mortality in under-five children attributable to this disorder, despite tremendous technological advances in last three decades.

This chapter focuses on principles and strategies for management of MAM children and also highlights the community based approach and challenges faced in the management of these cases in low and middle income countries.

## 12.2 BURDEN OF MODERATE ACUTE MALNUTRITION

In low and middle income countries, MAM has been reported to affect around 10% of children under-five years of age. According to the World Health Statistics report,[5] a "global total of 52 million under-five children could be classified as having acute malnutrition in 2012, of which 33 million had MAM. Thus, MAM affects roughly 1 in 10 children under 5 years of age in the least developed countries.[6] Prevalence of MAM (assessed by wasting with weight for height between −2 Z-score and −3 Z-score) in under-five children as of 2013 in 10 most affected countries is depicted in **Table 12.1**.[7] India and Nigeria are the top two countries with highest burden in terms of total number of children with MAM.

### MAM and Under-five Mortality

MAM is an intermediate stage of worsening nutritional status which invariably leads to severe acute malnutrition (SAM) if timely and adequate nutritional support is not provided. It is a potential pathway to death trap indirectly by worsening of a child's nutritional status to SAM or directly in the presence of inter-current serious childhood illnesses. The

**Table 12.1** Prevalence of Moderate Acute Malnutrition (MAM) among Under-five Children (2012)[7]

| Ranked by prevalence (2007-2011) | Country | Year | Number of Children with MAM and SAM | MAM Prevalence (%) |
|---|---|---|---|---|
| 1 | South Sudan | 2010 | 3,38,000 | 23 |
| 2 | India | 2005-2006 | 20 625,461,000 | 20 |
| 3 | Timor-Leste | 2009-2010 | 38,000 | 19 |
| 4 | Sudan | 2010 | 817,000 | 16 |
| 5 | Bangladesh | 2011 | 2,251,000 | 16 |
| 6 | Chad | 2010 | 320,000 | 16 |
| 7 | Pakistan | 2011 | 3,339,000 | 15 |
| 8 | Sri Lanka | 2006-2007 | 277,000 | 15 |
| 9 | Nigeria | 2008 | 3,783,000 | 14 |
| 10 | Indonesia | 2010 | 2,820,000 | 13 |

*Source:* United Nations Children's Fund, World Health Organization, The World Bank, UNICEF-WHO-World Bank Joint Child Malnutrition Estimates, 2013.uploads/2012/07/GHA_Report_2012-Websingle.pdf.

duration of untreated MAM leading to SAM has been reported to be shorter among younger children aged less than 35 months.[8] There is a high risk of reverting back to MAM and even worsening to SAM after successful treatment if not appropriately followed up, resulting in high mortality.[9]

## 12.3 WHAT CAUSES MODERATE ACUTE MALNUTRITION?

Apart from poverty and food crises, the root causes of malnutrition, several triggers related to disruption of food production and distribution networks, faltering of state structures, the absence of basic services, the complete breakdown of public health infrastructure and sanitation systems etc. impact the nutritional status of young children. Rapid loss of weight resulting in wasting is usually a direct impact of combination of infection and feeding on diets that do not satisfy nutritional needs. The main underlying causes of wasting have been outlined in **Box 12.1**.[10]

Wasting has a strong relationship with causes which lead to rapid weight loss. Poor diet leads to weight loss and increased risk of infection. Infection, in turn, adversely affects the nutritional status of the child and this initiates a vicious cycle. A previously healthy

**Box 12.1 Underlying Causes of Moderate Acute Malnutrition**[10]
- "Poor access to appropriate, timely and affordable health care
- Inadequate caring and feeding practices (e.g. failure of exclusive breastfeeding or low quantity and quality of complementary foods)
- Poor food security – not only in humanitarian situations, but also an ongoing lack of food quantity and diversity, characterized in many resource-poor settings by a monotonous diets with low nutrient density, together with inadequate knowledge of patterns of food storage, preparation and consumption
- Lack of a sanitary environment, including access to safe water, sanitation, and hygiene services."

child can quickly become wasted following an episode of severe infection. This is generally associated with loss of appetite. As wasting worsens, children become more susceptible to infections.

Episodes of diarrheal diseases, low birth weight and small for gestational age are the other suggested risk factors for wasting in childhood.

## 12.4 CHALLENGES IN MANAGEMENT OF MODERATE ACUTE MALNUTRITION[11]

1. Despite a large case load and associated mortality risk, MAM is not given the

attention it deserves partly because of lack of consensus on programmatic guidance on case definition, admission and discharge criteria, management approaches, and treatment protocols. Inconsistent definitions also lead to difficulty in evaluation and comparison of effectiveness of the nutritional programs for MAM.

2. Approaches intended to address MAM have predominantly focused on targeted or blanket supplementary feeding. Both are product driven and do not always take in to account the underlying cause of malnutrition. Therefore beneficiaries often have a risk of relapse because underlying reasons may not be addressed.

3. There is a huge evidence gap, related to effectiveness of nutrition counseling (in both facility and community management of MAM), cost effectiveness of various interventions, and appropriate comparison of products. Most of the experience is primarily from Africa with limited data from other settings.

4. There is limited understanding of requirements of various nutrients in children with MAM, who live in unhealthy and insanitary environments.

5. There are several areas with lack of consensus on MAM management protocols e.g. management of MAM and diarrhea, MUAC for monitoring, integration of guidelines with other child health programs, etc.

6. In the management programs there is a deficiency of basic medical treatment guidelines for children who are referred for MAM management.

7. Monitoring and reporting of MAM management data has limitations with a weak link to formal health information systems which is a barrier in analysis of data for the purpose of decision making.

Over the years, approach to nutritional management of children with MAM has remained suboptimum in contrast to children suffering from life-threatening SAM. The key

**Box 12.2 How Management of MAM Differs from SAM[12]**

1. Experiences from management of SAM are not necessarily transferable to MAM. Transferring the same treatment model from SAM to MAM may overburden the healthcare system.

2. Medical and nutritional treatments may differ due to their clinical differences. Moreover, resource implications for supply of specialized supplementary feeding products for MAM might be substantial.

3. Integrating MAM treatment into workload of community health workers (CHW) requires different and broader expertise.

4. Treatment needs to align more closely to prevention as compared to SAM, where the emphasis is on immediate recovery and prevent death.

5. Multi-sector approaches may be needed for the prevention and treatment of MAM.

issues which need to be considered are listed in **Box 12.2**.[12]

## 12.5 PRINCIPLES OF NUTRITIONAL MANAGEMENT OF MAM

Nutritional management of MAM requires to follow certain basic principles on nutritional support in terms of recommended nutrient intakes, quantity, nutrient density, presence of anti-nutrients, supplementary foods, mineral component, and hygiene standards along with essential nutrition actions, counseling, and other activities that identify and prevent underlying causes of malnutrition, including nutrition insecurity. There are summarized in **Box 12.3**.[13]

### 1. Recommended Nutrient Intakes (RNIs)

In order to allow catch-up growth in weight and height in children with MAM it is imperative that Recommended Nutrient Intakes (RNIs) of these children are known. If these requirements are adequately met, deaths resulting from malnutrition can be prevented, their resistance to infection can be strengthened, and convalescence from prior illness and catch up growth can be ensured.

**Box 12.3 Principles of Nutritional Management of MAM[13]**

- Every child needs to receive nutrition of sufficient quality and quantity to enable normal growth and development.
- Management of MAM children between 6–59 months should include essential nutrition actions such as breastfeeding promotion and support, education and nutrition counselling for families, and other activities that identify and prevent underlying causes of malnutrition, including nutrition insecurity.
- Children 6–59 months of age with MAM need to receive nutrient-dense foods to meet their extra needs for weight and height gain and functional recovery.
- Nutrient-dense foods enable children to consume and maximize the absorption of nutrients in order to fulfill their requirements of energy and all essential nutrients. Animal-source foods are more likely to meet the amino acid and other nutrient needs of recovering children. Plant-source foods, in particular legumens or a combination of cereal and legumes, also have high-quality proteins, although they also contain some anti-nutrients such as phytates, tannins or inhibitors of digestive enzymes, which may limit the absorption of some micronutrients, particularly minerals.
- The amonuts of anti-nutrient compounds and naturally occurring toxins, cyanogens, alkaloids or other potentially poisonous or deleterious ingredients can be minimized by using appropriate food-processing methods, such as soaking, germination, malting and fermentation.
- Supplementary foods, particularly when they represent the main source of energy, need to provide nutrients at levels that do not cause adverse efects in MAM children when consumed for several months.
- The amount of supplementary food that needs to be given to a MAM child requires consideration of the availability and nutrient content of the child's habitual diet, including whether the child is being breastfed, the likelihood of sharing of the supplemental food within and beyond the household, and access to other foods.
- The formulation of supplementary food should be safe and effective, particularly where MAM children use this food as their only source of energy.
- The mineral component should be authorized by a regulatory body.
- Hygiene standards should comply with the *Codex Alimentarius* for infant and yound children's food.

Whereas RNIs are set for healthy individuals living in clean environments, there are no generally accepted RNIs for those with moderate malnutrition who live in poor environments.

Two sets of recommendations for nutrient intakes have been proposed **(Table 12.2)**. First are the minimum nutrient requirements for those MAM children who are using appropriately processed locally-available foods[14] and second are the proposed optimum requirements for those children with MAM who require specialized formulations of complementary, supplementary, or rehabilitation foods.[15]

## 1. Choice of Foods and Ingredients

Knowledge pertaining to the nutritional qualities of foods and ingredients considered suitable for nutritional needs of children with

MAM children is important for suggesting cost-effective nutritional interventions, particularly to treat infants and young children with MAM who consume cereal-based diets. It is necessary to know energy density, the nutritional values of the main food groups, the special beneficial qualities of animal-source foods, macronutrient content and quality, minerals and vitamins etc. **Box 12.4** summarizes important characteristics of diets appropriate forchildren with MAM.[11]

## 2. Concept of Anti-nutritional Factors

Food constituents that have a negative impact on the solubility or digestibility of required nutrients and thereby reduce the amounts of bioavailable nutrients and available energy in the foods are considered 'Anti-nutritional'. However, food constituents with anti-nutrient properties may also have beneficial health

**Table 12.2** Proposed Recommended Nutrient Intake (RNI) for Children with Moderate Acute Malnutrition Living in Poor Environments Expressed as Nutrient Energy Densities[11,14,15]

| Nutrient | Unit | Locally available foods | Specially formulated foods | Nutrient | Unit | Locally available foods | Specially formulated foods |
|---|---|---|---|---|---|---|---|
| *Protein* | | | | *Water Soluble Vitamins* | | | |
| Protein | grams | 24 | 26 | Thiamine | mg | 600 | 1000 |
| *Minerals* | | | | Riboflavin | mg | 800 | 1800 |
| Sodium | mg | 550 | 550 | Pyridoxine | mg | 800 | 1800 |
| Potassium | mg | 1400 | 1600 | Cobalamin | mg | 1000 | 2600 |
| Magnesium | mg | 200 | 300 | Folate | mg | 220 | 350 |
| Phosphorous | mg | 600 | 900 | Niacin | mg | 8.5 | 18 |
| Sulphur | mg | 0 | 200 | Ascorbate | mg | 75 | 100 |
| Zinc | mg | 13 | 20 | Pantothenic acid | mg | 2.7 | 3 |
| Calcium | mg | 600 | 840 | Biotin | mg | 10 | 13 |
| Copper | mg | 680 | 890 | *Fat Soluble Vitamins* | | | |
| Iron | mg | 9 | 18 | Retinol | mg | 960 | 1900 |
| Iodine | mg | 200 | 200 | Cholecalci-feral | mg | 7.4 | 11 |
| Selenium | mg | 30 | 55 | Tocopheral | mg | 11.5 | 22 |
| Manganese | mg | 12 | 12 | Phytomena-dione | mg | 20 | 40 |
| Chromium | mg | 0 | 11 | *Essential Fatty Acids* | | | |
| Molybdenum | mg | 0 | 0 | N-6 fatty acid | grams | 5 | 5 |
| | | | | N-3 fatty acid | grams | 0.85 | 0.85 |

**Box 12.4 Recommendations on Diets Suitable for Children with MAM[11]**

- Energy requirements of moderately malnourished children increase in relation to the rate of weight-gain during catch-up growth. Energy requirements also depend on the type of tissue deposition.
- A low weight-gain in relation to energy intake may be due to preferential fat deposition as a result of an inadequate supply of nutrients needed for the accumulation of lean tissue.
- The diets of children recovering from moderate wasting should provide at least 30% of their energy as fat and 10–15% as protein.
- Diets of moderately malnourished HIV-infected children are increased by 20–30% in comparison with those non-HIV-infected children who are growing well. There is no evidence for increased protein requirements in relation to energy; i.e. 10% to 15% of the total energy intake is sufficient, as for non-HIV-infected children with moderate malnutrition.
- The nutritional requirements of moderately malnourished children probably fall somewhere between the nutritional requirements for healthy children and those for children with SAM during the catch-up growth phase.

properties, and the significance of each anti-nutritional factor has to be considered in the context of the specific diets and the specific nutritional problems in a population.

Phytates and polyphenol compounds are two important anti-nutritional food constituent in diets in low-income countries which can have a negative nutritional impact. These compounds inhibit the absorption of proteins and minerals, in particular iron, zinc, and calcium, or lead to complex formation with iron and other metals and cause precipitation of protein, which reduces absorbability. Therefore anti-nutritional properties of food items need to be considered while choosing a combination of food items.

## 3. Dietary Counseling

Dietary counseling of mothers or caregivers of MAM children is the most important component of managing these children. However, dietary counseling alone does not have a significant role in the recovery from MAM.[16] The outcome also depends on who provides dietary counseling and where.

- Results after three months of dietary counseling on "seven basic messages (breastfeeding, good complementary feeding, meal frequency, hand washing, birth spacing, and prenatal nutrition) provided by doctors at home and in clinic and helped by nurses in the clinic, recorded that approximately 50% of the children had moved from MAM to mildly malnourished or well-nourished category."[17]

- Comparison of two nutrition education intervention groups (with and without food supplementation) showed significant improvement in weight-for-age as compared to control group but results within the two intervention groups did not suggest any significant difference implying that the food supplement provided no added benefit.[18]

Though published data regarding the effectiveness of dietary counseling to mothers of moderately malnourished children are limited, the results suggest that weight gain tends to be slow even with counseling interventions. Recurrent infections, associated with poor living conditions and poor appetite during illness, may have an important role to play. Advocacy for improved complementary feeding and for utilizing family foods for catch-up growth remains weak but dietary counseling can be effective when done well.

Frequent, regular exposure to a few simple, uniform, age-appropriate messages, together with an opportunity for interaction between caregiver and counselor, has been found to be beneficial. Counseling of a mother/care taker often needs to be tailored keeping in mind real life situation like competing demands on mothers' time. Therefore it requires significant skill and insight on the part of a counselor to strike a balance between delivering uniform messages and negotiating compromises. But nutrition counseling is often left to minimally trained personnel or volunteers with poor knowledge and communication skills making it difficult to achieve a desired level of success.

## 12.6 PREVENTION AND TREATMENT STRATEGIES

Management of MAM can be broadly categorized into prevention and treatment strategies. Generally, wasting in these children results in a loss of body mass relative to height. Therefore the standard practice has been to provide the child with additional energy and nutrient-dense foods to promote weight gain. The selection of the particular management approach is related to underlying situation and food security.

- *Strategies for prevention* Well known public health strategies including promotion of appropriate breastfeeding and complementary feeding practices, access to appropriate health care for the prevention and treatment of disease, and improved sanitation and hygiene practices, complement efforts to prevent MAM. Multiple-micronutrient powders, small-quantity lipid based nutrient supplementation (LNS), and single-nutrient supplements are used to augment the nutritional content of the home diet.

- *Strategies for treatment* Over the years, emphasis on exploring optimal food-based treatments for MAM has increased.[11] WHO technical note on supplementary foods for managing MAM in children ages 6–59 months calls for "providing locally available, nutrient-dense foods to improve nutritional status and prevent SAM."[13] The guidelines suggest that "an energy intake of 25 kcal/kg/d in addition to the standard nutrient requirements of a non-malnourished child would support a reasonable rate of weight gain without promoting obesity." However, there is no evidence-informed recommendation for the composition of specially formulated foods for treatment.[18]

Strategies for prevention and treatment of MAM also need to consider food security of the population, apart from considering underlying factors responsible for causing MAM. Food security depends upon several factors including seasonal factors.

## 1. Counseling for Food: Secure Populations

In food-secure populations, caregivers can be counseled and supported in using high-quality, home-available foods to promote recovery in acutely malnourished children.[19] This can be coupled with general health-promotion approaches to mitigate the underlying factors contributing to acute malnutrition for example, WASH and health-seeking behaviors. Two systematic reviews[20, 21] find no significant differences in mortality between the provision of any type of specially formulated food and standard care, which consists of medical care and counseling without food supplementation. The mean weight gain was reported to be significantly higher in Ready to Use Therapeutic Food (RUTF) group than in the standard care group in which mothers were taught to prepare a high-calorie cereal milk.[22]

## 2. Counseling for Food: Insecure Populations

Integrated approaches are needed for provision of supplemental food under situations of food insecurity. Under such circumstances it is critical to address the immediate need for an improved diet which can treat MAM and prevent the progression to SAM. It should simultaneously address the underlying factors for causing malnutrition. Livelihood diversification, social protection schemes, and conditional cash transfers are some of the approaches being explored in these contexts.[19]

## 3. Supplemental Feeding Programs

Supplemental feeding programs (SFPs) are generally implemented in food-insecure populations, including humanitarian emergency contexts. The aim in these situations is to reduce mortality and prevent further deterioration of children's nutritional status. These SFPs are classified as targeted SFPs or blanket SFPs, depending on the recipients. Blanket SFP provides supplemental food to everyone within a defined population, regardless of whether children are acutely malnourished while a targeted approach provides supplemental rations only for malnourished children meeting program cut-off criteria.

### Supplemental Foods

The standard practice for SFPs is to provide a ration of staple food, such as fortified blended foods (FBF), commonly Supercereal or Supercereal Plus.[11] However, some of the available RUTFs have been developed specifically for treating MAM. Two commonly used nutritional supplementations are lipid based nutrient supplementation (LNS) and blended foods. Both of these have been tried as a full daily dose or in a low dose given as a complement to the usual diet. Commercially available products containing LNS as well as blended foods are effective in treating children with MAM. Although LNS is reported to have greater weight gains and recovery rate than those treated with locally produced cereal-legume products,[23] it has not resulted in reduction of mortality or risk of default or progression to SAM.[20] Blended foods such as corn soy blend (CSB) +++ may be equally effective and cheaper than LNS.[20, 21] No significant differences were seen when Supercereal Plus was compared with LNS.

However, there are no studies evaluating interventions to improve the quality of home diet (soaking, germination, malting, fermentation), an approach that needs to be evaluated in areas where food is available but cultural habits and lack of awareness about nutrition are the main determinants of malnutrition. MAM is most prevalent in Asia but there are hardly any studies from this region.

## 4. Seasonal Supplementation

Seasonal feeding supplementation programs, aimed at tackling expected increase in malnutrition, provide blanket feeding programs in chronically food-insecure settings. A spike in the incidence of MAM and SAM is seen in these settings in the period before the harvest, known as the "lean season." Seasonal SFPs, include all children who either have, or are at risk for, MAM. The evidence remains limited on the effectiveness or cost-effectiveness of such approaches for prevention. However, RUTF supplementation for non-wasted children has been reported to reduce seasonal increase in prevalence rates of wasting.[24,25] Introduction of one packet of RUTF per day for children in the intervention group led to an estimated 36% difference in the incidence of wasting and a 58 percent difference in the incidence of severe wasting in Niger.[25]

## 12.7 COMMUNITY-BASED MANAGEMENT OF MAM

Management issues peculiar to children with MAM are not clearly understood and therefore standard treatment guidelines are yet to be established because of numerous inconsistent findings pertaining to effectiveness of management approaches.[20,21,25] Low coverage, non-compliance, and high associated costs are some of the limitations of targeted SFPs in emergencies.[25] Therefore, there is a growing interest in developing evidence base for effective interventions for management of children detected to have MAM. Community-based management of acute malnutrition (CMAM), also sometimes known as Community-based Therapeutic Care (CTC) or Integrated Management of Acute Malnutrition (IMAM) is a concept which promotes new management practices.

## CMAM Guidelines

Community-based management of acute malnutrition (CMAM) was primarily introduced to provide care to the majority of children with uncomplicated SAM as outpatients, so as to take care of the inherent limitations in facility-based care. CMAM approach has now also been proposed to prevent and treat MAM and in the process prevent SAM by timely management of MAM at community level. CMAM Forum provides guidelines for diets suitable for children with MAM, approaches to counseling caregivers, and a decision-making framework for selecting appropriate supplementary feeding program (SFP) approaches.[11]

### For Infants below 6 Months of Age with MAM

Exclusive breastfeeding for first 6 months is recommended. These infants are not admitted in to SFPs but managed by providing supplementary food and skilled support to the mothers to enable continued breastfeeding. The infants need to be monitored for weight gain. Lactating mothers of infants with MAM should be admitted to SFP regardless of their own nutritional status. Mothers of infants who have stopped breastfeeding due to any reason should be supported to re-establish exclusive breastfeeding wherever possible.[20]

### Children between 6–59 Months with MAM

They should be managed with CMAM guidelines and some of them need to be included in supplementation depending upon extent of food security. Unlike children suffering from SAM, there is no need to feed highly fortified therapeutic foods to all the children between 6–59 months age detected to have MAM.

Two broad approaches commonly used for community based management of MAM children in this age group focus on (a) dietary counseling to educate families on appropriate feeding practices; and (b) to address the problem of food security.

- *Dietary counseling* This approach is guided by the assumption that the families have access to all foods needed for feeding their children but it is the lack of knowledge and ignorance about how best the available foods can be used.
- *Food insecurity* Insufficient access to nutrient-dense foods can be addressed by providing food supplements, usually fortified blended flours.

However, review of these approaches has revealed that the dietary advice given to families is often nonspecific, *i.e.* not really different from the advice given to well-nourished children. Therefore the impact of nutrition programs focusing on improving nutrition related knowledge and efficacy of supplementary feeding programs using blended flours remains uncertain.[26-28]

## Lack of Efficacy of Nutritional Programs

Low nutritional density of the diets recommended as part of nutritional counseling has been regarded as one of the major reasons to explain the apparent lack of efficacy of some of the nutritional programs. The recommended nutrient-dense foods are generally expensive therefore in actual situations food supplements are usually made with the cheapest sources of energy (cereals) and proteins (legumes) and often have no added fat. Such supplements often have a nutritional profile (high protein, low fat, and high dietary fiber and anti-nutrient content) that does not seem the best adapted to promote rapid growth of malnourished children.[29]

The current understanding is that "children with moderate malnutrition should get the foods that provide all the nutrients they need for full recovery, not just the food choice that represents the cheapest option to provide them energy and proteins. Efficacy of the chosen foods to promote recovery and their accessibility must be the first criteria to consider when making a choice."[30]

The CMAM model integrates community engagement with the treatment of SAM as well as MAM. But despite more than 60 countries implementing CMAM, coverage remains a big constraint, with only 10% of SAM cases able to access treatment. MAM cases also lack access to basic medical treatment and growth monitoring, further emphasizing the need for scaling up CMAM.[11]

## 12.8 DIAGNOSIS AND MANAGEMENT OF MAM

Moderate acute malnutrition can be diagnosed by using weight-for-height Z-scores, measuring mid-upper arm circumference (MUAC), and checking for bilateral pedal edema **(Fig. 12.1)**. Active screening for assessment of nutritional status of children can be done by frontline workers in community/healthcare providers in health facilities using Integrated Management of Neonatal and Childhood illness (IMNCI) guidelines.[31] Passive screening can be done during village health and nutrition days, immunization sessions, and hospital visits.

Nutrition counseling and education, and supplementary feeding are the two essential components of management of MAM.

## 1. Nutrition Counseling and Education

The concept of nutrition counseling and education is expected to be effective in situations where caregivers have access to affordable food but do not have sufficient awareness of how to combine foods into appropriate diets for feeding malnourished or at-risk children. This approach focuses on educating caregivers how to increase dietary diversity and meet nutritional requirements so as to improve feeding practices.

## 2. Supplementary Feeding

Supplementary feeding *i.e.* the provision of specially formulated supplementary foods, has for long been provided to vulnerable children in areas with food insecurity and as a part of emergency food aid interventions to

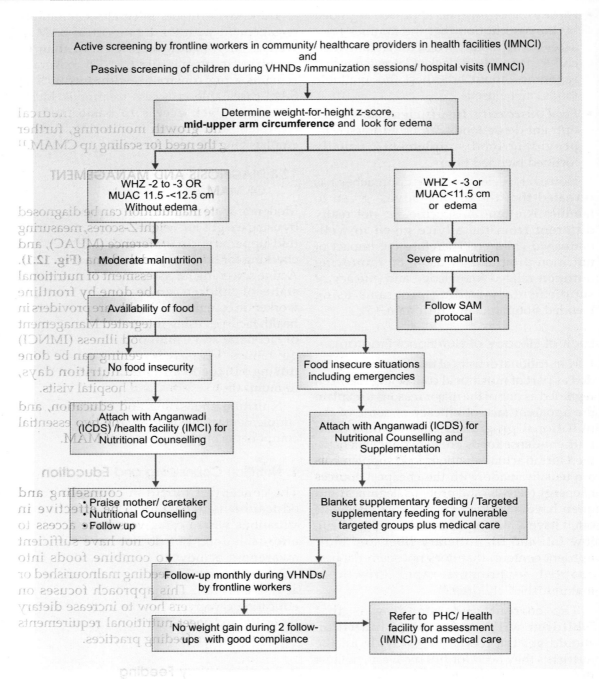

Fig. 12.1 Diagnosis and management algorithm for MAM in Children 6–59 Months

treat moderately malnourished children or to prevent a deterioration of nutrition among at-risk populations. As also discussed earlier, blanket supplementary feeding programs (BSFP) and targeted supplementary feeding (TSF) are two types of supplementary feeding programs for management of children with MAM.

- *Blanket supplementary feeding program* Supplementary food rations and/or micronutrient supplements are distributed to all target vulnerable families in food insecure situations. This approach has been used when MAM prevalence rates exceed 20% (or when it is >15% in the context of aggravating circumstances, such as epidemics). The objective of a BSFP is to prevent and control widespread malnutrition and to reduce excess mortality among those at risk. The beneficiaries are children, pregnant and lactating women, the elderly, and chronically ill in the affected areas.

- *Targeted supplementary feeding program* This is implemented in food insecure situations, including in emergencies. The aim is to treat MAM and to prevent children with MAM from going down to the category of SAM. TSF should ideally be run in conjunction with a general food distribution (GFD).

The management involves adding a nutrient rich supplemental food that provides the daily recommended dietary allowance of all micronutrients in addition to child's regular diet. A cereal and legume blended flour that provides about half of the total energy requirement for catch-up growth, 75 kcal/kg/day is generally used for nutritional supplementation. Ready to use fortified spreads have been successfully used to treat MAM children in Africa.[32] Experience from Ethiopia suggests high rates of deterioration and no improvement in children with MAM who did not have access to supplementary feeding.[33]

*Specialized foods used for Supplementary Feeding*

Traditionally specialized food products, including fortified blended foods (FBF), have been used as food aid products. These special foods have also been developed to provide food supplements for prevention and treatment of MAM. Various formulations of corn soy blends (CSB) and wheat soy blends (WSB) have been used as specialized foods. Over time, these foods are evolving with the advances in scientific evidence of their nutritional value and impact.

### 3. Other Interventions

While nutrition counseling and education and supplementary feeding are the two essential components of MAM management, there is a need to focus on other related contexts for broader complementary actions aimed at disease prevention, psychosocial care, shelter, etc.

Depending upon the situation of food security a child with MAM can be managed in Anganwadi/health center with dietary counseling for the use of quality, locally available dietary diverse foods at outpatient/community level in case availability of food is not a problem. In situations of food insecurity, including emergencies, children with MAM need supplementary feeding apart from nutritional counseling which is possible in an Anganwadi setting. In both situations, monthly follow up during VHNDs/ hospital visits is critical to ensure proper growth of the child.

After ensuring compliance, if there is no weight gain during 2 follow-ups, the child should be referred to a health facility for assessment of associated illnesses and management as per IMNCI treatment guidelines.

### 12.9 MAM AND SUSTAINABLE DEVELOPMENT GOALS

Undernutrition figured as an indicator (prevalence of underweight children under five years of age) rather than a target of Goal 1 of Millennium Development Goals (MDGs) (*Eradicate extreme hunger and poverty*).[34] That could be one of the reasons that during the last two decades a lot of attention was given to eradication of poverty rather than invest on effective interventions to combat undernutrition.[35] Consequently, several low and middle income countries have achieved Goal

1 without making a significant dent in the burden of undernutrition. Fortunately, Sustainable Development Goals (SDGs) relate undernutrition more to hunger than poverty. Therefore Goal 2 of SDGs (*End hunger, achieve food security and improved nutrition and promote sustainable agriculture*) has following two important targets assigned to it which address the problem of undernutrition.[36]

- "By 2030, end hunger and ensure access by all people, in particular the poor and people in vulnerable situations, including infants, to safe, nutritious and sufficient food all year round".
- By 2030, end all forms of malnutrition, including achieving, by 2025, the internationally agreed targets on stunting and wasting in children under 5 years of age, and address the nutritional needs of adolescent girls, pregnant and lactating women, and older persons.

## References

1. Black RE, Allen LH, Bhutta ZA, *et al*. Maternal and Child Undernutrition Study Group. Maternal and child undernutrition: global and regional exposures and health consequences. Lancet. 2008;371:243–260.
2. World Health Organization. Global and regional trend estimates for child malnutrition. WHO global database on child growth and development. Geneva, World Health Organization; 2012. From:http://www.who.int/nutgrowthdb/estimates/ en/index.html.Accessed16 September 2016.
3. The Millennium Development Goals Report 2015. New York: United Nations;2015.
4. World Health Organization. Consultation on the Dietary Management of Moderate Malnutrition. 30 September to 3 October 2008. Geneva: WHO;2010.
5. World Health Organization. World Health Statistics 2013, Geneva:WHO;2013.
6. United Nations Children's Fund. The state of the World's Children 2014 In Numbers: Revealing Disparities, Advancing Children's Rights. New York:UNICEF;2014.
7. United Nation Children's Fund, World Health Organization, The World Bank.UNICEF-WHO-World Bank Joint Child Malnutrition Estimates-

Levels and trends.From: http://www.who.int/nutgrowthdb/estimates/en/#.Accessed on 17 September 2016.
8. Isanaka S, Grais RF, Briend A, Checchi F. Estimates of the duration of untreated acute malnutrition in children from Niger. Am J Epidemiol. 2011;173:932–40.
9. Chang CY, Trehan I, Wang RJ, Thakwalakwa C, Maleta K, Deitchler M, Manary MJ. Children successfully treated for moderate acute malnutrition remain at risk for malnutrition and death in the subsequent year after recovery.J Nut. 2013;143:215–20.
10. World Health Organization/UNICEF/World Food Program. Global Nutrition Targets 2025: wasting policy brief (WHO/NMH/ NHD/ 14.8 targets). Geneva : World Health Organization; 2014. From: http://www.who.int/nutrition/topics/globaltargets_wasting_policybrief.pdf?ua=1.Accessed on 30 October 2016.
11. Annan RA, Webb P, Brown R. Management of Acute Malnutrition (MAM): Current knowledge and practice. CMAM Forum Technical Brief. September 2014. European Commission and UNICEF. From: http://www.cmamforum.org/Pool/Resources/MAM-management-CMAM-Forum-Technical-Brief-Sept-2014.pdf.Accessed on 17 September 2016.
12. Becic T, Moktar N. International symposium: Understanding Moderate malnutrition in Children fore Effective Interventions. Sight and Life 2014;28:91-96. From: http://www.sightandlife.org/fileadmin/data/Magazine/2014/28_2_2014/17_Congress_report_malnutrition.pdf.Accessed on 17 September 2016.
13. World Health Organization. Technical note :Supplementary foods for the management of moderate acute malnutrition in infants and children 6-59 months of age.2012, WHO, Geneva. From: http://apps.who.int/iris/bitstream/10665/75836/1/9789241504423_eng.pdf.Accessed on 17 September 2016.
14. Golden MH. Proposed nutrient densities for moderately malnourished children. Food and NutritionBulletin, 2009;30:S267-342. From: http://www.who.int/nutrition/publications/moderate_malnutrition/FNBv30n3_suppl_paper1.pdf.Accessed on 17 September 2016.
15. Maternal, Infant and Young child Nutrition Working group (Formulation Subgroup). Formulations for fortified complementary foods and supplements: review of success products for

improving the nutritional status of infants and young children - Ten Year Strategy to Reduce Vitamin and Mineral Deficiencies. Food and Nutrition Bulletin, 2009; 30: 2239- 55.From: http://fnb.sagepub.com/content/30/2_suppl2/S239.full.pdf. Accessed on 17 September 2016.

16. Glatthaar II, Fehrsen GS, Irwig LM, Reinach SG. Protein-energy malnutrition: The role of nutrition education in rehabilitation. Hum Nutr Clin Nutr. 1986;40C:271–85.

17. Fernandes-Concha D, Gilman RH, Gilman IB. A nutritional rehabilitation program in Peruvian peri-urban shanty town (pueblo joven). Trans R Soc Trop Med Hyg. 1991;85:809–13.

18. Roy SK, Fuchs GJ, Mahmud Z, Ara G, Islam S, Shafique S, Akbar SS, Chakraborty B. Intensive nutrition education with or without supplementary feeding improves the nutritional status of moderately-malnourished children in Bangladesh. J Health Popul Nutr. 2005,23:320–30.

19. Bhutta ZA, Das JK, Rizvi A, et al. Evidence-based interventions for improvement of maternal and child nutrition: what can be done and at what cost? Paper 2. Lancet Maternal and Child Nutrition Series. Lancet. 2013;382:452–77.

20. Lazzerini M, Rubert L, Pani P. Specially formulated foods for treating children with moderate acute malnutrition in low- and middle-income countries. Cochrane Database Syst Rev. 2013;(6):CD009584.

21. Lenters LM, Wazny K, Webb P, Ahmed T, Bhutta ZA. Treatment of severe and moderate acute malnutrition in low-and middle-income settings: a systemic review, meta- analysis and Delphi process. BMC Public Health. 2013;13 (Suppl 3):S3-S23.

22. Singh ADS, Kang G, Ramachandran A, Sarkar R, Peter P, Bose A. Locally made ready to use therapeutic food for treatment of malnutrition: a randomized controlled trial. Indian Pediatr. 2010;47:679–86.

23. Ackatia-Armah RS, McDonald CM, Doumbia S, Erhardt JG, Hamer DH. Malian children with moderate acute malnutrition who are treated with lipid-based dietary supplements have greater weight gains and recovery rates than those treated with locally produced cereal-legume products: a community-based, cluster-randomized trial. Am J Clin Nutr. 2015;101:632–45.

24. Defourny, Seroux G, Abdelkader, Harczi G. Management of moderate acute malnutrition with RUTF in Niger. Emergency Nutrition Network, Field Exchange Issue, 2007,31:2–8.

25. Navarro-Colorado C. A retrospective study of emergency supplementary feeding programs. Save the Children/ ENN, June 2007. Available at: http://www.ennonline.net/pool/files/research/Retrospective_Study_of_Emergency_Supplementary_Feeding_Programs_June%2007.pdf. Accessed 30 May 2009.

26. Isanaka S, Nombela N, Djibo A, et al. Effect of preventive supplementation with ready-to-use therapeutic food on the nutritional status, mortality, and morbidity of children aged 6 to 60 months in Niger: a cluster randomized trial. JAMA. 2009; 301:277–85.

27. Ashworth A, Ferguson E. Dietary counseling in the management of moderate malnourishment in children. Food Nutr Bull. 2009;30:S406–33.

28. Beaton GH, Ghassemi H. Supplementary feeding programs for young children in developing countries. Am J Clin Nutr. 1982;35(4 suppl):863–916.

29. de Pee S, Bloem MW. Current and potential role of specially formulated foods and food supplements for preventing malnutrition among 6- to 23-month old children and for treating moderate malnutrition among 6- to 59-month-old children. Food Nutr Bull. 2009;30:S434–63.

30. Briend A, Prinzo ZW. Dietary management of moderate malnutrition: time for change. Food and Nutrition Bulletin. 2009;30:S265–6.

31. Ministry of Health and Family Welfare. Integrated Management of Neonatal and Childhood Illness. Training Modules for Physicians. Chartbooklet. New Delhi: Govt. of India;2009.

32. Manary MJ, Sandige HL. Management of acute moderate and severe childhood malnutrition. BMJ. 2008;337:1227–30.

33. James P, Sadler K, Wondafrash M,Argaw A, Luo H, Geleta B, et al. Children with moderate acute malnutrition with no access to supplementary feeding programs experience high rates of deterioration and no improvement: results from a prospective cohort study in rural Ethiopia. PloS One. 2016;11(4):e0153530.

34. United Nations. Millennium Project. Goals, targets and indicators. From: http://www.unmillenniumproject.org/goals/gti.htm.Accessed on 17th September 2016.

35. Patwari AK. Millennium development goals and child undernutrition. Indian Pediatr. 2013;50:449–52.

36. Sustainable Development Goals. United Nations. Available from: http://www.un.org/sustainabledevelopment/hunger/.Accessed on 17 September 2016.

# Management of Severe Acute Malnutrition in Special Situations

S Manazir Ali, Praveen Kumar

Severe acute malnutrition (SAM) may have co-morbidities like diarrhea, HIV, tuberculosis, pneumonia, malaria etc. Management outcome is better in an uncomplicated child compared to a child having these co-morbidities. Adherence to WHO recommended management protocol decreases the risk of death in children with severe acute malnutrition (SAM), however certain modifications may have to be done in special situations. In this chapter, we will discuss management of children with few of these important co-morbidities, where the standard management may need modification.

## 13.1 MANAGEMENT OF SEVERE ACUTE MALNUTRITION WITH DIARRHEA

Diarrhea is one of the most common co-morbidity with which SAM children may present to a health facility. A descriptive study from Colombia reported diarrhea in 68% of malnourished children at admission.[1] The relationship between malnutrition and diarrhea is bidirectional. Malnutrition predisposes children to a greater incidence and duration of diarrhea,[2] and malnutrition can be triggered or worsened by significant diarrhea.[2,3] Several studies in children with SAM have shown that mortality is significantly higher in those with diarrhea than in those without diarrhea.[4] Children with

SAM may present with any of the following types of diarrhea: acute diarrhea, persistent diarrhea, and chronic diarrhea.

## A. Acute Diarrhea

Misdiagnosis and misclassification of dehydration is common in SAM children. Challenges of assessment of dehydration and fluid therapy including choice of ORS have been already discussed in Chapter 9. A child with severe acute malnutrition with acute diarrhea usually improves on 2 hourly therapeutic feed (F-75). However if number of stools remain high (>10 stools/day) along with weight loss or episodes of dehydration, change in feeding protocol is required.

## B. Continued or Persistent Diarrhea

Broad principles of management of persistent diarrhea remain same as described earlier. All children should be assessed for dehydration and managed as described in Chapter 9. Children with severe acute malnutrition have reduced capacity to absorb carbohydrates due to reduced level of disaccharidases in gut.[5-7] This can result in prolongation of acute diarrhea. Several tests have been used to identify carbohydrate malabsorption but none of them can be treated as gold standard. A few tests are discussed below:

a. *Carbohydrate tolerance test* This is a screening test where the child receives 2 g/kg of glucose as 10% solution after 6 hours of fast and blood sugar is monitored every 30 minutes for 2 hours. If blood sugar rise is less than 30 mg, it is taken as evidence of intolerance. Rise of blood sugar less than 20 mg/kg is considered diagnostic of malabsorption.[8]

b. *Fecal markers of carbohydrate malabsorption* A stool pH less than 5.5 (normal pH ranges between 7 and 7.5) and the presence of reducing substances in the feces are indicative of carbohydrate intolerance and malabsorption as a result of villous atrophy. A higher mean stool weight and higher lactic acid content are also consistent with carbohydrate malabsorption.[9]

c. *Intestinal biopsy* Small bowel biopsy showing reduced levels of disaccharidases is another method for determining carbohydrate malabsorption.

All SAM children with persistent diarrhea should also be investigated for associated co-morbidities including pneumonia, urinary tract infection, HIV, and tuberculosis.

### Re-feeding Diarrhea

Carbohydrate intolerance is usually the result of villous atrophy and small bowel bacterial overgrowth, which are common in malnourished patients when they enter rehabilative phase. Diarrhea occurs promptly after milk feeds (F-100) are begun. The diarrhea clearly improves when milk intake is reduced or stopped, and reoccurs when milk is given again.

### Dietary Management of Continued/ Persistent Diarrhea

Children who have continued diarrhea may require some changes in dietary protocol described in Chapter 9. These children may be given starter feed (F-75) more frequently and lesser volume per feed to decrease lactose load - 1 hourly along with measures to prevent /treat dehydration. If diarrhea still continues, then these children should be shifted on

lactose free diet with reduced starch **(Fig. 13.1)**. Response to therapeutic diet is adjudged as shown in **Box 13.1**. **Tables 13.1** and **13.2** show the lactose free starter diet, and lactose free catch-up diet, respectively, for use in children with prolonged diarrhea and lactose intolerance.

A systematic review examined therapeutic feeding approaches for children with persistent diarrhea and severe acute malnutrition.[10-15] Three randomized controlled trials were done in inpatient settings. In Mexico, investigators compared a chicken-based diet, a soy-based diet, and an elemental diet), all provided by nasogastric tube. There was no significant difference in the time to

---

**Box 13.1 Criteria for Response to Lactose-free diet for Persistent Diarrhea in Severe Acute Malnutrition**

A. *Good response to therapy*
   1. Weight gain >5 g/kg/day after 48–72 hours on therapeutic diet
   2. Fewer diarrheal stools (<6 stools/24 hours)
   3. Absence of fever and better activity
B. *Poor response:* Failure of therapeutic diet
   1. An increase in stool frequency ( usually to >10 watery stools a day), often with a return of signs of dehydration
   2. Failure to establish  weight gain within 7 days

---

**Table 13.1** Recipe of Lactose free (Reduced Starch) Starter Diet

| Contents per 100 mL | Amount |
|---|---|
| Egg white* (g) | 5 |
| Glucose (g) | 3.5 |
| Cereal flour: powdered puffed rice** (g) | 7 |
| Vegetable oil (g) | 4 |
| Water to make (mL) | 100 |
| Energy (kcal/100 mL) | 75 |
| Protein (kcal/100 mL) | 1 |
| Lactose (kcal/100 mL) | - |

*Egg white may be replaced by 3 g of chicken. Egg white or chicken may be replaced with commercially available pure protein like casein. Whole egg could be used and the vegetable oil may be adjusted accordingly.

**Other proteins that can be used are ground nut, soy or locally used pulses: however, they can increase the viscosity of the diets and need cooking.

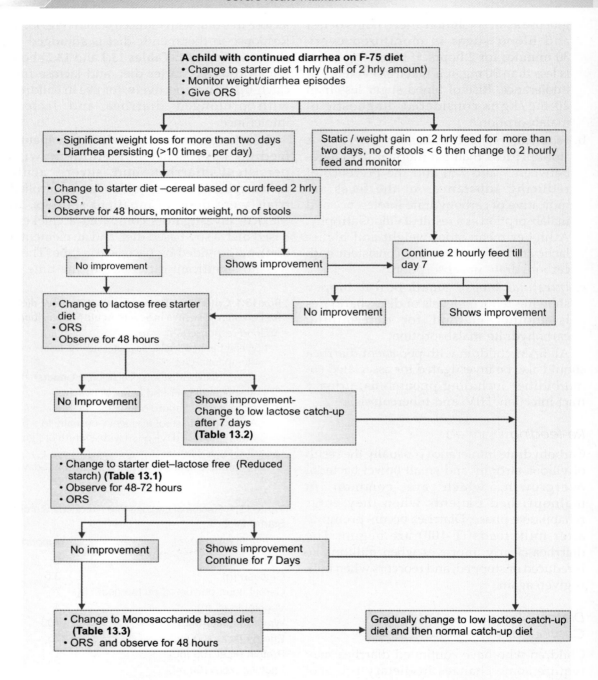

Fig. 13.1 Algorithm of management of continued /persistent diarrhea in SAM

recovery from diarrhea or in mortality.[11] In another study in Pakistan that compared a full-strength soy diet to half-strength buffalo milk with rice/lentil and yoghurt, there was no difference in the time to recovery, measured as time to cessation of diarrhea; stool volume and frequency were not different-mortality was not reported.[12] In

**Table 13.2** Recipe of Low Lactose Catch up Diet

| Contents (per 100 mL) | Egg based |
|---|---|
| Milk (cow's milk or toned dairy milk (mL) | 25 |
| Egg white* (g) | 12 |
| Vegetable oil (g) | 4 |
| Cereal flour: powdered puffed rice** (g) | 12 |
| Energy (kcal/100 mL) | 100 |
| Protein (g/100 mL) | 2.9 |
| Lactose (g/100 mL) | 1 |

*Egg white may be replaced by 7.2 g of chicken or commercially available pure protein like casein.
**Powdered puffed rice may be replaced by commercial pre-cooked rice preparations (in same amounts).

Zambia, an amino-acid-based infant formula was compared to a standard skimmed milk diet. This was the only trial that followed WHO guidelines for the treatment of persistent diarrhea, but it used the Wellcome classification of malnutrition.[13] In summary, none of the diets evaluated in these trials produced statistically significant improvements in measures of persistent diarrhea in children with severe acute malnutrition.

Also, there is no evidence of utility of probiotics in children with SAM. Few researchers have tried pancreatic supplements in children who fail to respond, but the results are not consistent.

## 13.2 MANAGEMENT OF SAM IN HIV INFECTED CHILDREN

HIV-infected children with severe acute malnutrition are nearly three times more likely to die while on nutritional rehabilitation therapy, compared to their HIV-negative counterparts.[14] HIV weakens the body's natural defence system; as a result of which the body's ability to fight infection is greatly reduced. Frequent infections and diseases make the body weaker and accelerate progression from a symptomatic HIV infection to AIDS. HIV and frequent infections further increase the nutrition needs of a child

with severe acute malnutrition. HIV should be suspected in a child with SAM in presence of following:

- Death or prolonged illnesses in parents
- Oral thrush
- Generalized lymphadenopathy
- Tuberculosis
- Parotid enlargement
- Recurrent pneumonia
- Persistent diarrhea

The basic principles and steps of management of SAM in these children are similar. Initiation of anti-retroviral therapy (ART) and other long-term treatment of illnesses that are not immediately lethal should be delayed until the metabolism of major organs has improved through nutritional therapy. NACO (National AIDS Control Organization) recommends that all under-five children diagnosed as HIV infected should be started on antiretroviral drug treatment, irrespective of clinical and immunological staging.

- For severe pneumonia in HIV infected children, children should receive an antibiotic which has anti-staphylococcal and Gram-negative coverage (e.g. amoxiclav and gentamicin).
- For pneumonia with severe hypoxia, consider *Pneumocystis pneumonia* and add a high dose of co-trimoxazole, 6-hourly for 3 weeks.
- Other opportunistic infections like tuberculosis should be treated as per the NACO guidelines.

**Table 13.3** Recipe of Monosaccharide Based Diet

| Contents(per 100 mL) | Egg based |
|---|---|
| Egg white (g)* | 25 |
| Glucose (g)** | 3 |
| Vegetable oil (g) | 4 |
| Water to make (mL) | 100 |

*Egg white may be replaced by 12g of chicken or commercially available pure protein like casein.
**Jaggery may be used instead of glucose/sugar.

- In children who rapidly gain weight because of adequate nutrition and ART, dosages of ARVs should be frequently reviewed.
- The recurrence of severe malnutrition that is not caused by a lack of food in children receiving ART may indicate treatment failure and the need to switch therapy.

## WHO Guidelines 2013 for Management of SAM with HIV[16]

- Children with severe acute malnutrition who are HIV infected and who qualify for lifelong antiretroviral therapy should be started on antiretroviral drug treatment as soon as possible after stabilization of metabolic complications and sepsis. This would be indicated by return of appetite and resolution of severe edema.
- HIV-infected children with severe acute malnutrition should be given the same antiretroviral drug treatment regimens, in the same doses, as children with HIV who do not have severe acute malnutrition.
- HIV-infected children with severe acute malnutrition who are started on antiretroviral drug treatment should be monitored closely (inpatient and outpatient) in the first 6–8 weeks following initiation of antiretroviral therapy, to identify early metabolic complications and opportunistic infections.
- Children with severe acute malnutrition who are HIV infected should be managed with the same therapeutic feeding approaches as children with severe acute malnutrition who are not HIV infected.
- HIV-infected children with severe acute malnutrition should receive a high dose of vitamin A on admission and zinc for management of diarrhea as indicated for other children with severe acute malnutrition, unless they are already receiving commercial F-75, F-100 or ready-to-use therapeutic food, which contain adequate vitamin A and zinc.

- HIV-infected children with severe acute malnutrition in whom persistent diarrhea does not resolve with standard management should be investigated to exclude carbohydrate intolerance and infective causes, which may require different management, such as modification of fluid and feed intake, or antibiotics.

## 13.3 MANAGEMENT OF MALARIA IN SAM

Malaria is a common febrile illness in many tropical areas. The prevalence of malaria amongst children with SAM depends on the local transmission intensity of malaria. Cerebral malaria is the most dreaded form of malaria in severely malnourished children.

The clinical diagnosis of severe malaria is unreliable because the signs and symptoms of malaria overlap with other common febrile illnesses such as pneumonia, meningitis, and sepsis. Current guidelines do not recommend blanket treatment with antimalarials, in children with SAM.

### Diagnosis of Malaria

Diagnosis is by microscopic blood slide examination or rapid diagnostic tests (RDT) that detect parasite antigens. The sensitivity of both types of test increases with increasing blood parasite density. Microscopy may detect malaria parasite densities as low as 5 to 10 parasites/$\mu$L of blood, but this is highly dependent on the skill and experience of the technologist, the care taken in preparing the slide, and examining sufficient high power fields. In practice, false positives are common. In general, *Plasmodium falciparum* histidine-rich-protein 2 (PfHRP$_2$) based RDTs are more sensitive than lactate dehydrogenase (LDH) based RDTs. A significant risk of presumptively treating a febrile child for malaria without a malaria test result (or worse, with a false positive result), is that the treatment for the true cause of the illness may have been omitted. On the other hand, in high transmission areas, it should be recognized that children may have coincidental parasitemia and so there may still be another cause of illness that also needs to be treated.

Extensive evaluations of the sensitivity and specificity of RDTs, their effectiveness in various health care settings have been undertaken, but none has specifically tested their diagnostic performance in relation to SAM.

## Treatment of Malaria in SAM

Artemisinin-based antimalarials are very safe in comparison to other antimalarials. Artemisinin combination therapy (ACT) is recommended by the WHO for treating *Plasmodium falciparum* malaria.[17]

Some of the drugs used in treating malaria are potentially more toxic in the malnourished child than in well-nourished children and should be avoided if possible. Combinations containing amodiaquine should be avoided in the severely malnourished. Quinine should also be avoided as this is less effective and it can induce prolonged and dangerous hypotension, hypoglycemia, arrhythmia, and cardiac arrest.

## 13.4 MANAGEMENT OF SAM WITH TUBERCULOSIS

Tuberculosis itself or often in combination of HIV/AIDS is common in malnourished children due to immune system dysfunction. RNTCP guidelines should be followed for investigations and treatment.

Children with pulmonary TB are often unable to produce sputum and infections tend to be paucibacillary (low numbers of bacilli), meaning that false negatives are common. TB diagnosis in children should be based on clinical features, supported by culture and microscopy, chest radiograph and tuberculin skin test. Children often catch TB from adults at home, and siblings may be infected as well. When a child is started on treatment, it is important to offer screening to all household contacts.

Four drug regimen i.e. rifampicin (10 mg/kg), isoniazid (10 mg/kg), pyrazinamide (30 mg/kg) and ethambutol (20 mg/kg) should be started for initial two months during the intensive phase. This should be followed by rifampicin (10 mg/kg), isoniazid (10 mg/kg) and ethambutol (20 mg/kg) for four months maintenance phase along with pyridoxine supplementation. Pyridoxine should be given (throughout treatment with isoniazid) at 5–10 mg/day in a single dose to prevent isoniazid-induced polyneuropathy.

## 13.5 MANAGEMENT OF FEVER IN SAM

Children with SAM should be managed conservatively unless child has high fever as paracetamol administration may be toxic because of prolonged half-life of paracetamol, even in the absence of liver abnormality. Moderate fever up to 38.5°C does not need to be treated actively. These children should be managed by exposing the body, nursing in a ventilated place; and encouraging oral intake of fluids. A severely malnourished child with temperature >39°C can be offered antipyretic therapy. Cooling can be dangerous. It should only be resorted to children with hyperpyrexia.

## 13.6 MANAGEMENT OF ANEMIA IN SAM

Anemia remains an important co-morbidity with severe acute malnutrition.[16] In a cross sectional study which included 131 cases of severe acute malnutrition aged 6 months to 5 years, 67.3% children reported having severe anemia (<7 g/dL); 13.8% had moderate anemia. The most common type of anemia was microcytic (38.6%) followed by megaloblastic (30.5%). Nearly two-thirds of patients with megaloblastic anemia had folic acid deficiency, 12% had vitamin $B_{12}$ deficiency, and 8% had both vitamin $B_{12}$ and folic acid deficiency.[18]

## Indication for Blood Transfusions

Packed cell transfusion is indicated if the hemoglobin concentration is less than 4 g/dL or the hematocrit is less than 12% in the first 24 hours after admission. Blood transfusion can be given to critically ill SAM children if they have Hb between 4–6 g/dL.

- Give 10 mL per kg body weight of packed red cells or whole blood slowly over 3 hours.
- These children should not receive feed during and for at least 3 hours after a blood transfusion.

Transfusion is not advised during 48 h to 14 days (after hospitalization) even if hemoglobin is found to be less than 4 g/dL unless there is an evidence of ongoing loss. If there is heart failure with very severe anemia, exchange transfusion should be carried.

Folic acid is started from day 1 while iron supplementation should be started only when the child enters rehabilitative phase. Vitamin $B_{12}$ should be supplemented if peripheral smear shows macrocytosis or serum vitamin $B_{12}$ level is low.

## References

1. Bernal C, Velasquez C, Botero J. Treatment of severe malnutrition in children: Experience in implementing the world health organization guidelines in turbo, Colombia. J Pediatr Gastroenterol Nutr. 2008;46:322–8.
2. Brewster DR. Critical appraisal of the management of severe malnutrition J Paediatr Child Health. 2006;42:583–593.
3. Talbert A, Thuo N, Karisa J, Chesaro C, Ohuma E, Ignas J, et al. Diarrhoea complicating severe acute malnutrition in Kenyan children: a prospective descriptive study of risk factor and outcome. PLoS One. 2012;7:e38321.
4. Maitland K, Berkley JA, Shebbe M, Peshu N, English M, Newton CR. Children with severe malnutrition: can those at higher risk of death be identified with the WHO protocol? PLoS Med.2006;3:e500.
5. Bandsma RH, Spoelstra MN, Mari A, et al. Impaired glucose absorption in children with severe acute malnutrition J Pediatr.2011;158:282–7.
6. Hammer HF, Hammer J. Diarrhea caused by carbohydrate malabsorption. Gastroenterol Clin North Am. 2012;41:611–27.
7. Greene HL, McCabe DR, Merenstein GB. Protracted diarrhea and malnutrition in infancy: Changes in intestinal morphology and disaccharidase activities during treatment with total intravenous nutrition or oral elemental diets. J Pediatr. 1975;87:695–704.
8. Nyeko R, Kalyesubula I, Mworozi E, Bachou H. Lactose intolerance among severely malnourished children with diarrhoea admitted to the nutrition unit, Mulago hospital, Uganda. BMC Pediatr. 2010;10:31.
9. Brewster D. Inpatient management of severe malnutrition: time for a change in protocol and practice. Ann Trop Paediatr. 2011;31:97–107.
10. Brewster D, Kukuruzovic R. Milk formulas in acute gastroenteritis and malnutrition: a randomized trial. J Pediatr Child Health. 2002;38:571–7.
11. Sauniere JF, Sarles H. Exocrine pancreatic function and protein calorie malnutrition in Dakar and Abidjan (West Africa): silent pancreatic insufficiency. Am J Clin Nutr. 1988;48:1233–8.
12. Beau JP, Fontaine O, Garenne M. Management of malnourished children with acute diarrhoea and sugar intolerance. J Trop Pediatr. 1989;35:281–4.
13. Nurko S, Garcia-Aranda JA, Fishbein E, Perez-Zuniga MI. Successful use of a chicken-based diet for the treatment of severely malnourished children with persistent diarrhoea: a prospective randomised study. J Pediatr. 1997;131:405–12.
14. Bhutta Z, Molla AM, Issani Z, Badruddin S, Hendricks K, Snyder JD. Nutrient absorption and weight gain in persistent diarrhoea: comparison of a traditional rice-lentil/yoghurt/milk diet with soy formula. J Pediatr Gastroenterol Nutr. 1994;18:45–52.
15. Amadi B. Role of food antigen elimination in treating children with persistent diarrhea and malnutrition in Zambia. J Pediatr Gastroenterol Nutr. 2002;34:S54–S56.
16. WHO. Guideline: Updates on the management of severe acute malnutrition in infants and children. Geneva: World Health Organization; 2013.
17. Makanga M, Premji Z, Falade C, Karbwang J, Mueller EA, Andraiono K, et al. Efficacy and safety of the six-dose regimen of artemether-lumefantrine in pediatrics with uncomplicated Plasmodium falciparum malaria: A pooled analysis of individual patient data. Am J Trop Med Hyg. 2006;74:991–8.
18. Thakur N, Chandra J, Pemde H, Singh V. Anemia in severe acute malnutrition. Nutrition. 2014; 30:440–2.

# Stunting

Karanveer Singh

## 14.1 DEFINITION

Stunting occurs as a result of long-standing (chronic) undernutrition, resulting in linear growth retardation.Stunting is defined as "height for age" less than –2 Z-scores below the median height-for-age (and sex) on the WHO Child Growth Standards.[1]

## First 1000 Days and Stunting

Most of the stunting occurs due to insult during first 1000 days of life (starting from conception till the child is 24 months of age). When nutrient requirements for growth are not met over a long period of time during this critical phase of life, stunting occurs. First 1000 days of life is also critical as maximum brain development takes place during this phase.It is from conception through the first two years of life when critical physical and mental development takes place, although additional linear growth faltering may still happen after the first two years of life.[2] Development during pregnancy and first two years of life determines the individual's potential for life in terms of risks of morbidity and mortality, school achievement, income earning potential, physical strength, and risk of chronic disease.[3] Due to this importance, this period is called the 1000 days window of opportunity.

## Consequences of Stunting

Undernutrition is directly or indirectly responsible for nearly half of all child deaths, globally. As per estimates, a stunted child is approximately five times more likely to die from diarrhea than a non-stunted child. Stunted children are more likely to die from other childhood illnesses such as pneumonia, measles, malaria or HIV/AIDS.[4] Stunting alone is responsible for approximately 15% of all under-five mortality worldwide and 400,000 deaths in South Asia.[4]

A stunted child may be only few inches shorter than what he or she could have been, but this is not simply an issue of height. Stunting also impairs brain/cognitive development, their productivity, intelligence, development of society and country. Stunted children have poor learning capacity and poor school performances thus leading to reduced earnings. It also increases risk of nutrition related chronic diseases such as diabetes, hypertension, and obesity. There are strong evidences showing adverse effect of low stature mothers on birthweight and length of their children.

## 14.2 ETIOLOGY OF STUNTING

Child undernutrition is caused not only due to food scarcity, but also by recurrent illness; poor hygiene and sanitation practices at the household and community level; inappropriate feeding and care practices; and lack of access to health and other social services.

UNICEF's conceptual framework of child undernutrition **(Fig. 14.1)** described the multifactorial determinants of malnutrition more than two decades ago.[5] Causes are classified as immediate, underlying, and basic.

- *Immediate causes* include inadequate dietary intake and disease;
- *Underlying causes* include household food insecurity (lack of availability of, access to, and/or utilization of a diverse diet), lack of education and social factors leading to inadequate care and inappropriate feeding practices, poor household, and surrounding environment.
- *Basic causes* include the societal structures and processes that neglect human rights and perpetuate poverty, limiting or denying the access of vulnerable populations to essential resources. Social, economic, and political factors have a long-term influence on maternal and childhood undernutrition.

Undernutrition thus traps children, families, communities and nations in an intergenerational cycle of undernutrition, illness and poverty.

## Pathophysiology

Stunting in childhood is attributed to multiple factors that are often inter-linked and these range from biological, social and environmental spheres. Stunting occurs when the nutrient intake does not meet nutrient needs of the child for a long duration. Further, nutrient needs may be increased by illnesses; recurrent illnesses also reduces appetite and interferes with nutrient utilization, resulting in an imbalance between nutrient needs with existing nutrient intakes. Other contributing factors include poor maternal health and nutrition, inappropriate infant and young child feeding practices, and infection. Maternal nutritional status and care before, during, and after pregnancy has major influence on early growth and development, beginning in the womb.[4] As per estimates,

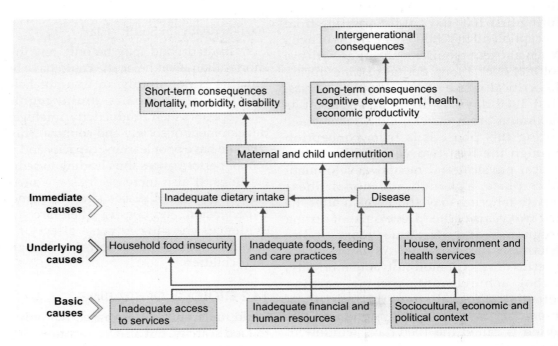

Fig.14.1 UNICEF conceptual framework of undernutrition (adapted)

intrauterine growth restriction due to maternal poor nutritional status accounts for 20% of childhood stunting.[6] Other maternal factors contributing to stunting include short stature, short birth spacing, and adolescent pregnancy, which interfere with nutrient availability to the fetus (owing to the competing demands of ongoing maternal growth).

- Suboptimal infant and young child feeding practices like lack of exclusive breast-feeding, diluted milk, delayed introduction and inappropriate amount and quality of complementary feeding have major impact on growth and development.
- Micronutrient deficiency and lack of food diversity is important which may not always occur due to food scarcity.
- Infectious diseases like diarrhea which is more common when feeding practices are suboptimal may have long-term consequences for linear growth, depending on the severity, duration, and recurrence, particularly if there is insufficient nourishment to support recovery.
- Subclinical infections, resulting from unsafe water, exposure to contaminated environments and poor hygiene, causes nutrient malabsorption and reduced gut immunity against disease-causing organisms.[7]

The growth and development of a child is thus negatively influenced by food scarcity due to household poverty, suboptimal feeding practices, maternal education, surrounding environment, quality of water,and inadequate child stimulation.

## Economic Growth and Stunting

There is an emerging consensus that economic growth of population can have a positive impact on reducing stunting. However, the relationship between economic growth and stunting is not always a straight forward one. Although, India experienced a period of sustained economic growth rates greater than 7% between 1994 and 1997 and about 8% or

greater rate in 2004 and 2005,[8] but this was not associated with significant reduction of child stunting between 1993-2006. This poor correlation may be explained by the fact that economic growth during this period did not lead to significant increase in public development expenditure, considerable reductions in poverty, and/or increased equity.[9]

## 14.3 LEVELS AND TRENDS OF STUNTING

### Global Trends

The Global Nutrition Report 2016 states that globally there are 156 million under 5 children who are stunted.[10] The global trend in the prevalence of stunting and numbers of children affected is decreasing but not fast enough.Between 1990 and 2015, stunting prevalence declined from 39.6% to 23.8% and numbers affected declined from 255 million to 156 million.

Since 2000, while Asia as a whole has reduced stunting by almost half, from 38% in 2000 to 24% in 2015, but the progress among sub-regions within Asia has been uneven. Stunting rates in Eastern Asia have dropped by more than two thirds since 2000, compared with Southern Asia, where stunting declined by less than one third during the same period.In 2015, more than half of all stunted under-5 children lived in Asia (88 million) and more than one third lived in Africa. Since 2000, Africa has made only a limited progress, reducing the prevalence rates of stunting from 38% to 32 % in 2015.

According to a recent report, 38% of South Asia's under- five children are stunted. Levels of child stunting in South Asia are comparable to those in sub-Saharan Africa (37%) and three times higher than those in East Asia and the Pacific (12%) or Latin America (11%).[11]

### Stunting in India

India contributes about one-third of world's stunted children. According to the Global Nutrition Report 2016,[6] India ranks 114 (out of 132 countries for whom data were available) for prevalence of stunting and ranks 120 for prevalence of wasting.

Stunting reduced by 19.4% over the last eight years from 48% (NFHS-3) in 2005-2006 to 38.7% (RSoC) in 2013-2014. But, 46.8 million children still face a diminished life due to stunting–53% of which come from four states– Uttar Pradesh, Bihar, Madhya Pradesh, and Maharashtra. The average annual rate of reduction in stunting between NFHS-3 and RSoC is 2.4% which is below India's target rate of 3.7% annual decline (needed to meet the global commitment of a 40% reduction in the number of stunted children less than 5 years of age from the 2010 levels by 2030).

## 14.4 STUNTING—AN IMPEDIMENT TO HUMAN DEVELOPMENT

A recent multi-country longitudinal study of children from Brazil, Guatemala, India, the Philippines, and South Africa has shown relation between stunting with a reduction in schooling. Adults who were stunted at age 2 completed nearly one year less school than non-stunted individuals.[12]

Another study of Guatemalan adults found that those adults who were stunted during childhood had less total schooling, lower test performances, lower household per capita expenditure and a greater likelihood of living in poverty.[13] Stunting is thus an enormous drain on economic productivity and growth. Economists estimate that stunting can reduce a country's gross domestic product by up to 3%.

Economic analysis has shown that annual GDP losses from low weight, poor child growth, and micronutrient deficiencies is approximately 11% in Asia and Africa[14] and preventing malnutrition delivers $16 in returns on investment for every $1 spent. Survey conducted in eight low-income and middle-income countries has shown that interventions which cause 1 cm of additional height have potential to increase in median

hourly wages by 4.5%[14] and 0.55% from a study of eight high-income countries.[14]

For women, stunting in early life was also seen to be associated with a lower age at first conception and a higher number of pregnancies and children. According to World Bank estimates, a 1% loss in adult height due to childhood stunting is associated with a 1.4% loss in economic productivity.[16] It is estimated that stunted children earn 20% less as adults compared to non-stunted individuals.[17]

## 14.5 ACTIONS FOR REDUCING STUNTING IN A POPULATION

To accelerate progress in reducing stunting, multiple efforts are needed that reach beyond the nutrition sector. Nutrition interventions, by themselves, may not result in the desired impact if the target population suffers from frequent infection like diarrhea and pneumonia. Food security, poverty alleviation, sanitation, safe drinking water, improved household and outdoor environments are equally important.

Growth failure often begins *in utero* and continues after birth due to poor nutritional status of mothers, inappropriate IYCF practices, and infections. Therefore, focusing on the critical 1000-day window from a woman's pregnancy to her child's second birthday is critically important. Actions that can be taken across multiple areas to reduce rates of stunting are discussed below:

## 1. Improving Nutritional Status of Adolescent Girls

Improving nutritional status of school going and out of school adolescent girls is important. Dietary counseling must be undertaken to promote dietary diversity and ensuring that their diets have adequate energy, protein and micronutrient that meets their daily requirements. The dietary counseling must be complemented by weekly iron and folic acid supplementation as the prevalence of anemia among adolescent girls is very high. Several states have started weekly iron and folic acid supplementation, and twice yearly (six months apart) deworming prophylaxis for improving their hemoglobin status. In food insecure areas of the country, these steps must be augmented by provision of micronutrient fortified supplementary foods.

## 2. Improving Nutritional Status of Pregnant and Lactating Mothers

It is important to have targeted interventions to improve nutritional status of pregnant and lactating women. Meeting the high nutrient needs of pregnant and lactating women may be challenging due to food scarcity, lack of education, social taboos and lack of health services. In South Asia, staple diets are often low in energy density and micronutrient deficient. Thus, it is important to improve diets by dietary diversification and increased intake of locally available nutrient-rich foods and better service utilization.Women in reproductive age must have access to foods adequate in quality and quantity, particularly during pregnancy and lactation, including access to and consumption of fortified foods, iodized salt, iron and folic acid supplements. In food insecure settings, women should be provided supplementary foods to improve their well-being and pregnancy and lactation outcomes.

## 3. Antenatal Care

All pregnant women should have access to antenatal care. Antenatal care visits provides opportunity to identify high risk pregnancy, detect and prevent intrauterine growth retardation, improving compliance with IFA tablets intake, and food supplementation in form of take home ration.

## 4. Improving Early Initiation and Sustaining Exclusive Breastfeeding for Six Months

There is strong scientific evidence to suggest that early initiation and exclusive breast-feeding for six months improves nutritional status of infants by providing optimal nutrition, preventing infections like diarrhea, pneumonia, and providing growth factors. In resource-poor settings, lack of breastfeeding is associated with undernutrition, because breastmilk is displaced, or replaced, by less nutritious foods like diluted animal milk or formula. Breastfeeding continues to provide significant amount of energy, good quality proteins,and micronutrients in second year of life also. Hence, interventions to support mothers in continuing breastfeeding will protect them from stunting. This is even more important in resource poor countries where quality of complementary food is often suboptimal.

## 5. Improved Complementary Feeding Practices

Improving complementary practices which include timely introduction, adequate amount, and good quality of complementary feeding (which has diversity, good quality of protein and rich in micronutrients) is one of the most effective interventions for preventing stunting among children. Evidence suggests that greater dietary diversity[18] and the consumption of foods from animal sources are associated with improved linear growth.[18,19]

## 6. Improving WASH Practices

Stunting is contributed by several household, environmental, socioeconomic, and cultural factors. Infections are more common and recurrent if WASH (Water, Sanitation and Hygiene) practices are poor. Promoting hand washing by soap before cooking, feeding infants, and keep surrounding clean are capable of preventing infections like diarrhea and pneumonia. Measures to make community understand the importance and practice is critical in achieving reduction in stunting. However, this will be successful only when measures are taken to make safe water available to the population and community is able to afford soap (socioeconomic status).

## 7. Agriculture and Food Policies

Household food security, food diversity, and food safety are other factors which contribute to reduction of stunting. Emphasis should be placed to work in the area of Agriculture and Food Security, so that mothers and young children get suitable foods which are of good quality, and has diversity. Agriculture systems have a crucial role in provision of food, livelihoods, and income.[20] For long term reductions in poverty, hunger, and stunting it would be crucial to focus on investments to enhance agriculture productivity and boost global food supply.

## 8. Social Safety Nets

Social safety net are measures that provide regular and predictable support to the poor, under-privileged and vulnerable population. Such programs reduce poverty and protect population by targeting reduction of nutrition vulnerability and supporting livelihoods among the poor and socially disadvantaged populations. The main goal of social protection programs is to augment income. Transfers can be in the form of cash or food, although with improved technology for tracking income transfers, cash transfers are increasingly the preferred means to support chronically poor households. Between 0.75 and 1.0 billion people in low-income and middle-income countries currently, receive cash support.[21]

## 9. Political Leadership and Commitment

Political commitments to ensure good quality food at affordable price is important. Employment opportunities, political stability, equity and minimal gap in rural and urban income are other factors which influence food security at household level. Equity-driven nutrition-sensitive programs that have the ability to improve vulnerable populations' access to and utilization of services, achieve high reductions in the national average prevalence of stunting. Such programs also close gaps between the wealthier and poorer population segments. Political commitment, multi-sectoral collaboration, integrated service delivery, and community involvement in program activities are all common elements that contribute to success.

## 10. Education

Education policies that keep girls in school throughout adolescence may also have an impact on delaying marriage and childbearing and are associated with positive economic and health outcomes. Increases in parental schooling, especially maternal education have contributed to reduction in stunting.[22]

## 14.6 CONCLUSIONS

Stunting in children is a powerful marker of failed development. Prevalence of stunting in a country is a marker of sensitivity towards children. Stunting has both short and long term implications. It increases morbidities, mortality, decreases cognitive development, increases health expenditure, obesity related morbidities, and work capacities as adults. Causes are multifactorial which includes women's illiteracy, adolescent marriage and pregnancy, nutritional status of adolescent girls and pregnant women, quality of complementary foods, WASH practices. To ensure good physical growth and brain development thus reducing stunting would need improved child feeding practices, good hygiene, and appropriate physical activity. We need to ensure age-appropriate foods for infants and young children and appropriate physical activity for older children. This and improved household hygiene and sanitation practices that include access to safe water and sanitation can help achieve optimal height.

### References

1. WHO. Nutrition Landscape Information System; Country Profile Indicators, Interpretation Guide. Geneva:WHO;2010.
2. Leroy JF, Ruel M, Habicht JP, Frongillo EA. Linear growth deficit continues to accumulate beyond the first 1000 days in low and middle-income

countries. Global evidence from 51 national surveys. J Nutr. 2014;144:1460–6.

3. Victora CG, Adair L, Fall C, Hallal PC, Martorell R, Richter L, Sachdev HS: Maternal and Child Undernutrition Study Group. Maternal and child undernutrition: consequences for adult health and human capital. Lancet. 2008; 371:340–57.

4. Black RE, Victora CG, Walker SP, Bhutta ZA, Christian P, de Onis M, et al. Maternal and Child Nutrition Study Group. Maternal and child undernutrition and overweight in low-income and middle-income countries. Lancet. 2013; 382(9890):427–51.

5. Harmonised Training Package (HTP): Resource Material for Training on Nutrition in Emergencies; Module 5:.Italy: United Nations System Standing Committee on Nutrition, 2011.

6. Gluckman PD, Pinal CS. Regulation of fetal growth by the somatotrophic axis. J Nutr. 2003;133(5 Suppl 2):1741S-1746S.

7. Prendergast AJ, Rukobo S, Chasekwa B, Mutasa K, Ntozini R, et al. Stunting is characterized by chronic inflammation in Zimbabwean infants. PLoS One. 2014 Feb 18;9:e86928.

8. Basu K, Maertens A. The pattern and causes of economic growth in India. Oxford Review Economic Policy 2007;23: 143–67.

9. Joe W, Rajaram R and Subramanian SV. Understanding the null-to-small association between increased macroeconomic growth and reducing child undernutrition in India: role of development expenditures and poverty alleviation. Maternal and Child Nutrition 12(Suppl. 1)(2016): 196–209.

10. Global Nutrition Report: From Promise to Impact, Ending Malnutrition by 2030.

11. Aguayo VM, Menon P. Stop stunting: improving child feeding, women's nutrition and household sanitation in South Asia. Matern Child Nutr. 2016;12 Suppl. 1:3–11.

12. Martorell R, Horta BL, Adair LS, Stein AD, Richter L, et. al. Consortium on Health Orientated Research in Transitional Societies Group. Weight gain in the first two years of life is an important predictor of schooling outcomes in pooled analyses from fivebirth cohorts from low- and middle-income countries. J Nutr. 2010;140:348–54.

13. Hoddinott J, Behrman JR, Maluccio JA, Melgar P, Quisumbing AR, et al. Adult consequences of growth failure in early childhood. Am J Clin Nutr. 2013;98:1170–8.

14. Horton S, Steckel R. Global economic losses attributable to malnutrition 1900-2000 and projections to 2050. In: Lomborg B.The Economics of Human Challenges. Cambridge, UK: Cambridge University Press; 2013.

15. Gao W, Smyth R. Health human capital, height and wages in China. Journal of Development Studies 2010;46: 466–84.

16. World Bank. Repositioning Nutrition as Central to Development: A Strategy for Large-Scale Action. Washington, D.C.: The World Bank Group; 2006.

17. Grantham-McGregor S, Cheung YB, Cueto S, Glewwe P, Richter L, Strupp B. International Child Development Steering Group.. Developmental potential in the first 5 years for children in developing countries. Lancet. 2007;369:60–70.

18. Arimond M, Ruel MT. Dietary diversity is associated with child nutritionalstatus: evidence from 11 demographic and health surveys. J Nutr. 2004;134:2579–85.

19. Sari M, de Pee S, Bloem MW, Sun K, Thorne-Lyman AL, et al. Higher household expenditure on animal-source and nongrain foods lowers the risk of stunting among children 0-59 months old in Indonesia: implications of rising food prices. J Nutr. 2010;140:195S-200S.

20. Pinstrup-Andersen P. The African food system and its interactions with human health and nutrition. Ithaca: Cornell University Press; 2010.

21. DFID. Cash transfer evidence paper. London: Department for International Development Policy Division; 2011.

22. Ruel MT, Alderman H; Maternal and Child Nutrition Study Group.Nutrition-sensitive interventions and programmes: how can they help to accelerate progress in improving maternal and child nutrition? Lancet. 2013;382(9891):536–51.

# Prevention of Severe Acute Malnutrition

JP Dadhich

## 15.1 INTRODUCTION

The Global Nutrition Targets for 2025[1] and the Sustainable Development Goals (SDGs) have expressed global desire to reduce the burden of severe acute malnutrition.[2] Globally high burden countries (like India) need to look into prevalence and underlying determinants of wasting; set annual targets for reduction of wasting; make available required resources; and achieve reduction of wasting through systemic planning and implementation.[3]

### What Causes Severe Acute Malnutrition?

Conceptual framework of undernutrition developed by UNICEF[4] (*see* Chapter 2) provides a holistic view of factors causing malnutrition. The framework is a general description of causative factors of malnutrition and includes basic causes; underlying causes; and immediate causes. All these factors need to be kept in mind while planning prevention of severe acute malnutrition. Rapid weight loss may also happen due to combined effect of infections and inadequate diet. Severe infectious diseases in early childhood—such as measles, diarrhea, pneumonia, meningitis, and malaria—can also cause acute wasting and have long-term effects on linear growth.[3–5]

The first year of life is a crucial period as growth is very rapid and simultaneously a nutrition transition is also happening. Growth faltering is most evident during first two years of life, particularly during the first phase of complementary feeding (6 to 12 months) when rates of diarrheal illness due to food contamination are at their highest.[6] An analysis of 39 nationally representative datasets from developing countries revealed that growth faltering in weight for length/height is restricted to the first 15 months of life, followed by rapid improvement.[7]

### Interventions for Prevention of Sever Acute Malnutrition (SAM)

Prevention is the key to achieve a reduction in the number of children with wasting as envisaged in various global commitments and goals. Interventions for preventing SAM may be nutrition-specific or nutrition-sensitive.

Nutrition-specific interventions address the immediate causes of undernutrition, like inadequate dietary intake as well as some of the underlying causes like feeding practices and access to food. As the first line of prevention, interventions to reduce wasting should address the nutrition needs of infants and young children by enhancing optimal Infant and Young Child Feeding (IYCF) practices.[8] Interventions should include enhancing optimal breastfeeding and a focus on improving complementary feeding through increased affordability and accessibility of locally available nutritious foods. Ensuring food security is equally important as underlined by documentation of higher post-treatment relapse and non-recovery from SAM during food insecurity in studies from India and China.[9,10]

Nutrition-sensitive interventions are important to tackle underlying and basic causes of malnutrition and may help in delivering nutrition-specific interventions.[5] It is important to strengthen nutrition-sensitive interventions to prevent malnutrition.[11]

## 15.2 GROWTH MONITORING: EARLY IDENTIFICATION

Growth monitoring consists of routine measurements to detect abnormal growth, combined with some action when this is detected.[12] Growth monitoring with periodic assessment of the weight and length/height of the child or measuring mid-arm circumference is vital for detecting growth faltering at an early stage, identifying possible causes, and responding to the situation thereby preventing progression to moderate and severe acute malnutrition.

National programs in India are increasingly realizing the importance of growth monitoring as an important component of nutrition interventions. The integrated child development services (ICDS) has adopted the WHO growth standards in the joint mother and child protection card. The ICDS mission document has included monthly child growth monitoring during the village health and nutrition days as a core intervention and envisaged linking one to one counseling for optimal breastfeeding practices with growth monitoring. In the quest to focus on the children under 3 years, ICDS mission has included monthly weighing of all children 0–3 years, identification of growth faltering, and reinforcement of appropriate counseling of caregivers on optimal IYCF and health care by the anganwadi worker cum nutrition counselor, as a service. During the growth

monitoring sessions, malnourished children in need of medical attention are referred to health facilities.[13]

Ministry of Health, Government of India has also envisaged in-service orientation of ASHAs and ANMs on growth monitoring and identification of children with SAM using MUAC.[14]

## Anthropometric Methods to Identify SAM

Several studies have found variations in the sensitivity and specificity of methods for identifying SAM and international guidelines have provided varied views about the ideal tool to detect wasting.

A study analyzing anthropometric data from 47 countries recommends that the MUAC and weight for height are not alternative measures of the loss of body tissue but complementary variables. Both should be used independently to guide admission for treatment of malnourished children.[15] Another study which analyzed data from 16 cross-sectional nutritional surveys in South Sudan, the Philippines, Chad, and Bangladesh concluded that MUAC <125 mm should not be used as a stand-alone criterion of acute malnutrition given its strong association with age, sex, and stunting, and its low sensitivity to detect slim children.[16] One more study, which looked into the effect of age and gender on MUAC cut-offs, found that optimal cut-off values increased with age and varied with gender. The study highlights a need for a global reference value for MUAC cut-offs for different age and gender groups for detecting severe acute malnutrition at community level.[17]

A Joint Statement on Community-Based Management of Severe Acute Malnutrition by United Nation (2007) suggested using mid-arm circumference (MUAC) < 110 cm as the criteria to detect SAM.[18] This was modified by WHO in 2013 in guidelines on "Updates on the management of severe acute malnutrition in infants and children" that suggests a mid-arm circumference of < 115 cm or a weight-for-height/length <–3 Z-score of the WHO growth standards as cut-offs for identification and diagnosis of severe acute malnutrition.[19]

## 15.3 OPTIMAL INFANT AND YOUNG CHILD FEEDING PRACTICES

Child malnutrition is intimately related to inappropriate infant and young child feeding practices and occurs entirely during the first two years.[20] Optimal IYCF practices include initiating breastfeeding within one hour after birth, exclusive breastfeeding for the first six months, and appropriate complementary feeding thereafter with continuation of breastfeeding till two years of age or beyond.[21]

Optimal IYCF practices are not only important for ensuring optimum nutritional status but are equally important to reduce childhood morbidity particularly infectious diseases like diarrhea and pneumonia and improve child survival.[22] There is strong evidence for the positive effects of optimal IYCF practices as provided in the Global Strategy for Infant and Young Child Feeding and guiding principles for complementary feeding of the breastfed child on growth of infants and young children.[23]

## A. Advantages of Early and Exclusive Breastfeeding

Breastmilk not only contains all the nutrients like carbohydrates, fats including fatty acids, proteins, minerals, vitamins, and water necessary for growth and development but it is also rich in anti-microbial factors like antibodies, cytokines and anti-inflammatory factors, digestive enzymes, hormones, and transporters which play an important role in preventing diseases especially infections.[24] It provides all the energy required by an infant in the first six months of life and remains an important source of energy, proteins, and other nutrients beyond six months of age. In the second year of life, 500 mL of breastmilk provides 37% of energy, 55% of proteins, 76% of vitamin A, and 98% of vitamin C requirements of the child[25] **(Fig. 15.1)**.

Early initiation of breastfeeding prevents neonatal infections. A study from Nigeria using demographic and health survey data found that prevalence of diarrhea was higher among children whose mothers did not initiate breastfeeding within the first hour of birth.[26] Another study from Uganda states that first hour initiation and exclusive breastfeeding

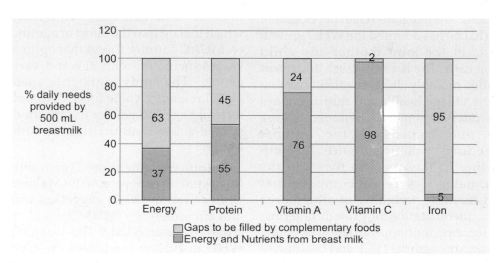

**Fig. 15.1** Nutrition provided by breastmilk in second year of life (Adapted from WHO (2009). Infant and young child feeding: Model Chapter)

reduced the probability occurrence of both diarrhea and ARI.[27] Preventive effect of exclusive breastfeeding on major childhood morbidities like diarrhea and pneumonia is well documented. A systematic review observed that relative risk for prevalence of diarrhea was 1.26 and 1.68, while for pneumonia it was 1.79 and 2.48 for predominant and partial breastfeeding children, respectively as compared to exclusive breastfeeding.[5] Another systematic review has concluded that exclusively breastfed neonates have a significantly lower risk of sepsis, diarrhea, and respiratory infections compared with those partially breastfed.[28]

### B. Role of Optimal IYCF in Preventing Wasting

Evidence shows positive role of optimal IYCF in preventing wasting. A cross-sectional study from India, which looked into relationship of infant feeding practices and undernutrition found that standardized IYCF score was significantly lower in undernourished children than those with normal grades. The study concluded that per unit increase in standardized IYCF score may reduce underweight, stunting, and wasting prevalence by 2–3%.[29]

Another study from Bangladesh found that universalization of early initiation of breastfeeding and exclusive breastfeeding up to 6 months achieved through community-based peer counseling, prevents growth faltering below 6 months of age.[30]

The risk of undernutrition and growth faltering is reported to be higher in formula fed infants than in breastfed infants. The incidence and prevalence of diarrhea, an important contributory factor for under-nutrition, was almost double in formula-fed infants than in breastfed infants and at 6 months, breast-fed infants were heavier and tended to be taller than infants fed formula.[31] A study from Israel has found beneficial effect of exclusive breastfeeding on weight gain in the first 3 months of life in comparison to exclusive bottle-feeding or mixed feeding.[32]

### 15.4 INTERVENTIONS FOR ENHANCING OPTIMAL INFANT FEEDING PRACTICES

IYCF practices may be enhanced sustainably if the Global Strategy for IYCF is implemented in its' entirety. A study looking into trends in exclusive breastfeeding rates in 22 countries over a period of 20 years stated that countries with policies and programs most consistent with the global strategy have a better annual rate of rise in exclusive breastfeeding.[33] Important determinants for optimal IYCF practices, as envisaged in the Global Strategy for IYCF include helpful hospital practices, protection of mother from the commercial influence of formula manufacturers, maternity protection, family support to the mother, correct information, and access to counseling and support services.

We will now discuss some of the important evidence based interventions for enhancing IYCF practices. Trends in IYCF practices in India over past 2 decades are shown in **Table 15.1**.

### A. IYCF Counseling

Mother's perception of not having enough milk is a major reason for adding supplemen-

**Table 15.1** Trends in Infant and Young Child Feeding Practices in India

| Indicators | NFHS-1 (1992-93) | NFHS-2 (1998-99) | NFHS-3 (2005-06) | RSOC (2013-14) |
|---|---|---|---|---|
| Initiation of breastfeeding within one hour of birth (%) | 9.5 | 15.8 | 23.4 | 44.6 |
| Exclusive breastfeeding < 6 months (%) | 51.0* | 41.2* | 46.0 | 64.9 |
| Children 6–9 months receiving solid or semi-solid food (%) | 31.4 | 33.5 | 55.8 | 50.5 |

* Exclusive breastfeeding < 4 months. NFHS: National Family Health Survey; RSOC: Rapid Survey on Children

tary foods leading to mixed or non-exclusive breastfeeding.[34] Many of other preventable lactation difficulties also contribute to stopping of breastfeeding prematurely. Enough scientific evidence is now available which suggests that counseling, either one-to-one or in groups, is an effective tools to improve duration of IYCF practices.[35]

- In the WHO Child Growth Standards study, trained lactation counselors supported the mothers to prevent and manage breastfeeding difficulties from soon after birth and at specified times during the first year after birth. By using this strategy, good compliance to exclusive breastfeeding was achieved in all the participating countries.[36]
- A Cochrane review on support for breastfeeding mothers, concluded that training on infant and young child feeding, which in turn led to more qualified professional and lay support to the mothers, resulted in prolonged breastfeeding duration.[37]
- A systematic review assessing the effects of promotional interventions on breastfeeding concluded that counseling or educational interventions can increase exclusive breastfeeding by 43% at day 1, by 30% till 1 month, and by 90% from 1–5 months.[38]
- In the Promotion of Breastfeeding Intervention Trial (PROBIT), skilled counseling provided by trained and skilled care provider led to improvement in exclusive breastfeeding rates.[39]
- Antenatal and postnatal counseling provided by community-based trained peer counselors can effectively increase the initiation and duration of exclusive breastfeeding.[40]

*Community-based Counseling*

Counseling provided by trained community level counselors including traditional birth attendants, anganwadi workers, and auxiliary nurse midwives (ANM) has also resulted in improved rates of exclusive breastfeeding and reduction of diarrhea.[41] Community-based interventions, including group counseling or education and social mobilization, with or without mass media, were similarly effective, increasing timely breastfeeding initiation by 86% and exclusive breastfeeding by 20%.[42]

A community-based intervention in India using peer counseling by mother support groups (MSG's) resulted in improving the infant and young child feeding (IYCF) practices significantly.[43]

A study from Bangladesh[44] reported that intensive nutrition education with or without supplementary feeding significantly improves the complementary feeding practices resulting in improved status of moderately malnourished children. Components of intervention included (*a*) nutritional counseling on breastfeeding, complementary food and introducing *khichuri* as complementary food; (*b*) disease control with identification of diseases, home management of common childhood diseases and proper referral of the sick children based on IMCI criteria; and (*c*) appropriate caring practices like child stimulation, personal hygiene and sanitation, allocation of extra time and care during illness and diseases.

## B. Baby Friendly Hospital Initiative

Routine use of early formula supplementation leads to reduced suckling on breast by infant causing inhibition of milk secretion and undermining of mother's confidence about sufficiency of her milk supply. All these factors lead to decreased duration of exclusive breastfeeding.

Adherence to the 10 steps of Baby Friendly Hospital Initiative (BFHI) **(Box 15.1)** has a positive impact on breastfeeding practices. There is a dose-response relationship between the number of BFHI steps women are exposed to and the likelihood of improved early breastfeeding initiation, exclusive breastfeeding at hospital discharge, and

**Box 15.1 Baby Friendly Hospital Initiative: 10 Steps to Successful Breastfeeding**

Every facility providing maternity services and care for newborn infants should:

1. Have a written breastfeeding policy that is routinely communicated to all health care staff.
2. Train all health care staff in skills necessary to implement this policy.
3. Inform all pregnant women about the benefits and management of breastfeeding.
4. Help mothers initiate breastfeeding within half an hour of birth.
5. Show mothers how to breastfeed, and how to maintain lactation even if they should be separated from their infants.
6. Give newborn infants no food or drink other than breast milk, unless medically indicated.
7. Practice rooming-in-that is, allow mothers and infants to remain together—24 hours a day.
8. Encourage breastfeeding on demand.
9. Give no artificial teats or pacifiers (also called dummies or soothers) to breastfeeding infants.
10. Foster the establishment of breastfeeding support groups and refer mothers to them on discharge from the hospital or clinic.

**Source**: *Protecting, Promoting and Supporting Breastfeeding: The Special Role of Maternity Services*, a joint WHO/UNICEF statement published by the World Health Organization.

exclusive breastfeeding duration.[45] Step 3 (prenatal education) and Step 10 (postnatal breastfeeding support) are the most difficult steps to implement, although these steps are crucial in impacting maternal breastfeeding decisions[46], especially, practicing exclusive breastfeeding.[47]

## C. Maternity Protection

For the mother to practice breastfeeding, the baby and mother duo should remain together. This is a challenge for the women particularly who are employed outside the home. Provision of maternity entitlements in the form of adequate leave and worksite facilities like crèches, breastfeeding rooms, breastfeeding breaks etc provide a conducive environment for breastfeeding. There are evidence suggesting that provision of maternity leave

results in increased duration of breastfeeding and lesser maternal separation anxiety and optimal maternal infant attachment.[48]

## D. Protection from Commercial Influence of Formula Manufacturers

Marketing tactics of formula manufacturers to promote their products directly to the public and through the health care system compete with breastfeeding. Regulation of such practices help mothers to make appropriate and informed decisions.[49] For regulating the marketing of breastmilk substitutes, World Health Assembly (WHA) adopted a resolution for International Code of Marketing of Breastmilk Substitutes. Countries have to enact and implement a national legislation based on the provisions of the Code.

Several studies have highlighted negative effects of promotional activities of formula manufacturers on breastfeeding practices.

- A study from Philippines has found that children were more likely to be given formula if their mother were exposed to advertising messages or products were suggested by a doctor. Mothers who were using formula were 6.4 times more likely to stop breastfeeding before 12 month.[50]
- Another study reported that distribution of free samples of infant formula at discharge negatively impact duration and exclusivity of breastfeeding.[51]
- A randomized controlled trial revealed that educational materials on breastfeeding produced by manufacturers of infant formula and distributed to pregnant women intending to breastfeed had a substantially negative effect on the exclusivity and duration of breastfeeding.[52]

## E. Interventions to Improve Maternal Nutrition during Pregnancy and Lactation

Maternal body-mass index has been found an important determinant for all categories of child undernutrition including wasting.[53] Maternal undernutrition increases risk of wasting in children many fold.[54] Nutritional interventions including dietary advice to pregnant women, provision of balanced energy protein supplements, and high protein or isocaloric protein supplementation has been found useful in addressing maternal undernutirtion.[55]

## 15.5 OTHER INTERVENTIONS

### A. Improvement in Basic Health Care Facilities

Access to health services is important as timely intervention in childhood diseases like diarrhea and respiratory infections is crucial to prevent wasting.[56] Barriers for utilization of health care facility include long distance to health facility; long waiting times; lack of medicines and supplies; negative attitude of health workers; suboptimal examination of the sick child; and high cost of healthcare.[57] Effective primary health care system should address each of these factors.

### B. Food Security at Household Level

Household food security is an important determinant of optimal nutritional status in children. A qualitative study from India has found fragile food security or seasonal food paucity as one of the important cause of child undernutrition. Adequate employment opportunities, equitable distribution of resources, control over inflation and food prices, appropriate food supplementation program, and appropriate social security are some of the measures to ensure household food security.

### C. Improvement in Water, Sanitation, and Hygiene

Water, sanitation, and hygiene (WASH) interventions are important to reduce infectious diseases in children. Safe water supply, presence of toilet in the household, hand-washing with soap and water after defecation and before feeding are important measures to prevent infectious diseases like diarrhea. Apart from the physical infra-structure, safe WASH practices require behavior change interventions.[58-60]

## 15.6 INNOVATIVE COMMUNITY INTERVENTIONS FOR MANAGING SEVERE WASTING

### A. Action Against Malnutrition (AAM): Experiences from Tribal India[61]

Action Against Malnutrition (AAM) is a comprehensive, multi-strategy community based management of malnutrition (CMAM) program implemented in 7 blocks of rural India (in the state of Jharkhand, Bihar, Odisha, Chhattisgarh) with an objective to reduce malnutrition among children 0–3 years through community mobilization and community based management of malnutrition using local foods and food production.[61] The programis built upon community participation to achieve a sustainable awareness of child nutrition in the community, and aimed to prevent as well as manage malnutrition.

### Intervention Areas

The program included three interventions areas with different interventions:

*Area 1:* Only intervention was strengthening of systems.

*Area 2:* Interventions included participatory learning activity (PLA) along with the systems strengthening. PLA Meetings created platform that built knowledge on IYCF practices, catering to women of all age groups. Identified women were followed up by home visits.

*Area 3:* Interventions included Creche facility along with the Participatory Learning Activity (PLA) and systems strengthening. Crèches catered children from 6 months to 3 years. Crèches provided spaces for working mothers who went to work freely and then came to breastfeed their children at regular intervals. Complementary feeding of children was also taken care of where meals were provided

3 times a day and for children who were undernourished 5 times a day with an increase in the amount of cooking oil. Crèche provided up to 868 kcal (70% of daily nutritional requirements)+ 15.4 g protein per day with a menu based on local foods containing energy dense foods with 350–500 kcal/100 g.

In the intervention group with Crèche, impact on wasting (over a period of 4–6 months and a cohort of 587 children), was significant. Among the severely malnourished children, 49% shifted to moderate malnutrition and 36% became normal. Among the moderately malnourished children, 67% became normal. All the children in the cohort, who were normal at the beginning of the program, maintained the status. These results suggest that a comprehensive set of intervention incorporating sustainable solutions can be helpful not only in treating but preventing the severe acute malnutrition.

## B. Rajmata Jijau Mother-Child Health and Nutrition Mission-Maharashtra- An Innovative Intervention to Reduce the Prevalence of Severe Wasting[62]

Maharashtra was able to reduce Wasting from 19.9% in 2006 to 15.5% in 2012, a percentage point change of–4.4% and a decline of 22.1% (CNSM, 2012). Similarly, Severe Wasting reduced from 7.81% in 2006 to 4.16 in 2012, a percentage point change of –3.65 and a decline of 46.7% (http://www.ids.ac.ukl).

This was achieved through innovative interventions like addressing the malnutrition issue through a mission; focused approach to improve coverage, and weighing of all children; awareness generation about the importance of 10 essential interventions including breastfeeding etc; conducting regular training programs on child care, nutrition, care during illness etc.; and treating Severe Acute Malnutrition (SAM) and Moderate Acute Malnutrition (MAM) using a three tier system— through Village Child Development Center (VCDC) in Anganwadi Centers for community management at village level, Child Treatment Center (CTC) for facility based management of SAM and MAM children (at PHC level), and Nutrition Rehabilitation Center (NRC) for facility based management (at the level of rural hospital/district hospital).

This model contributed to substantial reduction in wasting and child mortality.[62]

## 15.7 CONCLUSIONS

Reducing the burden of severe acute malnutrition, as envisaged in the global nutrition commitments requires tackling of complex social and political challenges with comprehensive measures. It requires equitable access to food and health care, policies and programs to enhance breastfeeding and optimal IYCF practices, universal access to safe drinking water, universal access to sanitation, surveillance system for quickly detecting and responding to growth faltering, and putting system in place for prompt action to thwart food shortages particularly ensuring food adequacy during the emergencies. It is important to note the crucial role of optimal IYCF practices in prevention and management of SAM. Any intervention for management of severe acute malnutrition should have a strong component on enhancing optimal IYCF practices for sustainable results.[63]

This is prudent to conclude that prevention leading to a sustainable decrease in the burden of severe acute malnutrition can only be achieved through a comprehensive plan to tackle all the causative and underlying determinants. It cannot be achieved simply through providing commercial fortified food products to infants and children.

## REFERENCES

1. World Health Organization. Nutrition - Global targets 2025. Available from: www.who.int/ nutrition/topics/ nutrition_globaltargets2025/ en/. Accessed on 16 August 2016.
2. United Nations. Sustainable Developmental Goals - Goal 2: End hunger, achieve food security and improved nutrition and promote sustainable

agriculture. Available from: http://www.un.org/sustainabledevelopment/hunger. Accessed on 24 August, 2016.

3. WHO. Global Nutrition Targets 2025- Wasting Policy Brief. Available from: http://www.who.int/nutrition/publications/globaltargets2025_policybrief_wasting/en/. Accessed on 27 August 2016.

4. UNICEF (1990). Strategy for improved nutrition of children and women in developing countries. Available from: http://www.ceecis.org/iodine/01_global/01_pl/01_01_other_1992_unicef.pdf. Accessed on 5 September, 2016.

5. Black RE, Victora CG, Walker SP, Bhutta ZA, Christian P, de Onis M, Ezzati M, Grantham-McGregor S, Katz J, Martorell R, Uauy R. Maternal and Child Nutrition Study Group. Maternal and child undernutrition and overweight in low-income and middle-income countries. Lancet. 20133;382:427–51.

6. Dewey KG. Tackling the double burden of malnutrition: What actions are needed at the individual and family level. UN Steering Committee on Nutrition. SCN News. 2006;32:16–20.

7. Shrimpton R, Victora CG, de Onis M, Lima RC, Blössner M, Clugston G. Worldwide timing of growth faltering: implications for nutritional interventions. Pediatrics. 2001;107:E75.

8. WHO. Global Strategy for Infant and Young Child Feeding. Available from: http://www.who.int/nutrition/topics/global_strategy_iycf/en/. Accessed on 4 September 2016.

9. Burza S, Mahajan R, Marino E, Sunyoto T, Shandilya C, Tabrez M, et al. Seasonal effect and long-term nutritional status following exit from a community-based management of severe acute malnutrition program in Bihar, India. Eur J Clin Nutr. 2016;70:437–44.

10. Shen X, Gao X, Tang W, Mao X, Huang J, Cai W. Food insecurity and malnutrition in Chinese elementary school students. Br J Nutr. 2015;114:952–8.

11. UNICEF (2015). Prevention and Treatment of Severe Acute Malnutrition in East Asia and the Pacific Report of a Regional Consultation, Bangkok, Thailand, June 24-26, 2015. Available from:http://www.unicef.org/eapro/UNICEF_EAPRO_SAM_consultation_2015_report.pdf. Accessed on 20 August 2016.

12. Panpanich R, Garner P. Growth monitoring in children. Cochrane Database Syst Rev. 2000;2: CD001443.

13. Ministry of Women and Child Development, Government of India (2012). ICDS mission - the broad framework for implementation. Available from: http://wcdsc.ap.nic.in/ICDS/References/IcdsMission.pdf. Accessed on October 17, 2016.

14. Ministry of Health and Family Welfare, Government of India (2011). Operational guidelines on facility based management of children with severe acute malnutrition. Available from: http://nrhm.gov.in/images/pdf/programmes/child-health/guidelines/operational_guidelines_on_fbmc_with_sam.pdf. Accessed on October 17, 2016.

15. Grellety E, Golden MH. Weight-for-height and mid-upper-arm circumference should be used independently to diagnose acute malnutrition: policy implications. BMC. 2016;2:10.

16. Roberfroid D, Huybregts L, Lachat C, Vrijens F, Kolsteren P, Guesdon B. Inconsistent diagnosis of acute malnutrition by weight-for-height and mid-upper arm circumference: contributors in 16 cross-sectional surveys from South Sudan, the Philippines, Chad, and Bangladesh. Nutr J. 2015;14:86.

17. Fiorentino M, Sophonneary P, Laillou A, Whitney S, de Groot R, Perignon M, et al. Current MUAC cut-offs to screen for acute malnutrition need to be adapted to gender and age: The example of Cambodia. PLoS One. 2016;11:e0146442.

18. WHO,UNICEF,WFP, UN SCN (2007). Community-based management of Severe Acute Malnutrition. Available from: http://apps.who.int/iris/bitstream/10665/44295/1/9789280641479_eng.pdf?ua=1&ua=1.Accessed on October 12, 2016.

19. WHO (2013). Guideline: Updates on the management of severe acute malnutrition in infants and children. Available from:http://apps.who.int/iris/bitstream/10665/95584/1/9789241506328_eng.pdf. Accessed on October 12, 2016.

20. Gupta A, Rohde JE. Infant and young child undernutrition- Where lie the solutions? Econ Pol Wkly. 2004:52;13–16.

21. UNICEF (2011). Programming guide - infant and young child feeding. Available from: http://www.unicef.org/nutrition/files/Final_IYCF_programming_guide_2011.pdf. Accessed on 4 September 2016.

22. Jones G, Steketee RW, Black RE, Bhutta ZA, Morris SS; Bellagio Child Survival Study Group. How many child deaths can we prevent this year? Lancet. 2003;362:65–71.

23. Saha KK, Frongillo EA, Alam DS, Arifeen SE, Persson LA, Rasmussen KM. Appropriate infant feeding practices result in better growth of infants and young children in rural Bangladesh. Am J Clin Nutr. 2008;87:1852–9.

24. Prentice A. Constituents of human milk. Available from: http://archive.unu.edu/unupress/food/8F174e/8F174E04.htm. Accessed on September 4, 2016.

25. WHO (2009). Infant and young child feeding: Model Chapter for textbooks for medical students and allied health professionals. Available from: http://apps.who.int/iris/bitstream/10665/44117/1/9789241597494_eng.pdf?ua=1. Accessed on 4 September 2016.

26. Ogbo FA, Page A, Idoko J, Claudio F, Agho KE. Diarrhoea and suboptimal feeding practices in Nigeria: Evidence from the national household surveys. Paediatr Perinat Epidemiol. 2016;30:346–55.

27. Bbaale E. Determinants of diarrhoea and acute respiratory infection among under-fives in Uganda. Australas Med J. 2011;4:400–9.

28. Khan J, Vesel L, Bahl R, Martines JC. Timing of breastfeeding initiation and exclusivity of breastfeeding during the first month of life: effects on neonatal mortality and morbidity--a systematic review and meta-analysis. Matern Child Health J. 2015;19:468–79.

29. Mukhopadhyay DK, Sinhababu A, Saren AB, Biswas AB. Association of child feeding practices with nutritional status of under-two slum dwelling children: a community-based study from West Bengal, India. Indian J Public Health. 2013;57:169–72.

30. Haider R, Saha KK. Breastfeeding and infant growth outcomes in the context of intensive peer counselling support in two communities in Bangladesh. Int Breastfeed J. 2016;11:18.

31. Villalpando S, López-Alarcón M. Growth faltering is prevented by breast-feeding in underprivileged infants from Mexico City. J Nutr. 2000;130:546–52.

32. Fawzi WW, Forman MR, Levy A, Graubard BI, Naggan L, Berendes HW. Maternal anthropometry and infant feeding practices in Israel in relation to growth in infancy: the North African Infant Feeding Study. Am J Clin Nutr. 1997;65:1731–7.

33. Lutter CK, Morrow AL. Protection, promotion, and support and global trends in breastfeeding. Adv Nutr. 2013;4:213-9.

34. Oommen A, Vatsa M, Paul VK, Aggarwal R. Breastfeeding practices of urban and rural mothers. Indian Pediatr. 2009;46:891–4.

35. Bhutta ZA, Ahmed T, Black RE, Cousens S, Dewey K, Giugliani E, et al. What works? Interventions for maternal and child under-nutrition and survival. Lancet. 2008; 371:417–40.

36. WHO Multicentre Growth Reference Study Group. Assessment of linear growth differences among populations in the WHO Multicentre Growth Reference Study. Acta Paediatr. 2006;450: 56–65.

37. Britton C, McCormick FM, Renfrew MJ, Wade A, King SE. Support for breastfeeding mothers. Cochrane Database System Rev. 2006;4: CD001141.

38. Bhutta ZA, Das JK, Rizvi A, Gaffey MF, Walker N, Horton S, Webb P, Lartey A, Black RE; Lancet Nutrition Interventions Review Group; Maternal and Child Nutrition Study Group. Evidence-based interventions for improvement of maternal and child nutrition: what can be done and at what cost? Lancet. 2013;382:452–77.

39. Kramer MS, Chalmers B, Hodnett ED, Sevkovskaya Z, Dzikovich I, Shapiro S, et al. Promotion of breastfeeding intervention trials (PROBIT): a randomised trial in the Republic of Belarus. JAMA. 2001;285:413–20.

40. Haider R, Ashworth A, Kabir I, Huttly SRA. Effect of community-based peer counsellors on exclusive breastfeeding practices in Dhaka, Bangladesh: a randomised controlled trial. Lancet. 2000;356:1643–7.

41. Bhandari N, Bahl R, Mazumdar S, Martines J, Black RE, Bhan MK(Infant Feeding Study Group). Effect of community-based promotion of exclusive breastfeeding on diarrhoeal illness and growth: a cluster randomized controlled trial. Lancet. 2003; 361:1418–23.

42. Rollins NC, Bhandari N, Hajeebhoy N, Horton S, Lutter CK, Martines JC, et al. Why invest, and what it will take to improve breastfeeding practices? Lancet. 2016;387:491–504.

43. Kushwaha KP, Sankar J, Sankar MJ, Gupta A, Dadhich JP, Gupta YP, et al. Effect of peer counselling by mother support groups on infant and young child feeding practices: the Lalitpur experience. PLoS One. 2014;9:e109181.

44. Roy SK, Fuchs GJ, Mahmud Z, Ara G, Islam S, Shafique S, Akter SS, Chakraborty B. Intensive nutrition education with or without supplementary feeding improves the nutritional status of moderately-malnourished children in Bangladesh. J Health Popul Nutr. 2005;23:320–30.

45. Pérez-Escamilla R, Martinez JL, Segura-Pérez S. Impact of the baby-friendly hospital initiative on breastfeeding and child health outcomes: a systematic review. Matern Child Nutr. 2016; 12:402–17.

46. Munn AC, Newman SD, Mueller M, Phillips SM, Taylor SN. The Impact in the United States of the baby-friendly hospital initiative on early infant health and breastfeeding outcomes. Breastfeed Med. 2016;11:222–30.

47. Yotebieng M, Labbok M, Soeters HM, ChalachalaJL, Lapika B, Vitta BS, Behets F. Ten steps to successful breastfeeding programme to promote early initiation and exclusive breastfeeding in DR Congo: a cluster-randomised controlled trial. Lancet Glob Health. 2015;3:e546–55.

48. Cooklin AR, Rowe HJ, Fisher JR. Paid parental leave supports breastfeeding and mother-infant relationship: a prospective investigation of maternal postpartum employment. Aust N Z J Public Health. 2012;36:249–56.

49. Shealy KR, Li R, Benton-Davis S, Grummer-Strawn LM. The CDC Guide to Breastfeeding Interventions. Atlanta: U.S. Department of Health and Human Services, Centers for Disease Control and Prevention, 2005. Available from: https://www.cdc.gov/breastfeeding/pdf/breastfeeding_interventions.pdf. Accessed on 1 September, 2016.

50. Sobel HL, Iellamo A, Raya RR, Padilla AA, Olivé JM, Nyunt-US. Is unimpeded marketing for breast milk substitutes responsible for the decline in breastfeeding in the Philippines? An exploratory survey and focus group analysis. Soc Sci Med. 2011;73:1445–8.

51. Donnelly A, Snowden HM, Renfrew MJ, Woolridge MW. Commercial hospital discharge packs for breastfeeding women. Cochrane Database Syst Rev. 2000;2:CD002075.

52. Howard C, Howard F, Lawrence R, Andresen E, DeBlieck E, Weitzman M. Office prenatal formula advertising and its effect on breast-feeding patterns. Obstet Gynecol. 2000;95:296–303.

53. Choudhury N, Raihan MJ, Sultana S, Mahmud Z, Farzana FD, Haque MA, et al. Determinants of age-specific undernutrition in children aged less than 2 years-the Bangladesh context. Matern Child Nutr. 2016 Oct 12.

54. Senbanjo IO, Olayiwola IO, Afolabi WA, Senbanjo OC. Maternal and child under-nutrition in rural and urban communities of Lagos state, Nigeria: the relationship and risk factors. BMC Res Notes. 2013;6:286.

55. Bhutta ZA, Das JK, Rizvi A, Gaffey MF, Walker N, Horton S, Webb P, Lartey A,Black RE; Lancet Nutrition Interventions Review Group; Maternal and Child Nutrition Study Group. Evidence-based interventions for improvement of maternal and child nutrition: what can be done and at what cost? Lancet. 2013;382:452–77.

56. Kavosi E, Rostami ZH, Kavosi Z, Nasihatkon A, Moghadami M, Heidari M. Prevalence and determinants of under-nutrition among children under six: A cross-sectional survey in Fars province, Iran. Int J Health Policy Manag. 2014;3:71–6.

57. Lungu EA, Biesma R, Chirwa M, Darker C. Healthcare seeking practices and barriers to accessing under-five child health services in urban slums in Malawi: a qualitative study. BMC Health Serv Res. 201619;16:410.

58. Dangour AD, Watson L, Cumming O, Boisson S, Che Y, Velleman Y, et al. Interventions to improve water quality and supply, sanitation and hygiene practices, and their effects on the nutritional status of children. Cochrane Database Syst Rev. 2013;8:CD009382.

59. Aheto JM, Keegan TJ, Taylor BM, Diggle PJ. Childhood malnutrition and its determinants among under-five children in Ghana. Paediatr Perinat Epidemiol. 2015;29:552–61.

60. Schlegelmilch MP, Lakhani A, Saunders LD, JhangriGS. Evaluation of water, sanitation and hygiene program outcomes shows knowledge-behavior gaps in Coast Province, Kenya. Pan Afr Med J. 201630;23:145.

61. Action Against Malnutrition (AAM): Experiences and Outcomes of a Comprehensive Community Based Programme to Address Malnutrition in Tribal India. Int J Child Health Nutr. 2015;4:151–62.

62. Rajmata Jijau Mother Child Nutrition Mission–Government of Maharashtra. Available from: http://www.mahnm.in.Accessed January 20, 2017.

63. UNICEF (2015). Management of Severe Acute Malnutrition in children: Working towards results at scale. Available from: http://www.unicef.org/eapro/UNICEF_program_guidance_on_manangement_of_SAM_2015.pdf. Accessed on 9 September 2016.

# 16 Progress, Programs, and Policies for Managing and Preventing Severe Acute Malnutrition

Amir Maroof Khan

Undernutrition is a major cause of child mortality and childhood morbidity. The Sustainable Development Goal 2.2 states to end all forms of malnutrition by 2030, and to achieve the internationally agreed targets on stunting and wasting in children under five years of age by 2025.

Global Nutrition Report 2016 ranks India at 114 of the 132 positions regarding prevalence of stunting and ranks 120 out of 130 nations regarding wasting, which is a dismal figure for the nation.[1] The cycle of undernutrition continues with poorly nourished adolescents and child marriages leading to pregnancies which are often multiple and result in low birth weight babies.

Comparing the recent data on child undernutrition from Rapid Survey on Children (RSoC, 2013-14) with another national level data from National Family Health Survey (NFHS-3) conducted around a decade back, we observe that there has been a decline in prevalence of wasting (19.8 to 15.1%), underweight (42.5 to 29.4%) and stunting (48 to 38.7%).[2,3] On the other hand, the India Health Report on Nutrition 2015 reports that the pace of improvement in the nutritional status of children is not in tune with the significantly rapid growth observed in Gross Domestic Product of the country.[4]

## 16.1 INDICATORS OF SEVERE ACUTE MALNUTRITION AT COMMUNITY LEVEL

Severe acute undernutrition constitutes a specific and unique subset of the malnutrition phenomenon. It requires immediate detection and rapid action to prevent its harmful effects on the health and development of the children.

To measure the impact of nutrition and nutrition related programs on SAM at the national and state levels requires nutritional surveillance data. But there are two issues with regards to the available nutrition data and its incompatibility with SAM related data.

i. The largest program related to child nutrition Integrated Child Development Scheme (ICDS) does not measure height of children and mid upper arm circumference (MUAC) which are the bases for identifying SAM. Its growth monitoring mechanism consists of measuring weight and age of the child, which misses SAM affected children.

ii. The prevalence data generated by various surveys such as NFHS and others have their own deficiencies and inappropriate-ness for estimating SAM. SAM is acute and associated with high mortality, and thus its estimation is a complex issue. Even if an attempt is made to find out the prevalence of SAM by piggy riding on these surveys, it would be hardly accurate due to the seasonal fluctuations, geographical variations, and the feasibility aspects of the varying definitions of SAM at field level.

The IAP recommends MUAC measurement for earlier detection of SAM in community settings. This is a feasible and implementable option to screen the children for SAM; and those detected may be further assessed for deciding their management stratgies.[5] However, there is some upcoming evidence which shows that MUAC and weight-for-height Z-scores (WHZ) may not identify the same individual child with SAM, using either of the two methods in isolation will fail to detect a certain proportion of SAM affected children.[6] More research is needed to decide about the validity and feasibility of using single or more than one method for detecting acute malnutrition in community settings.

The indicator, 'Geographic coverage' of SAM treatment is vulnerable to misinterpretations because of the possibility of variation in the understandings of the numerator and the denominator. For example; 'geographic coverage' may either be interpreted as the population covered by the SAM management facilities or the proportion of SAM children who were managed for SAM. In order to avoid such misinterpretations, it is important to report about SAM treatment coverage in unambiguous and exact terms. Indicators for SAM treatment coverage as recommended by UNICEF[7] are given in **Table 16.1**.

In spite of so many surveys, tracking child nutrition status is a challenging, task with lack of regular, consistent, and reliable anthropometric data. Data on SAM would be more contextual, season-specific, region-specific, and highly dynamic due to the higher mortality rates associated with it thus leading to a risk of underestimating its prevalence estimates. Apart from setting up a mechanism of generating regular national surveys every 3–5 years, it would be pragmatic to enhance the quality and reliability of the data being generated from the already existing ICDS and leveraging it for generating SAM related data too.

**Table 16.1** Indicators for Treatment Coverage of Severe Acute Malnutrition[7]

| Indicator | Definition | Explanation |
|---|---|---|
| Facilities geographical coverage | Number of facilities delivering community based management of acute malnutrition (CMAM)/all primary healthcare facilities | This indicator does not represent the spatial coverage, as the facilities may not be covering the whole population |
| Treatment coverage | Cases admitted within a given period/estimated burden for the same period | This treatment coverage can be either national treatment coverage for countries with national programs for SAM and target area treatment coverage for countries where SAM programs are not operating at the national level |
| Program implementation progress | Number of admissions/target case load | This can be used to measure the progress of a program in a target based approach. There is lack of SAM related data from India which makes it challenging for policy makers to develop evidence based policies and implement SAM related programs at the national and state levels |

## 16.2 MANAGEMENT OF SEVERE ACUTE MALNUTRITION: COMMUNITY LEVEL INITIATIVES

### Initiatives at International Level

- World Health Organization (WHO) defines 'Integrated management of SAM' as one of the basic health services to which child has access and it is embedded into a broader set of nutrition activities like infant and young child feeding (IYCF), nutritional supplementation and integrated into a multisectoral approach to tackling the determinants of undernutrition.

- World Bank has listed management of SAM among the top 13 cost effective interventions to tackle undernutrition.

- The Renewed Efforts against Child Hunger and Undernutrition (REACH) initiative and the Scaling up Nutrition (SUN) movement with a major push from UNICEF place emphasis on country led initiatives to be developed and implemented to combat SAM. It strives to help countries in developing SAM detection and management strategies within their routine child health care services.

- Community-based Management of Acute Malnutrition (CMAM) is an integrated approach combining nutrition sensitive interventions and nutrition specific interventions focusing on the first 1000 days of a child's life. CMAM approach to manage SAM and MAM in under-five children is directly implemented in more than 70 countries.[8]

### The 1000 Days Approach

The 1000 days from conception to the child attaining two years of age is of prime importance in laying the nutritional foundation for a children's future health.[9] Essential interventions of this approach are listed in **Box 16.1**. These form the basis for comprehensive child nutrition related programs in India.

**Box 16.1 The 10 Interventions of the 1000 Days Approach**

1. Timely initiation of breastfeeding within one hour of birth
2. Exclusive breastfeeding for six months
3. Timely introduction of complementary foods
4. Age appropriate complementary feeding for children 6 to 23 months of age
5. Safe handling and hygienic complementary feeding practices
6. Full immunization, six monthly vitamin A supplementation and deworming
7. Frequent and active feeding with ORS and zinc during diarrhea
8. Timely and therapeutic feeding for children affected with SAM
9. Improved food and nutrient intake for adolescent girls to prevent anemia and marriage, and pregnancy delayed till 18 years
10. Improved food and nutrient intake for women particularly during pregnancy and lactation.

### Initiatives in India

The discussions on SAM started around 2006-07 in India. Certain pilot initiatives took off mainly spearheaded by UNICEF using imported and patented (PlumpyNut) ready to use therapeutic foods (RUTF) for management of SAM children. This strategy faced opposition from some sectors, the main argument being that use of RUTF will discourage the comprehensive and preventive efforts to manage undernutrition. Another concern was the high cost of the patented RUTF. In 2009, the Government of India banned the import of this RUTF. By that time various community groups in certain states, *e.g.* Chattisgarh, had started pilot projects on community based management of severe acute malnutrition (CSAM) using local foods instead of RUTF. On the other hand, nutrition rehabilitation center (NRCs) had been initiated by many states alongside these projects thus formally institutionalizing SAM management.

The international conference on CMAM 2011 in Addis Ababa gave impetus to policy makers and opinion leaders in various key sectors *e.g.* NRHM, Ministry of Women and

Child Development, right-to-food activists, UNICEF, and other donors. A decision was taken to formulate and adopt a locally produced, not-for-profit, energy rich and nutrient dense therapeutic food in Indian settings. Madhya Pradesh and Odisha, the two states which represented India at the international CMAM conference took lead in piloting CSAM programs in India. For both these states, Anganwadi centers of ICDS have been the focal point for delivering CSAM. Madhya Pradesh attempted to provide and assess an integrated model for the management of SAM in India which includes using facility and community based therapeutic care as a continuum of care approach. It also attempts to assess the cost-effectiveness of out-patient care through CSAM to the inpatient treatment being provided using NRCs. Odisha attempted to study the following modes of SAM treatment:

a. Different hot cooked meals at fixed intervals;

b. A special fortified variant of the dry Take Home Ration (THR); and

c. Milk based energy rich, nutrient dense therapeutic food as THR.

Studies have shown that CMAM is cost effective and cost-effectiveness ratios for CMAM are similar to that for other priority child health interventions.[10,11] The Indian Academy of Pediatrics (IAP) Consensus Statement 2013 suggests hospitalization for children less than 6 months and home based therapy with either locally prepared foods or RUTF for older children. (IAP 2013) Hospitalized children less than 6 months are not given RUTF, but exclusive breastfeeding is practiced.[5]

Based upon whether the nutrition interventions focus on the direct or indirect causes of undernutrition, the existing nutrition interventions in India can be divided into two broad categories:

1. *Direct causes of undernutrition among mothers and children:* Nutrition specific interventions such as ICDS and mid-day meal and those under the NRHM targeting micronutrient deficiencies such as distribution of iron folic acid, along with establishing convergence between water, sanitation, education, nutrition, and health programs.

2. *Indirect causes of undernutrition:* National Rural Employment Guarantee Act (NREGA) and public distribution system (food security for the poor).

However, it is disappointing to note that the Union budget for food and nutrition security as a proportion of total budget has declined from 12.5% (2014-15 revised estimates) to 10.9% (2015-16 estimation). Even the food and nutrition security as a proportion of GDP has declined from 1.7% to 1.4% during the same period.

## 16.3 NUTRITIONAL REHABILITATION CENTERS

Under the National Health Mission, *Bal Shakti Yojana* was launched in Madhya Pradesh (MP) to manage SAM. Other states followed MP and established similar network of Nutritional Rehabilitation Centers (NRC).

Currently, the only model of SAM management approved at the national level is 'inpatient treatment of SAM'. This is being carried out by the Nutritional Rehabilitation Centers or Malnutrition Treatment Center set up in health facilities for management of SAM children with counseling of mothers for proper feeding and regular follow up. The Child Health Division of Ministry of Health and Family Welfare (MOHFW) has published and disseminated the operational guidelines for facility based management of children with SAM. In 2013-14, the central government received proposals from 23 states requesting to establish 1007 NRCs and funds were provided for the same under the National Health Mission. Available data shows that 872 NRCs were operational out of the 1007 already approved centers up to December 2014 in India.[12]

The community and peripheral health facilities identify SAM and refer to NRCs for medical management and institutional rehabilitation. Between April 2013 to December 2014, around one lakh children were admitted in NRCs all over India and around 55% of them were discharged successfully *i.e.* with a target weight gain. The funds for the NRCs are not provided separately as a scheme but under the Reproductive, Maternal, Newborn, Child Health and Adolescents (RMNCH+A) strategic approach adopted under the National Health Mission. These funds are for establishing NRCs, and covering the operational and the human resource costs. The Center also provides technical assistance to states, by way of developing trainer of trainers, developing guidelines, training modules, improving upon the protocols for SAM management, and also monitoring and reviewing the NRCs performance.

Desk reviews of reports received and field visits to the NRCs by supervisory teams at the Center led to the following salient recommendations:
1. The admission and discharge criteria need to be more strictly followed.
2. Treatment and nutritional protocols need to be adhered to the standard treatment guidelines.
3. Quality of care needs to be focused on by training medical officers, nurses, and deployment of nutritionists.
4. There is a need for improvising the linkages between NRCs, health facilities, and anganwadi centers for better referral and follow up.

Studies on NRCs have reported lower recovery rates *i.e.* from 46.8% to 56.4%[13,14] when compared with the reference i.e. 75% cut off of SPHERE guidelines.[15] The mortality rates and child sickness rates are also lower despite these low recovery rates. This apparently paradoxical finding raises questions over the effectiveness of NRCs in having an impact on SAM.

Experts opine that, in India, severe chronic malnutrition (SCM) due to chronic poverty and hunger is being managed as a vertical approach of NRCs and hence the desired results are not being produced. A horizontal approach with multisectoral approach, focusing on improving local diet, food security, infant and young child feeding (IYCF) practices, sustaining livelihood of mothers is needed to tackle the problem of predominant undernutrition *i.e.* SCM in the country. Even the erstwhile Planning Commissions of Government of India had recommended *Whole of Government* (WoG), *i.e.* intersectoral coordination between ministries, departments, policies, and programs, and *Whole of Society* (WoS), *i.e.* involvement of all key stake holders at the point of implementation for convergence, approach towards comprehensively addressing the issue of child malnutrition.

The not for profit organizations and certain state government have already started to implement and assess the impact of community based models but as of now there are no government policies or guidelines regarding these.

## 16.4 INTEGRATED CHILD DEVELOPMENT SERVICES (ICDS) SCHEME

This is the only institutionalized mechanism in India to directly tackle child undernutrition at the grass root level and the largest of its kind in the world. The primary functioning unit is anganwadi center (AWC) and anganwadi worker is the key functionary at the AWC.

All children less than 6 years, adolescent girls, pregnant and lactating women are eligible beneficiaries of ICDS. It was launched in 1975 with the objective of providing pre-school education, and supplementary nutrition to children less than six years. Being below the poverty line (BPL) cut-off is not a criterion for registration of beneficiaries under ICDS. There has been an increase in the number of aganwadi centers (AWCs) from 4891 AWCs in 33 blocks (projects) in 1975 to 13.46 lakh AWC and more than 7000 projects as on 31 March 2015.[16]

## Nutrition Components of ICDS

Under the revised nutrition and feeding norm of ICDS, state governments and union territories have been requested to provide 300 days of supplementary food in a year and more than one meal to children from 3–6 years who visit AWC. This consists of milk/banana/egg/seasonal fruits/micronutrient fortified food followed by a hot cooked meal (HCM). Children below 3 years, pregnant and lactating mothers are provided with pre-mixes/ready to eat foods in the form of Take Home Rations (THR). These comprise of dense energy foods and fortified blended mixtures for consumption.[16]

Food grains such as wheat, rice, maize, ragi are allocated at Below Poverty Line (BPL) rates to the states/UT through the department of food and public distribution for preparation of supplementary food under ICDS. In view of the Supplementary Nutrition Program (SNP), an essential component of ICDS, the provision of grains has been made as an entitlement under the National Food Security Act (NFSA 2013). Under the Act, the central government shall provide food grains in request of the entitlements to the state governments at prices specified in the Act.[17]

## Growth Monitoring in ICDS

Since the adoption of the new WHO Child Growth Charts in India from 2008, common Mother and Child Protection Card is being used both by the Ministry of Women and Child Development through ICDS as well as the Ministry of Health and Family Welfare through various health services. This change in reference has led to an increase in severely underweight children and in underweight children 0–6 months thus raising the demand for funds share of both Center and states.[18,19]

Some studies have shown that applying the WHO growth curves result in a higher prevalence of undernutrition as compared to the IAP references,[20,21] but other studies show that the prevalence is higher when IAP references are used.[18]

## Finances for ICDS

The revised financial norms provide for Rs. 6, Rs. 9 and Rs. 7 per day per child 6 months to 72 months, per severely malnourished child (6 mo–72 mo) and per pregnant and per-lactating mother, respectively. The funding pattern in terms of Center: State fund share was 90:10 between 2010-2015. The supplementary nutrition program component was 50:50 ratio. The North Eastern States have a 90:10 ratio. Since 2015, for all components of ICDS, the Center's share has been reduced making the share to 60:40. The ratio for SNP for all states and NE states however remain unchanged. The effect of the change in funding pattern in the effectiveness and functioning of ICDS is yet to be seen. The 12th Five Year Plan had allocated 1,23,580 crore. But up to 2016-17, Government of India allocated only 63% of the ICDS budget.

## Monitoring, Supervision, and Strengthening ICDS

The National Institute for Public Cooperation and Child Development (NIPCCD) under the Ministry of Women and Child Development (MWCD), Government of India conduct regular monitoring and supervision of ICDS scheme. The monitoring is carried out at the national, state, district, and community level.

The 12th Five Year Plan attempted to strengthen and restructure ICDS on three fronts:

### 1. Programmatic Reforms

These are regarding the strengthening of the package of services, focus on under three year children, nutrition counseling for mothers of under-3 children, management of severe and moderate underweight, through community based initiatives such as Sneha Shivir, and strengthening training and capacity building.

## 2. Management Reforms

Using Information and communication technology, web enabled management information system, provision of untied/flexi fund for promoting local innovations, anganwadi cum creches, and others.

## 3. Institutional Reforms

Delivery of quality services, mission mode of ICDS at district, state, and national levels, development of annual project implementation plans with states and union territories, and management support for ICDS at various levels are some of these. Due to the mission mode of ICDS, National Mission Steering Group (NMSG) and Empowered Program Committee (EPC) at National and state level for effective planning, implementation, monitoring and supervision of ICDS scheme has been constituted and creation of a separate ICDS mission budget has been recommended. Another major effort is towards the deployment of a nutrition counsellor cum additional worker in 200 high burden districts and link workers in other districts on demand by state governments.

The ICDS mission targets to attain three main outcomes listed in **Box 16.2**. Annual Health Survey (AHS) and District Level Household Survey (DLHS) data are to be used as baseline for evaluating the outcomes of ICDS mission.

---

**Box 16.2 Targets of ICDS Scheme**

1. Prevent and reduce young child under-nutrition (% underweight children 0-3 years) by 10 percentage point
2. Enhance early development and learning outcomes in all children 0-6 years of age
3. Improve care and nutrition of girls and women and reduce anaemia prevalence in young children, girls and women by one fifth.

---

## The Challenges for ICDS

There are some striking programmatic challenges and criticisms of ICDS. The system does not collect data on severe wasting and hence the burden of SAM cannot be known on a regular basis. Due to the provision of only one Anganwadi Worker (AWW), it is not possible for her to carry out the various activities such as nutrition counseling, pre-school education effectively. There is lack of convergence of ICDS with the health programs and other sectors of the government. It lays emphasis on 3–6 year old children and thereby neglects the 0–2 year age groups in which group undernutrition sets in at an early stage. ICDS is considered as a failure by many experts and policy makers in terms of its inability to show a visible reduction in the burden of child undernutrition in the country. As there is no national guideline on measurement of weight-by-height Z-scores (WHZ) or mid upper arm circumference, detection and management of SAM by the ICDS remains a distant reality.

## Sneha Shivir

Among the newer components added to ICDS under the restructured and strengthened ICDS scheme in 2012, one component was *Sneha Shivir*. It aimed to address the issue of moderate and severe undernutrition (Weight for age Z-scores of less than minus three) among children less than 6 years in a community based approach. In the first phase this has been launched in 200 high burden districts of various states of India. An additional anganwadi worker cum nutritional counsellor has been included to manage the added workload of these *Sneha Shivirs*.

## The Concept

The concept of *Sneha Shivirs* is based on the premise that some children thrive better than others because their care givers follow some positive care practices. These practices need to be promoted to convince mothers/care givers of undernourished children. Many such practices are rooted in local traditions and practices and are therefore culturally acceptable, affordable, and sustainable. Care behaviors are intrinsically linked and include infant and young child feeding, health, hygiene, psychosocial care, and care for girls and women.

## Goal and Strategies

Its overall goal is to ensure quick rehabilitation of undernourished children; enable families to sustain rehabilitation; and prevent future undernutrition by changing behaviors in child care, feeding and health seeking. Key strategies include the following:

  i. Orientation of anganwadi workers and supervisors;
 ii. 100% weight monitoring and tracking using growth charts and the Mother and Child Protection Card;
 iii. Involving the community in identification and management;
 iv. Showcasing positive practices; and
  v. Setting up of nutritional care and counseling sessions.

## Key Interventions

1. *12 day on site session:* This includes collection of severely and moderately undernourished children which should preferably be not more than 15 per session, orientation of mothers and caregivers of the selected children, weight monitoring, deworming, Iron Folic acid supplementation, hands on practice session for mothers and care givers to promote improved feeding and child care practices. It is learning by doing approach, with support from the peer group so that the mothers take accountability and are enabled to nutritionally rehabilitate their undernourished children. During these 12 days, an increase in weight by about 200–400 grams is expected to take place.

2. *18 day home based component:* The mother practices the things learnt during the on-site sessions, in their homes. This is supplemented by the follow up home visits by the AWW. Weight monitoring of the children registered for these SnehaShivirs have to be done and documented on days 0, 12 and 30.[16]

The ANM/doctor under the National Rural Health Mission (NRHM) is responsible for health check-up of all the underweight children reporting to SnehaShivirs. For those children who are attending the Shivir and still not showing signs of improvement, the ANM or a doctor is responsible for deciding on type of referral or treatment facilities required as well as linking the child to appropriate health care/treatment.

During the years 2013-14 and 2014-15, 1,61,665 and 2,07,189 *Sneha Shivir* camps have been sanctioned, respectively.[22]

## ICDS Systems Strengthening and Nutrition Improvement Project (ISSNIP)

*(Assisted by the International Development Agency (IDA)*

The World Bank has assisted ICDS projects aiming to improve the nutritional status of the children. The supports were intended to operationalize the projects and enhance their quality of content and delivery, and monitoring and evaluation. ISSNIP (earlier called as ICDS IV) aimed at adding value to the existing ICDS by attempting to pilot and assess more effective approaches to early childhood education (ECE) and incremental learning outcomes and further augment systems strengthening and convergence at different levels of implementation. In the first phase, 162 districts in eight states, having higher undernutrition rates will be covered. The list of proposed activities to be carried under ISSNIP has four broad components listed in **Table 16.2**.[23]

## 16.5 NATIONAL PLAN OF ACTION FOR CHILDREN (NPAC) 2016

The National Plan of Action for Children was launched in 2005 and is now succeeded by NPAC 2016.

**Table 16.2** Components of ICDS Systems Strengthening and Nutrition Improvement Project[23]

**Component 1:** *Strengthening and expanding ICDS monitoring systems*
- Review, harmonization and refinement of all existing guidelines in ICDS
- Strengthening and expanding ICDS monitoring systems
- Innovations in strengthening training and capacity building
- Strengthening convergence with health
- Institutional support for innovations and specific pilots
- Implementation support at district and block levels

**Component 2:** *Community Mobilization and Behavior Change Communication (BCC)*
- Piloting model(s) of community engagement
- Designing and piloting of social agreements and community monitoring (social audits) in ICDS
- Capacity Building of community based organizations (CBO) for engaging in ICDS
- Partnerships with local NGOs and review of existing models of PPP and piloting
- Designing and implementation of pilots and tools for strengthening home visits
- Designing and piloting use of Information, Communication and Technology (ICT) for communication and Management Information System (MIS)
- Design, pre-test and implement some mid-media initiatives such as folk theatre, film shows

**Component 3:** *Piloting Convergent Nutrition Actions*
- Developing conceptual frameworks and tools for facilitating multi-dimensional interventions
- Inter-sectoral nutrition action committee formation and consultations
- Development of state specific convergent nutrition action plans and designing and implementation of multi-sectoral pilots
- Documentation, evaluation and research on multi-sectoral pilots

**Component 4:** *Project Management, Technical Assistance Agency, Monitoring & Evaluation*
- Provision of Central Project Management Unit within MWCD and State Project Management Units (SPMUs)
- Technical Assistance Agency (at the central level)
- Establishment of a project monitoring system to monitor project activities and deliverables at all levels
- District Level Rapid Assessments and ongoing internal assessments at sector level using Lot Quality Assurance Sampling (LQAS) approach
- Conducting operations research studies; including documentation and dissemination of effective pilots
- Social assessments and ethnographic study in SC/ST/Minority areas
- Impact evaluation (including baseline and endline surveys)

NPAC 2005 was formulated for a five year period and covered 12 key areas which required immediate and sustained attention. However there was no formal evaluation of this program, and many of the program objectives are yet to be achieved. The new plan is set to carry forward this program with renewed impetus and modifications to realize its objectives.

NPAC 2016 takes into account the current priorities for children in India. It affirms the states responsibility to provide for all children in its territory before, during and after birth and provides for the their growth and development till they attain 18 years of age.

The focus is to serve its most vulnerable children first. Four key priority areas are identified:

1. Survival, Health and Nutrition;
2. Education and Development (including skill development);
3. Protection; and
4. Participation. NPAC sets target based approach towards achieving the desired changes.[24]

The salient features related to NPAC 2016 pertaining to child nutrition are as follows:
- Modernise AWCs as per the norms of restructured ICDS and link them with

digital database so as to monitor real-time data on services provided;

- Construction of anganwadi centers with adequate facilities in convergence with Mahatma Gandhi National Rural Employ-ment Guarantee Scheme (MGNREGS);
- Improve health and nutrition status of all parents-to-be, and pregnant and lactating mothers;
- Ensure adequate health care and nutrition support for the girl child;
- Key messages on childcare of pregnant and lactating women, nutrition, and sanitation delivered through mass media for behavior change and communication;
- Ensure availability of essential services, supports and provisions for nutritive attainment in a life cycle approach, including infant and young child feeding (IYCF) practices;
- Increased access and use of diverse and adequate nutritious food at household level
- Promote use of affordable, appropriate, and nutritious recipes based on local food resources and dietary practices;
- Implement 1000 days approach, infant and young child feeding (IYCF) practices;
- Reduce prevalence of micronutrient deficiency among women, children and adolescents;
- Strengthen referral mechanism and linkage between the community and Nutrition Rehabilitation Centers;
- Greater involvement of PRIs for leadership and steering role at grassroots level to identify severely malnourished children and mobilize parents to go to NRCs;
- Develop comprehensive strategy to detect and address undernutrition among boys and girls in the age group of 6–18 years;
- Strengthen nutrition management and information system through web-based Rapid Reporting System;
- Promote proper food handling, hygiene and sanitation practices at household and institutional level;

- Ensure that only child safe products and services are available in the country and put in place mechanisms to enforce safety standards; and
- Implement guidelines developed by the National Institute of Public Cooperation and Child Development (NIPCCD) to ban junk food (high fat, sugar, and salt).

## 16.6 MULTI-SECTORAL NUTRITION PROGRAM 2013

Earlier in 1993 and in 1995, the National Nutrition Policy and the National Nutrition Action Plan were devised to highlight specific roles and responsibilities of different government ministries/departments of the Government of India and state governments for addressing the challenge of undernutrition in the country and improve the nutritional status of the society.

The National Nutrition Mission was set up in 2003. It consisted of a two tiered supervisory structure, headed by the Prime Minister and included the concerned union ministers, chief ministers by rotation, academicians and technical experts and NGO representatives. Maharashtra was the first state to launch a nutrition mission in 2005 followed by Madhya Pradesh, Uttar Pradesh, Odisha, Gujarat, and Karnataka. The main focus has been intersectoral coordination.

The malnutrition problem in India is multidiensional, intergenerational set of inter related factors. The Prime Minister's National Council on India's Nutritional challenges in 2010 suggested and inter-alia decided that: "A multi-sectoral program to address the maternal and child malnutrition in selected 200 high burden districts would be prepared." The ministry of Women and Child Development was given the responsibility of preparing the multi sectoral program in consultation with the Planning Commission, MOHFW and other relevant ministries. Consequently a multi sectoral nutrition program was prepared. In 2013 it was decided by the Government of India that the Multi-sectoral Nutrition Program to address the maternal and child undernutrition will be implemented as a special intervention in 200 High Burden Districts across the country in a phased manner. The first phase will begin in 100 districts during the year 2013-14, while in the second phase, it will be scaled up to cover 200 districts during the year 2014-15. The National Mission Steering Group (NMSG) and Empowered Program Committee (M-EPC) constituted for ICDS Mission would be the highest administrative and technical bodies for ensuring effective planning, implementation, monitoring, and supervision.[25]

## The National Nutrition Mission

It has two components.

I. *Multi-sectoral Nutrition program to address maternal and child undernutrition* in 200 high-burden districts, which aims at prevention and reduction in child undernutrition (underweight prevalence in children under 3 years of age) and reduction in levels of anemia among young children, adolescent girls and women has been launched in January 2014.

II. *Information, Education, and Communication (IEC) campaign against malnutrition:* To create awareness about nutrition challenges and promote home-level feeding practices.

## Components

The Multi-sectoral Nutrition program would focus on the following components:

### 1. Nutrition Centric Planning

The District Nutrition Cell would act as the technical hub at the district level for all nutrition related interventions. The nutrition centric plan will be prepared in close consultation with the *Gram Panchayat*, Village Health, Sanitation and Nutrition Committees (VHSNCs), anganwadi level management and

support committee (ALMSC) and any other relevant agencies responsible for village to ensure active involvement of local representatives and community members in planning process.

### 2. Nutrition Centric/Sensitive Sectoral Interventions

In order to tackle the problem of under-nutrition, both direct and indirect nutrition interventions are essential. The Multi-sectoral Nutrition Program would focus on those specific roles and responsibilities for ensuring a strong coordinated approach for addressing undernutrition at the state, district, block, and village levels.

### 3. Nutrition Centric/Sensitive Gap Filling Support

The first priority would be to fill the existing gaps through resources from the sectoral plans/programs. However, even after this, if a relevant development deficit/gap remains uncovered/unfulfilled through existing sectoral interventions, and are identified through the rapid assessment, baseline and planning process, for improving the nutrition related indicators, gap-filling support would be provided under this program.

The schemes which have an overall bearing on nutrition and would be required to incorporate nutrition related interventions in their respective annual plans/annual project implementation plans and allocate required resources under the Multi-sectoral nutrition Program, with respect to the intended groups of beneficiaries in a life cycle approach are listed in **Table 16.3**.

As this ambitious program is in the process of roll out, some time will be required before its impact on the nutrition status of children in the community can be seen. The program would affect nutrition status at different stages of life, and in a life cycle approach, it will potentially affect the nutrition status of children of the country.[25]

**Table 16.3** Schemes Related to Nutrition, Govt. of India

| S. no | Target group | Schemes or programs |
|---|---|---|
| 1. | Pregnant and lactating | NRHM, Janani Suraksha Yojana (JSY) mothers and ICDS |
| 2. | Children 0–3 years | NRHM, Rajiv Gandhi National Creche Scheme (RGNCS), ICDS |
| 3. | Children 3–6 years | ICDS, NRHM, Janani Shishu Suraksha Karyakram (JSSK), RGNCS, Total Sanitation Campaign (TSC) |
| 4. | School Going Children 6–14 years | Mid-day meal, *Sarva Shiksha Abhiyan* |
| 5. | Adolescent girls 11–18 years | Rajiv Gandhi Scheme for the empowerment of adolescent girls (SABLA), Total Sanitation Campaign, National Rural Drinking Water Program |
| 6. | Adults | Mahatma Gandhi National Rural Employment Guarantee Scheme, Skill Development Mission, National Health Mission, National Iodine Deficiency Disorders Control Program, Bharat Nirman, Rashtriya Swasthya Bima Yojana |

## 16.7 NATIONAL FOOD SECURITY ACT (NFSA)

The Act passed in 2013 is one of the largest food safety programs in the world. It legislates provision of five kilograms of cereals per person per month at highly subsidized price of Rs. 1 to 3 per kg to around three fourths of the rural and half of the urban Indian population.

It is being primarily implemented by the Department of Food and Public Distribution under the Ministry of Consumer Affairs, Food and Public Distribution. It is expected that NFSA will provide nutrition support to the below poverty line families. This act also mandates provision of food grains to the supplementary nutrition program in various states, under ICDS. As various studies have pointed out towards the fallibility of Public Distribution System (PDS) and ICDS due to administrative and operational inefficiencies and riding on it, raises questions about the success of NFSA. Even though the NFSA doesn't in any way address the larger issues of nutrition such as dietary diversity, infant and young child feeding practices, it is a welcome step towards providing some sustenance to the very deprived sections of the society.[17]

Currently, 32 states/union territories are implementing this Act in a direct benefit transfer by giving direct cash transfer of food subsidy to the beneficiaries.

The Act also has a special focus on the nutritional support to women and children. Besides meal to pregnant women and lactating mothers during pregnancy and six months after the child birth, such women will also be entitled to receive maternity benefit of not less than Rs. 6,000. Children up to 14 years of age will be entitled to nutritious meals as per the prescribed nutritional standards. In case of non-supply of entitled food grains or meals, the beneficiaries will receive food security allowance. The Act also contains provisions for setting up of grievance redressal mechanism at the District and State levels. Separate provisions have also been made in the Act for ensuring transparency and accountability. The existing Antyodaya Anna Yojana (AAY) households, which constitute the poorest of the poor, will continue to receive 35 kg of food grains per household per month.[17]

## 16.8 MID-DAY MEAL SCHEME

With a view to enhance enrolment, retention and attendance and simultaneously improving nutritional levels among children, the National Program of Nutritional Support to Primary Education (NP-NSPE) was launched as a centrally sponsored scheme on 15th August 1995, initially in 2408 blocks in the country. By the year 1997-98 the NP-NSPE was introduced in all blocks of the country. In 2001 MDMS became a cooked Mid-day Meal Scheme under which every child in every Government and Government aided primary school was to be served a prepared mid-day meal with a minimum content of 300 calories of energy and 8–12 gram protein per day for a minimum of 200 days in a year. It was extended in 2002 to cover children studying in centers running under the Education Guarantee Scheme (EGS) and Alternative and Innovative Education (AIE) Scheme and Madarsas/Maktab. The scheme has been further extended to upper primary schools in 2006-07. A provision for serving mid-day meal during summer vacation in drought affected areas was also made. Since 2009-10 the scheme covers children studying in National Child Labour Project (NCLP) schools also.

Since its inception, the scheme has been revised from time to time. The per day calorie and protein provisions are as follows. For primary school children: 450 kcal and 12 gram of protein; and for upper primary: 700 kcal and 20 gram of protein.

It also supports for engagement of cook-cum-helpers, kitchen-cum-store and kitchen devices which are needed to sustain the mid-day meal scheme at the school level. The provision of micronutrients such as iron, folic acid, zinc, are to be through convergence with the school health and other programs of NRHM of the MOHFW.[26]

Guidelines to ensure quality, safety, and hygiene under the mid-day meal scheme are also in implementation. These include the setting up of management structure at various levels, tasting of the meal by at least one teacher, safe storage and proper supply of ingredients to the schools, capacity building,

testing of food samples to enhance quality and setting in place an emergency medical plan providing effective linkages with the health system, in case of any untoward incident.

## 16.9 RAJIV GANDHI SCHEME FOR EMPOWERMENT OF ADOLESCENT GIRLS (RGSEAG)—'SABLA'

A centrally-sponsored scheme in 205 districts selected from all the States/UTs. The scheme *Sabla* aims at empowering Adolescent Girls (AGs) (11–18 years) through nutrition, health care, and life skills education. It also aims towards mainstreaming out of school AGs into formal/non formal education. Nearly 100 lakh adolescent girls per annum are expected to be benefitted under the scheme. This scheme has two major components *viz.* nutrition and non-nutrition.

• Under the *nutrition component*, the out of school AGs in the age group of 11–14 years attending AWCs and all girls in the age group of 14–18 years are provided supplementary nutrition containing 600 calories, 18–20 grams of protein and micronutrients, per day for 300 days in a year.

• The *non-nutrition component* addresses the developmental needs of adolescent girls. Under this component, out of school adolescent girls of 11–18 years are being provided IFA supplementation, health check-up and referral services, nutrition and health education, Adolescent, Reproductive and Sexual Health (ARSH) counseling/guidance on family welfare, life skill education, guidance on accessing public services and vocational training (only 16–18 year old adolescent girls).[27]

The total number of beneficiaries under the scheme were 10228911 during 2014-15 and 4868553 in 2015-16 till the end of December 2015.[28]

A comparative multicentric study on adolescent girls has shown that there has been an improvement in the literacy status, awareness regarding onset of menstruation, use of sanitary napkins and indigenous pads using cotton and gauze, consultation with medical officers, anganwadi workers regarding vaginal infections, between 2007 and 2012. This points towards the effect of various programs, including SABLA, related to health of adolescent girls.[29]

## 16.10 VILLAGE HEALTH NUTRITION DAY (VHND)

The VHND is to be organized once every month (preferably on Wednesdays, and for those villages that have been left out, on any other day of the same month) at the AWC in the village. This will ensure uniformity in organizing the VHND. The AWC is identified as the hub for service provision in the Reproductive and Child Health Program (RCH-II), National Health Mission (NHM), and also as a platform for inter-sectoral convergence. VHND is also to be seen as a platform for interfacing between the community and the health system.

On the appointed day, Accredited Social Health Activisits (ASHAs), AWWs, and other will mobilize the villagers, especially women and children, to assemble at the nearest AWC. The ANM and other health personnel should be present on time; otherwise the villagers will be reluctant to attend the following monthly VHND. On the VHND, the villagers can interact freely with the health personnel and obtain basic services and information. They can also learn about the preventive and promotive aspects of health care, which will encourage them to seek health care at proper facilities. Since the VHND will be held at a site very close to their habitation, the villagers will not have to spend money or time on travel. Health services will be provided at their doorstep. The Village Health and Sanitation Committee (VHSC) comprising the ASHA, the AWW, the ANM, and the PRI representatives, if fully involved in organizing the event, can bring about dramatic changes in the way that people perceive health and health care

practices. The program managers have to provide supportive supervision regarding VHND.

The service directly linked to nutrition provided during these days are supplementary nutrition to underweight children, provision of vitamin A, weighing and plotting on growth chart to track malnutrition. VHND focuses on prevention of diseases due to nutritional deficiencies by giving information and counseling on:

- Healthy food habits;
- Hygienic and correct cooking practices;
- Checking for anemia, especially in adolescent girls and pregnant women; checking, advising, and referring;
- Weighing of infants and children;
- Importance of iron supplements, vitamins, and micronutrients;
- Food that can be grown locally; and
- Focus on adolescent pregnant women and infants aged 6 months to 2 years.

The issues directly linked to nutrition and discussed during VHND are: exclusive breastfeeding, complementary feeding, counseling for better nutrition, identification of cases that require special attention, children with grade III and IV level of malnutrition, children with severe anemia.

Organising a VHND requires prior preparation which includes activities such as: preparing a list of children who need care for malnutrition on the day, ASHA to ensure that malnourished children come for consultation with the auxiliary nurse midwife (ANM), the ANM to ensure that VHND is held and coordinate with AWW and ASHA regarding this, the Panchayati Raj Institution (PRI) to ensure that teachers and other PRI members are available and to provide support.

Sanitation, maternal health, child health, family planning, communicable diseases, gender, health promotion, are some of the services other than nutrition that are focused on during these days.

## Expected Outcomes of VHND

1. Increase in knowledge and awareness regarding the promotive and preventive interventions for health promotion and disease prevention increase in knowledge about the services available under national health and disease related programs.
2. Awareness about the social determinants of health enhanced community participation and involvement in decision making and improving health of the communities.
3. Enhancing coverage of preventive and promotive interventions for mothers, pregnant women, children and adolescents.[30]

## 16.11 JUNK FOOD GUIDELINES

Under the chairmanship of National Institute of Nutrition, a working group was constituted by the Ministry of Women and Child Development to formulate junk food guidelines pertaining to children. The group critically examined the guidelines of 23 countries and came out with their own recommendations. A comprehensive definition of 'junk food' has been formulated and all the food items which fall under this would be considered as junk food. These food items are those which are rich in sugar, in fat, or in salt. It recommends that vendors/street vendors should not sell the listed items within 200 metres of the school. Even those shops or restaurants which sell these items are not allowed to sell them to children in school uniforms. The report of the guidelines has also been sent to MOFHW for including the same in the guidelines of Food Safety Standards Authority of India (FSSAI).[31]

## References

1. International Food Policy Research Institute. 2016. Global Nutrition Report 2016: From Promise to Impact: Ending Malnutrition by 2030. Washington, DC Available from: www.ifpri.org/cdmref/p15738coll2/id/130354/filename/130565.pdf. Accessed October 29 2016.
2. Rapid Survey on Children 2013-2014. India Factsheet. Provisional. Ministry of Women and Child Development. Government of India. Available from: http://wcd.nic.in/issnip/National_Fact%20sheet_RSOC%20_02-07-2015.pdf. Accessed October 29 2016.
3. International Institute for Population Sciences and Macro International (2007). National Family Health Survey (NFHS-3), 2005-2006. India. Vol. I. Mumbai: IIPS. p. 537. Available from: http://pdf.usaid.gov/pdf_docs/PNADK385.pdf. Accessed October 29 2016.
4. Raykar N, Majumder M, Laxminarayan R, Menon P. 2015. India Health Report: Nutrition 2015. New Delhi, India: Public Health Foundation of India; 2015.
5. Indian Academy of Pediatrics, Dalwai S, Choudhury P, Bavdekar SB, Dalal R, Kapil U, Dubey AP, Ugra D, Agnani M, Sachdev HP; Indian Academy of Pediatrics. Consensus Statement of the Indian Academy of Pediatrics on integrated management of severe acute malnutrition. Indian Pediatr. 2013;50:399–404.
6. Laillou A, Prak S, de Grot R, Whitney S, Conkle J, Horton L, et al. Optimal screening of children with acute malnutrition requires a change in current WHO guidelines as MUAC and WHZ identify different patient groups. PloS One 2014; 9, e101159. Accessed October 28 2016.
7. UNICEF. Management of Severe Acute Malnutrition In Children: Working Towards Results At Large Scale. New York: UNICEF; 2015.
8. UNICEF. Global evaluation of community management of acute malnutrition (CMAM); Global Synthesis Report. New York: UNICEF; 2013.
9. Black RE, Allen LH, Bhutta ZA, Caulfield LE, de Onis M, Ezzati M, et al. for the Maternal and Child Undernutrition Study Group. Maternal and child undernutrition: global and regional exposures and health consequences. Lancet. 2008;371:243–60.
10. Puett C, Sadler K, Alderman H, Coates J, Fiedler JL, Myatt M, et al. Cost-effectiveness of the community-based management of severe acute malnutrition by community health workers in southern Bangladesh. Health Policy Plan. 2013. 28: 386–99.
11. Tekeste A, Wondafrash M, Azene G, Deribe K. Cost effectiveness of community-based and in-patient therapeutic feeding programs to treat severe acute malnutrition in Ethiopia. Cost Eff Resour Alloc. 2012; 10: 4. Available at: http://doi.org/10.1186/1478-7547-10-4. Accessed October 30 2016.

12. Press Information Bureau, Ministry of Health and Family Welfare, Government of India. Available at: http://pib.nic.in/newsite/PrintRelease.aspx?relid=107829. Accessed October 29 2016.

13. Singh K, Badgaiyan N, Ranjan A, Dixit HO, Kaushik A, Kuhwaha KP, Aguayo VM. Management of children with severe acute malnutrition: experience of Nutrition Rehabilitation Centers in Uttar Pradesh, India. Indian Pediatr. 2014;51:21–5.

14. Aguayo VM, Agarwal V, Agnani M, Agrawal D, Bhambhl S, Rawat AK, Gaur A, Garg A, Badgaiyan N, Singh K. Integrated program achieves good survival but moderate recovery rates among children with severe acute malnutrition in India. Am J Clin Nutr. 2013;98:1335–42.

15. Key Indicators. Management of acute malnutrition and micronutrient deficiencies standard 2: severe acute malnutrition. The Sphere project. Available at: http://www.spherehandbook.org/en/management-of-acute-malnutrition-and-micronutrient-deficiencies-standard-1-moderate-acute-malnutrition/. Accessed October 30 2016.

16. Integrated Child Development Scheme. Ministry of Women and Child Development, Government of India. Available from: http://icds-wcd.nic.in/icds/. Accessed September 26 2016.

17. National Food Security Act. Department of Food and Public Distribution, Ministry of Consumer Affairs, Food and Public Distribution, Government of India. Available from: http://dfpd.nic.in/nfsa-act.htm. Accessed September 26 2016.

18. Prinja S, Thakur JS, Bhatia SS. Pilot testing of WHO Child Growth Standards in Chandigarh: implications for India's child health programs. Bull World Health Organ. 2009;87:116–122.

19. de Onis M, Onyango AW, Borghi E, Garza C, Yang H; WHO Multicenter Growth Reference Study Group. Comparison of the World Health Organization (WHO) Child Growth Standards and the National Center for Health Statistics/WHO international growth reference: implications for child health programs. Public Health Nutrition. 2006;9:942–7.

20. Dhone AB, Chitnis UB, Jethani S. Comparison of WHO growth standards and Indian Academy of Pediatrics standards of under five children in an urban slum. Indian Journal of Community Health. 2013;25:277–80.

21. Aggarwal P, Kandpal SD, Negi KS. Comparative study on practical application, acceptability and feasibility of different types of growth monitoring charts. Indian J Prev Soc Med. 2012;43:332–8.

22. The government program to tackle malnutrition among children and women now in mission mode. Press Information Bureau, Government of India, Ministry of Women and Child Development. Available at: http://pib.nic.in/newsite/PrintRelease.aspx?relid=112666. Accessed October 30 2016.

23. ICDS Systems Strengthening and Nutrition Improvement Project (ISSNIP). Ministry of Women and Child Development, Government of India. Available from: http://icds-wcd.nic.in/issnip/home.htm. Accessed September 26 2016.

24. National Plan of Action for Children 2016. Ministry of Women and Child Development, Government of India. Available from: http://wcd.nic.in/acts/national-plan-action-children-2016. Accessed September 26 2016.

25. National Nutrition Mission. Ministry of Women and Child Development, Government of India. Available from: http://wcd.nic.in/documents/national-nutrition-mission-nnm. Accessed September 26 2016.

26. Mid-day Meal Scheme. Ministry of Human Resource Development, Government of India. Available from: http://mdm.nic.in/. Accessed September 26 2016.

27. Rajiv Gandhi Scheme for Empowerment of Adolescent Girls (RGSEAG)-SABLA (ENGLISH). Ministry of Women and Child Development, Government of India. Available from: http://wcd.nic.in/schemes/rajiv-gandhi-scheme-empowerment-adolescent-girls-rgseag-sabla. Accessed September 26 2016.

28. SABLA Scheme to benefit nearly 100 lakh adolescent girls per annum. Press Information Bureau, Government of India, Ministry of Women and Child Development. Available at: http://pib.nic.in/newsite/PrintRelease.aspx?relid=133064. Accessed November 20 2016.

29. Paul D, Patnaik R, Gopalakrishnan S. Improvement in knowledge and practices of adolescent girls on reproductive health with focus on hygiene during menstruation in five years. Health Popul Perspect Issues. 2014;37:1–14.

30. Village Health Nutrition Day. National Health Mission, Ministry of Health and Family Welfare, Government of India. Available from: http://nrhm.gov.in/communitisation/village-health-nutrition-day.html. Accessed October 30 2016.

31. Junk Food Guidelines. Press Information Bureau. Government of India; Ministry of Women and Child Development. December 28 2015. Available from: http://pib.nic.in/newsite/PrintRelease.aspx?relid=133957. Accessed September 26 2016.

# Index